Building *on a* Century *of* Caring

The Montreal Children's Hospital

1904 – 2004

L'Hôpital de Montréal pour enfants
The Montreal Children's Hospital

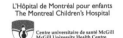

Centre universitaire de santé McGill
McGill University Health Centre

L'Hôpital de Montréal pour enfants 100 The Montreal Children's Hospital
1904-2004

Library and Archives Canada Cataloguing in Publication

Building on a Century of Caring: the Montreal Children's
Hospital, 1904–2004.

Includes index.
"Writers, Elizabeth Hirst ... [et al.]".
ISBN 1-896881-63-7 (bound).– ISBN 1-896881-65-3 (pbk.)

1. Montreal Children's Hospital – History.
I. Hirst, Elizabeth, 1949–

RA983.M62M66 2005 362.198'92'000971428
C2005-906115-4

Printed and bound in Canada

The writing and production of *Building on a Century of Caring: The Montreal Children's Hospital, 1904–2004,* were made possible thanks to the combined efforts of:

THE MONTREAL CHILDREN'S
HOSPITAL FOUNDATION

THE MCH CENTENNIAL COMMITTEE
(see list of members in Appendix IV)

THE EDITORIAL COMMITTEE
(see page xi)

THE WRITING, EDITING, DESIGN,
AND PRODUCTION TEAM

Authors
Elizabeth Hirst (also Project Manager
    for Hirst Communications)
Ellen Laughlin
Käthe Lieber
Janice Hamilton
Heather Pengelley

Coordinator
Francine Robillard

Editor
Donna Riley

Researchers/writers
Beth Bowers
Patricia Brown
Catherine Cunningham
Jode Lax
Daphnée Luck

Translator
Carole Pagé

Translation reviewer
Brigitte Morel-Nish

Copy Editor (French version)
Arlette Côté

Photographic research and new photography
MCH Medical Multimedia Services

Graphic design and layout
Ted Sancton/Studio Melrose

Foreword

It is with great pleasure that we write this foreword to *Building on a Century of Caring*.

As it happens, we are both third generation volunteers and supporters of The Montreal Children's Hospital. Earlier in our lifetimes, we heard stories from friends and relatives who helped launch it a hundred and one years ago, and more recently have seen its development into an absolutely top quality institution.

People, of course, are what make an institution what it is. The doctors, nurses, allied health professionals, non-clinical staff and volunteers have combined to achieve this reputation. Their collective dedication is inspiring, and to have been part of the centennial celebrations was both an honour and a pleasure.

Soon the hospital will be moving to a new home at the Glen site, the next step in its ongoing development as a major contributor to the health of the children of our community, far and wide.

HUGH AND MARTHA HALLWARD
CO-CHAIRMEN, MCH CENTENNIAL COMMITTEE

Message from the Associate Executive Director

As The Montreal Children's Hospital enters its second century of patient care, teaching, and research, I am both proud and privileged to assume the position of Associate Executive Director and to work with the dedicated staff and volunteers who have built this hospital's sterling reputation.

The enduring vision of all those who came before us at the Children's was to create and nurture a place where children of Quebec could receive medical services *par excellence*. Today, the people at our hospital keep that vision alive for future children, and link us truly to the hopes and aspirations of the past. We look ahead to our new home in the MUHC facility at the Glen site, and to the added strength of our association with our partners. We step forward into our new century with enthusiasm, and, as always, a smile for the children.

LINDA M. CHRISTMANN, MD, MBA
ASSOCIATE EXECUTIVE DIRECTOR
FOR THE PEDIATRIC MISSION, MUHC

Cover Photos

Of the many unique gifts made to the Montreal Children's Hospital, some of the most lasting come in the form of art—paintings, photography and sculptures that express the many and varied moods of the children and families who come through its doors.

For many years, a statue of a mother and children by sculptor Sybil Kennedy stood inside the main entrance to the hospital. Miss Kennedy was born in Montreal at the turn of the 20th century, just before the hospital's founding, and had a distinguished career as a sculptor both in Montreal and in New York City, where she exhibited at the Metropolitan Museum of Art. She died in 1986, back in her home town. She had no children of her own but, like many Montrealers, was moved by the work of the Children's.

A photo of her gentle statue appeared on the title page of the history published for the hospital's 75th anniversary, *The Montreal Children's Hospital, Years of Growth*, by Dr. Jessie Boyd Scriver. Dr. Scriver's description of it reads, in part: "At the front entrance hall today there stands a small bronze statue by Sybil Kennedy. It shows a mother holding her ill infant for examination. Beside her, a little boy secure at his mother's side is alert and appraising his surroundings . . . "

Unfortunately, several years after the book was published, the sculpture was stolen from the entrance hall. It has never been recovered.

However, it is still remembered by people connected with the Children's as, to use Dr. Scriver's words, "a pure and sensitive tribute to the work and atmosphere of the Montreal Children's Hospital."

The photo from Dr. Scriver's book appears on the back cover of this book, its successor.

A few years after the theft, an MCH physician travelling to Colorado came across "Flyin'"— a bronze statue of children tobogganing. The sculptor, Blair Muhlestein, like Sybil Kennedy, uses children as his inspiration, and the lively emotion in the faces of the children on their sled suggested this work of art as a worthy replacement for the statue whose loss had aroused such feeling in the hospital community.

Donated anonymously by that same physician, the new sculpture now sits outside the main entrance of The Montreal Children's Hospital, near a colourful mural by the Montreal Area Decorative Painters and a comfortable granite bench, enhancing the cosy and attractive outdoor space.

A message on the plaque below reads: "To the children, parents and staff of the Montreal Children's Hospital. April 1997. Keep flyin'."

A photo of "Flyin'" graces the front cover of this book, to underline that fitting message, and to express the excitement of looking forward into the hospital's next century.

Table of Contents

A Few Notes on Usage

When the Children's Memorial Hospital was re-named The Montreal Children's Hospital in 1955, special attention was given to the capitalization of the 'T' on the first word of the new name. This was a legal requirement to avoid confusion with an earlier Montreal Children's Hospital, also known as the Vipond Hospital, which had been absorbed into the Children's Memorial in 1940 but did not immediately relinquish its corporate identity. Over the years, the capital 'T' has been maintained in hospital documents and it was the intention of the writers and editors of this book to do the same. However, there are many places in the text where several hospital names of varying styles and vintages are used in the same paragraph. Therefore, to maintain consistency and readability, we have chosen, with apologies to traditionalists, to use a lower case 't' on all hospital names throughout the book, with the exception of photo credits.

For the same reason, we have also simplified some names and titles. For instance, The McGill University–Montreal Children's Hospital Research Institute, more recently, The McGill University–Montreal Children's Hospital Research Institute of the McGill University Health Centre (MUHC) Research Institute, is usually referred to more simply as, for example, "the MCH Research Institute." In the same vein, The Montreal Children's Hospital Foundation frequently becomes "the Children's Foundation," or simply "the Foundation." We have usually used the title "Executive Director" for the CEO of the Children's, even for references to years after the 1997 merger with the other MUHC institutions, when the title became "Associate Executive Director for the Pediatric Mission, MUHC."

THE WRITING AND EDITING TEAM

Acknowledgments

To borrow a well known phrase about raising children, it takes a village to write a book.

More than two hundred people were interviewed for *Building on a Century of Caring*, and many more provided additional facts, referred the writers to information sources, or reviewed drafts. The Editorial Committee provided solid support to the team of writers and editors, and contributed countless hours to advising, editing, and supplying additional information. It was particularly enjoyable for the writers to gather memories from retired staff members. Many were generous with their time and support, none more so than Drs. Elizabeth and Donald Hillman, who responded to countless requests for information and kindly reviewed several chapters and suggested useful changes.

The writing team is particularly indebted to Elisabeth Gibbon of the hospital's Public Relations Office, and Marcie Scheim, Centennial organizer and MCH Auxiliary President, who have been invaluable sources of information and links with other staff within the hospital. Administrative assistants throughout the Children's have been especially helpful, and three in particular have provided continual research and writing support throughout the project: Terry Séguin of Public Relations, Ginette Manseau of the Associate Executive Director's office, and Sylvie Sahyoun of the office of the Physician-in-Chief. Joanne Baird

and her staff at the MCH Medical Library have patiently guided writers and researchers through a sea of paper to the right answers. And the staff of the Research Institute and the Foundation have gone out of their way to help us dig up and verify facts.

The team is grateful to all of the contributors, but takes responsibility for any errors that may remain in the text despite their diligent assistance.

The writers and editors also owe a considerable debt of gratitude to Patricia Bryden for her research and writing in the early stages of this project.

The photographs and illustrations in the book tell the story of the Children's as well as the text, thanks to the creative talent of photographers Daniel Héon and Laurent Soussana and the diligent research and coordination of Jo-Anne Trempe, all of MCH Medical Multimedia Services.

We hope this book, the result of all our labours, is both informative and entertaining. And, while it was not designed as a comprehensive reference, we dare to hope that in decades to come, when someone else needs to re-tell the story of the Children's, our work will help them to carry forward the contributions, the achievements, and above all, the spirit of hope and caring that have always been at the heart of our institution.

ELIZABETH HIRST
for the writing team

Authors

Elizabeth Hirst is a public relations consultant and McGill University lecturer who has devoted the greater part of her career to strategic communications and writing in the field of health care and education.

Käthe Lieber, co-author of *Montreal: The International City,* is a writer and editor with a special interest in the history of Montreal's founding institutions, especially its universities and hospitals.

Ellen Laughlin is a freelance writer and consultant with a teaching background and 20 years' experience in the newspaper industry.

She has written articles and educational materials on topics as diverse as health, multiculturalism and media education.

Janice Hamilton has a background in news reporting and more than 20 years as a freelance writer. Specializing in science and health writing, she has also written non-fiction children's books and is currently at work on a book about the St. Lawrence River.

Heather Pengelley is a veteran medical writer and the editor of **Future Health** for Canadians for Health Research. She teaches writing at Concordia University's Journalism Department in Montreal.

Introduction

In 2004, the Montreal Children's Hospital celebrated the hundredth anniversary of its first admission. The occasion was celebrated with a wide variety of activities involving the staff, patients and their families, and the community at large, many of them described in this book. When planning the centennial program, the Centennial Committee decided that the occasion was also an excellent opportunity to re-acquaint all concerned with the unique story of the Children's. Its contributions have been celebrated in a number of publications, notably the history written by Dr. Jessie Boyd Scriver in 1979 for the hospital's 75th anniversary.

If the first 75 years of the Children's history were full, the succeeding 25 were overflowing. The identification of new conditions along with improved understanding of the causes and processes of known diseases; the development of more effective ways to treat, alleviate, and prevent illness and injury; the evolution of subspecialties and new professions; the proliferation of new technologies and medications; the growing complexity and regulation of the health care system; and the increasing speed of social change —all have produced new stories that would fill a multi-volume encyclopedia. Of necessity, we have not tried to cover all aspects of the hospital's history, nor attempted to identify everyone associated with them. Other types of publications, such as annual reports of the hospital, Research Institute, and MCH Foundation, are available to those seeking complete lists and comprehensive descriptions.

We wanted to bring the story up to date, and make it accessible and inviting to a wide variety of readers. Some may want to immerse themselves in it cover to cover. Others may be attracted to the theme of a particular chapter. Those more inclined toward browsing and discovery will find the boxes and sidebars on noteworthy characters, events, and achievements can be perused independently.

Our hope for this book is twofold: that readers associated with the Montreal Children's Hospital will recognize and remember their institution with pride; and that others, perhaps new to the Children's, will discover the caring, innovation, and excellence that have characterized this remarkable hospital since its founding and continue to do so as we move confidently into the future.

THE EDITORIAL COMMITTEE
BRUCE WILLIAMS, MD, CHAIRMAN
HARVEY GUYDA, MD
ELIZABETH HIRST
DEREK PRICE
MICHAEL PRICE
NICOLAS STEINMETZ, MD

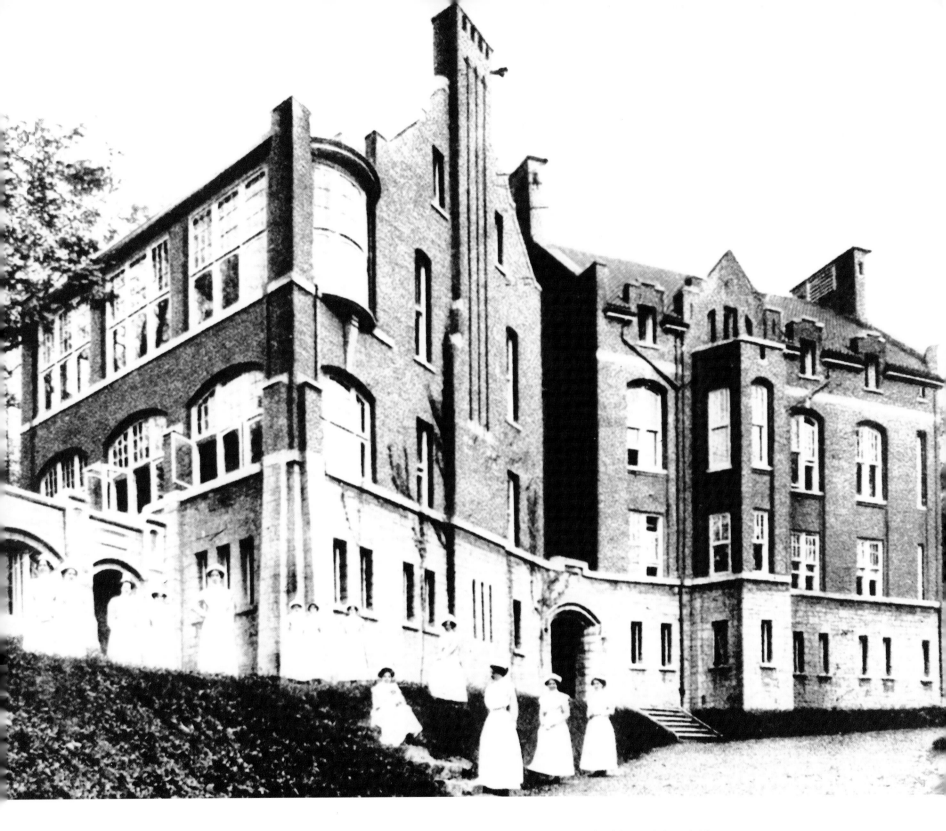

Nurses in front of the main building of the Children's
Memorial Hospital on Cedar Avenue, circa 1910

"As we look into the past, we find the story of the Montreal Children's Hospital a monument to faith, hope, and charity and to the indefatigable energy of those who believed in children."

DR. JESSIE BOYD SCRIVER, MCH PEDIATRICIAN
The Montreal Children's Hospital, Years of Growth, 1979

1

A History of Caring

The Montreal Children's Hospital (MCH) is an extraordinary place.

Place, of course, is an inexact word. Over the years, the physical space the hospital has occupied has evolved from an unimposing brick building on Guy Street in downtown Montreal, to a collection of cottages on the slopes of Mount Royal, to the current patchwork of old and more recent buildings on Tupper Street in the heart of the city. Its evolution will continue when the new McGill University Health Centre (MUHC) complex opens, with state-of-the-art facilities dedicated to the care of sick and injured children.

But what makes the Children's extraordinary is not bricks and mortar. Rather, it is the hospital's spirit—that unique blend of caring, innovation, uncompromising standards and public service that has characterized the institution since its inception. This spirit is a reflection of the countless individuals who have been part of the hospital's history, each contributing in some way to fulfilling its mission "to be a leader in the care and treatment of sick infants, children and adolescents, to be a source of support for their families, and to be an advocate for the right of all children to reach their full potential."

A NEW CENTURY'S VISION

At the turn of the 20th century, orthopedic surgeon Dr. Alexander Mackenzie Forbes, moved by the plight of crippled children begging in the streets of Montreal, mobilized a group of physicians and citizens to found a small hospital for youngsters suffering from bone tuberculosis, congenital defects, and complications from acute illness. The Children's Memorial Hospital (CMH), as it was called then, opened on January 30, 1904, with five children treated the first week.

A hundred years later, teams of highly specialized pediatric professionals at the Children's deal with more than 265,000 patient visits annually, using sophisticated equipment and techniques to treat increasingly complex cases. They transplant organs, correct heart defects at birth, and even prevent altogether many diseases and conditions that used to cripple or kill children in Dr. Forbes' time.

In the intervening century, countless doctors, nurses, technical specialists, support staff, families, and community members have been moved by the needs of children to build upon Dr. Forbes's original

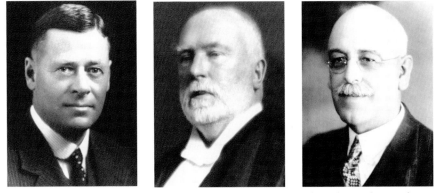

Dr. Alexander Mackenzie Forbes (left) was the hospital's founder and served as its Surgeon-in-Chief until 1929. Dr. Harold B. Cushing (centre) was the hospital's Physician-in-Chief from 1905 to 1938 and Sir Melbourne M. Tait, its first President (1902–1917).

vision. Together, they have developed the facilities, expertise, teamwork, and community support that enable today's staff to perform what in 1904 would have seemed feats of magic.

They have created a hospital that treats a wider range of conditions than Dr. Forbes could have imagined, with state-of-the-art technology and cutting-edge diagnostic and treatment procedures. Over the years, they have acquired a well-founded international reputation for excellence in patient care, research, and teaching.

"The vision of a young physician, the commitment of community-minded volunteers and the compassion of caregivers were essential to the creation of the Children's Memorial in 1904. All of these leadership qualities have allowed the Children's to grow and thrive during the last century, becoming the leader in many fields of pediatric care and research."

LOUISE DERY-GOLDBERG, PRESIDENT,
THE MONTREAL CHILDREN'S HOSPITAL FOUNDATION

Fresh air and sunshine were considered vital to children's recovery from such diseases as tuberculosis and poliomyelitis, but the rented 10-bed facility on Guy Street lacked outdoor space. When the Carsleys, who owned a large estate across the road, saw children playing on the hospital's steps and sidewalk, they offered to let them use their gardens during the warm months. Large tents were erected, and here 40 to 50 children lived from early spring until late fall. Most were sent home for the winter, as there were no indoor facilities for them, and their conditions were monitored on an outpatient basis until the following spring, when the tents went up again.

BURSTING AT THE SEAMS

It has not always been easy, for the years have brought an ever-widening array of challenges. Certainly the most persistent of these has been finding enough space.

From the beginning, the growing needs of sick children have put pressure on the hospital's physical facilities. When the original hospital opened at 500 Guy Street, the 10-bed facility was almost immediately filled to overflowing, even spilling out into tents on a neighbour's lawn during the summer.

When the hospital moved in 1909 to its new 45-bed building in the country-like setting above Cedar Avenue, the facilities seemed spacious at first. But as the hospital's work became better known, more and more families sought treatment for their children, and again the Children's had to expand. It did this by erecting a variety of outbuildings and taking over several smaller health-care facilities.

In 1956, the Children's moved to its current home on Tupper Street. The new space, about half of it purchased from the Montreal General Hospital and

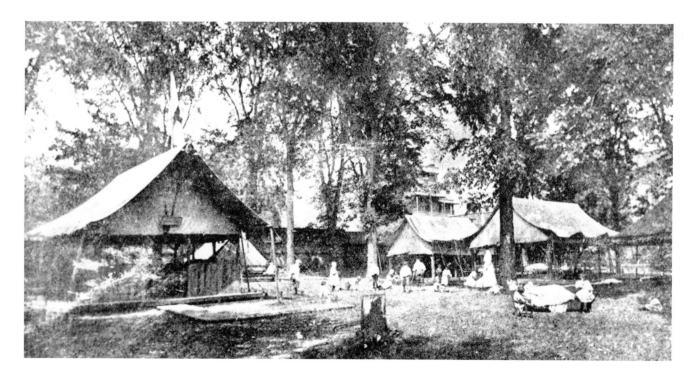

half newly constructed, provided sufficient space for inpatient, outpatient, diagnostic, laboratory, and research activities, as well as staff residences. But again, over the years, demand for services, as well as new technology and treatment programs, increased space needs beyond what the planners of the time could have envisaged.

In recent years, the Children's, housed in a complex of old and newer buildings and rented space nearby, has seemed at times to be bursting at the seams, calling upon all the creativity of its staff and supporters to continue implementing new programs and improving the care environment.

Today, staff and community alike look forward to the modern facilities of the planned MUHC complex. Using the latest planning and construction methods, the MUHC facilities are designed to provide more appropriate, long-term space solutions, in addition to providing much more flexibility for future growth.

A COMMUNITY OF SUPPORT

Like most hospitals, the Children's has dealt with financial concerns throughout its history. Until the 1960s, there was little government support and virtually all funds came from private donors and fundraising activities. Parents were billed for each hospital visit and procedure; however, most were unable to pay all or even part of the cost. As it was hospital policy to care for all children seeking treatment regardless of the family's economic situation, the hospital was constantly in need of funds.

In 1921, the Quebec Public Charities Act provided partial funding for hospitalization of the poorest patients, but funding for outpatient care, which was growing substantially, was not covered. The hospital's physicians—who volunteered their time at the Children's until the introduction of Medicare in 1970—often simply cancelled the bills of those who couldn't pay for hospital services. The hospital's survival depended literally upon the steady support of its community of private donors.

In 1961, the Quebec Hospital Insurance Plan ensured free inpatient care to all children—not just the indigent—but still there was no provision for outpatient services, nor for capital expenses, which together accounted for the largest portion of the hospital's deficit.

With the introduction of Medicare in 1970, "bad bills" became a thing of the past, as every member of society now had the right to publicly funded inpatient and outpatient care. Government responsibility for health care meant a steady source of funding for hospitals, ensuring some measure of financial security. However, it also entailed adherence to government policies. One of these was that no hospital be allowed to run an operating deficit—a tall order for the Children's at a time when the emergency room and outpatient clinics were overflowing, expansion plans were underway, and operating expenditures were spiralling due to increased costs of materials and labour.

Still, through a combination of cost-cutting measures and fundraising efforts, the hospital was able to put its financial status on an even keel for the first time in many years, attaining a balanced budget by 1972.

As it has been from the beginning, maintaining budgetary equilibrium is a yearly challenge. The Children's has had to prioritize services, ensuring necessary care to children while moving steadfastly forward in new directions. It has had to streamline its complement of staff while continuing to bring in new expertise. Being at the forefront of developing outpatient care and shorter hospital stays, in the current government-funded system, has ironically worked to the MCH's disadvantage, as the health-care system has not yet developed reliable formulas for measuring outpatient activity, and annual government funding is still based largely on the number of hospital beds and inpatient days.

Containing health-care costs requires the ongoing cooperation and commitment of staff in every department of the hospital and the continuing generosity of private donors. The Montreal Children's Hospital Foundation, established in 1973, administers funds from countless generous organizations and individuals to purchase specialized medical and surgical equipment, to support teaching and research activities, and to make possible special programs such as the Pain Management Service and the Autism Spectrum Disorders Program.

BRINGING IN THE PROFESSIONALS

At various times in its history, the MCH has also dealt with serious challenges to maintaining the necessary numbers of qualified personnel. Staff shortages were most severe during the two World Wars, when roughly a third of the hospital's doctors, nurses, and general staff volunteered for overseas service. During World War II, for instance, the hospital's medical staff consisted almost entirely of female interns.

Since the 1970s, there have been severe shortages of nurses, pediatric specialists, and other health-care professionals in Quebec. The reasons are many, including the reduced number of nursing graduates after the changeover from hospital nursing schools to CEGEP (*Collège d'enseignement général et pro-*

fessionnel) programs in the 1970s; a government-imposed limit on the number of places for medical students and residents in pediatric training programs; the necessity for out-of-province doctors to take Quebec exams before they can practise in the province; the requirement for clinical health professionals to pass French proficiency tests; a cap on the number of foreign physicians who can be recruited; an early retirement program for doctors and nurses in the late 1990s, intended by government as a cost-containment measure, that saw many senior staff members leave; and an overall reduction in graduates in other health-care professions.

Luckily, the Children's has always received applications from health-care trainees and professionals from around the world, attracted by the hospital's reputation for excellence in education, research, and patient care, and by the work of its world-renowned specialists in a variety of fields. Today, a great deal of time and energy must be devoted to recruiting and retaining high-calibre staff, but the efforts have met with great success.

DECADES OF CHANGE

One of the greatest ongoing challenges of the past hundred years has been keeping pace with increasingly rapid change in every area of the hospital's

Despite recent shortages of nurses, pediatric specialists, and other health-care professionals, the hospital has been extremely successful in recruiting high-calibre staff. (Left to right): nurse Maryse Duguay, assistant head nurse Lucie Jeanneau, and nurse Amanda Thompson

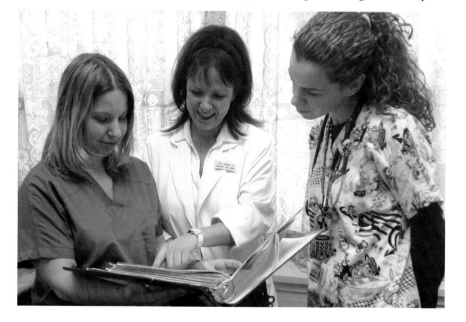

activities. Advances in knowledge, equipment, techniques, and philosophy of care—many of them spearheaded by the hospital itself—have made today's Montreal Children's very different from the Children's Memorial of 1904.

In its first 15 years, the hospital's activities expanded beyond orthopedic care into general patient care services, treating an ever-widening array of ailments. By the 1920s, pediatrics was developing as a specialty, and the Children's had become a teaching hospital of McGill University's Faculty of Medicine. Meanwhile, increased demand led to the construction of a new outpatient building.

In the 1930s, economic hardships brought greater numbers of children with malnutrition and its side effects, and the social service caseload increased dramatically. Rheumatic fever and tuberculosis were prevalent, and as knowledge about diseases grew, laboratory facilities were expanded.

The 1940s were a difficult time, with staff off to war and funds diverted to the war effort, but they were also exciting years. Antibiotics were discovered during the war and made available shortly thereafter, eliminating many serious illnesses and making others less severe. With the hospital's reputation spreading, patients were referred from throughout Canada and the northeastern United States, and applications for postgraduate studies came from around the world.

In the 1950s, families began to take a greater part in hospital life. There was increased awareness that children who were separated from their families during hospitalization often suffered psychological distress, which could compromise treatment and have long-lasting effects. As a result, visiting hours were extended and eventually eliminated, and families were encouraged to participate actively in their child's hospital care. The recognition that children tend to recover more quickly at home, that infections can spread more rapidly in a hospital setting, and that technological advances could reduce inpatient time, led to a shift away from hospitalization,

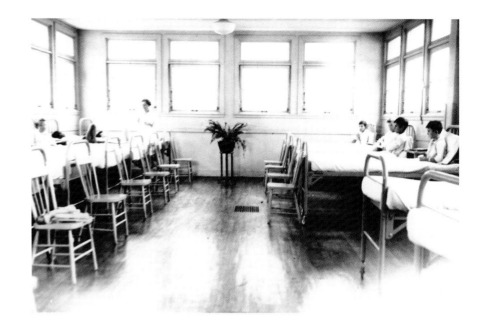

toward returning children to their homes as quickly as possible.

During the 1960s, the hospital became a leader in the development of outpatient services. Its home care program, launched in 1964, enabled many parents to care for chronically ill children at home with the hospital's support, and outpatient clinics, or ambulatory services, were developing at an increasing rate. Montreal's new metro system, with a station close to the Children's, made these and other hospital services more accessible than ever.

The 1970s brought publicly funded health care, which further increased the number of patients visiting the emergency room and ambulatory clinics. Research activities at the hospital flourished—even in less-than-perfect facilities—enhancing the hospital's reputation as a centre for learning and research. As specialists in a variety of fields worked together in the diagnosis and treatment of each child, this multidisciplinary team approach became a hallmark of the hospital's philosophy of care.

Day surgery, launched in the late 1970s, increased dramatically in the 1980s in an effort to return children to their families as quickly as possible. The shift

When the hospital was located above Cedar Avenue on the slopes of Mount Royal, hospitalized patients were housed in large wards, many located in "huts" away from the main building.

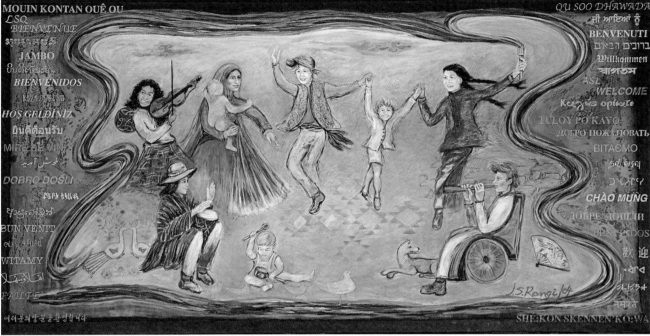

was made possible by advances in technology and expertise, along with well-developed follow-up programs. As only the most seriously ill children were now admitted, and as illnesses that previously claimed lives could now be treated, inpatients required more intensive, complex care than ever before.

The hospital responded to the growing diversity of Montreal's population in the mid-1980s with a pioneering multiculturalism program, which provided training programs for staff in dealing with cultural issues surrounding health, and a very active interpreter service. This decade also introduced computerization into every area of the hospital—including registration and admission of patients, scheduling, medication management, research, and record-keeping.

In the 1990s, the MCH's long-standing collaboration with other health-care institutions intensified, as did its involvement with community groups and outreach programs. In 1992, the MCH and four other McGill University teaching hospitals began exploring the possibility of combining forces to create

a stronger, unified medical centre, and in 1997 the McGill University Health Centre (MUHC) was born, with the Montreal Children's Hospital as a full partner.

As the MCH enters the 21st century, its commitment to the development of outpatient care remains strong, as does its investment in leading-edge surgery, trauma care, and the treatment of complex illnesses. Multidisciplinary teams are more important than ever in maintaining the standard of excellence the hospital's community has come to expect. The complexity of running today's modern children's hospital requires not only teams of health professionals, but also of specialists in other fields, such as housekeeping and building maintenance (both essential in infection control), food services, medical records, biomedical engineering and security, as well as administration, finance, computer systems, public relations, human resources—all of whom work together to ensure the best possible outcomes for children and their families. Collaborating with the other partners in the MUHC, with other Quebec health-care institutions, and with community groups is a vital part of the hospital's strategic evolution, as is the continued strengthening of relationships with government agencies at all levels.

A RECORD OF ACCOMPLISHMENTS

Despite, and often because of, the many challenges and developments over its century-long history, a tradition of innovation and excellence permeates all areas of the hospital, from the research laboratories to the laundry room.

The hospital's list of "firsts" is impressive. The hospital was the site of the first Canadian operation to repair a congenital heart defect in 1938, and MCH surgeons performed a heart transplant to the youngest recipient ever in Canada in 1988. In 1980, the first bone-marrow transplant in a Canadian pediatric setting took place at the Children's, and in 1990 MCH surgeons inserted the first bone-anchored hearing device in a child in Canada.

The Children's was the first pediatric hospital in Canada to open a speech therapy department (1933), a division of medical genetics (1949), a department of psychiatry (1950), a learning centre for children with learning disorders (1959), and a provincial centre for sudden infant death syndrome (SIDS) (1986). It launched the first pediatric burn unit (1971) and injury prevention program (1990) in a Quebec hospital.

These are just a few of the many initiatives that have had profound effects on the treatment and care of children not only at the MCH, but across Canada, and even in other parts of the world. There are advances and innovations, big and small, taking place

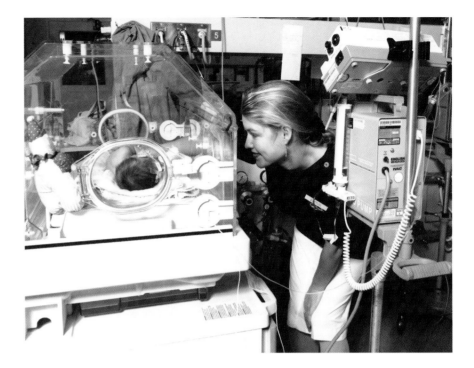

in every corner of the hospital virtually every day. It might be a new program for families of chronically ill children, or a new way to save money on cleaning supplies. It could be a groundbreaking research study, or a more effective way of performing a routine administrative task.

This book is full of stories of innovative techniques and programs, of excellence in the performance of daily duties, and of individuals who have inspired others to provide the very best in patient care, teaching, and research. These stories form the history of the Montreal Children's Hospital—a history of innovation, dedication, and caring that far exceeds the ambitions of the hospital's founders.

The hospital's founders would be astounded by the wide array of equipment, medications, and interventions available today to treat children of all ages.

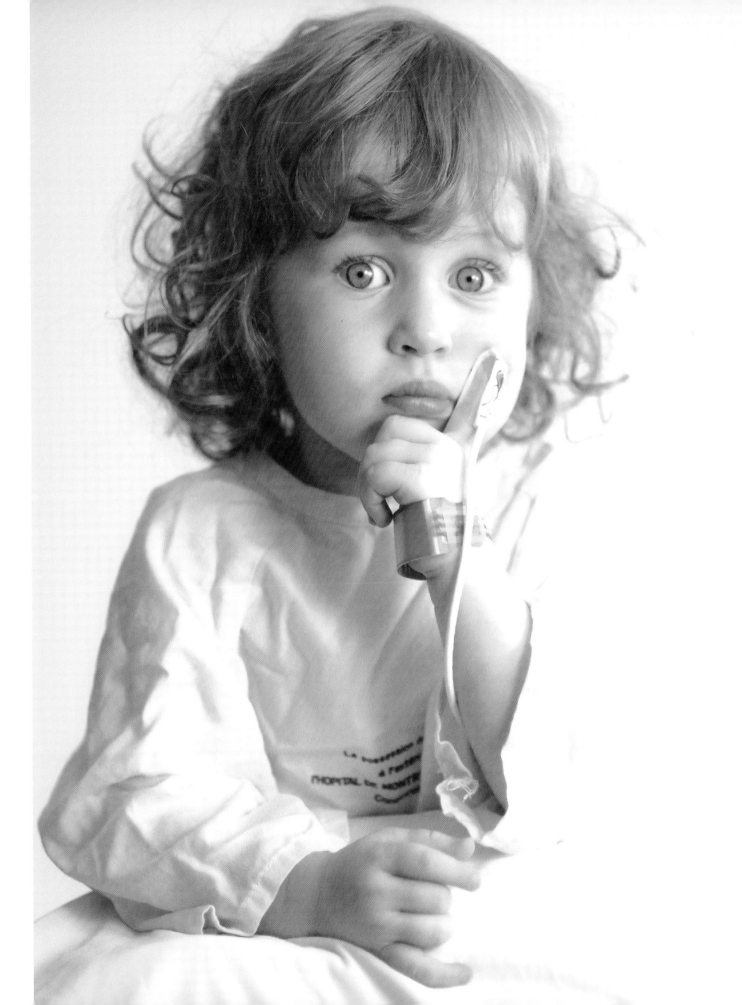

Noémi, the poster child for the 2002 MCH fundraising campaign, had more than a dozen middle ear infections (otitis media) before having day surgery to insert special tubes in her ears. The tubes improved air circulation in the ear and helped drain the infection, and Noémi has not had an ear infection since. Doctors at the Children's see more than 1,400 cases of otitis every year.

"Parents hold their children to be what they most value in the world. I think what makes the Children's special is that people here are conscious of the responsibility implied when parents confide a sick child to their care. Everyone involved with the Children's goes out of their way to honour that trust."

DR. NICOLAS STEINMETZ,
EXECUTIVE DIRECTOR, 1987–1995, 2003–2004

2

From Tots to Teens: Patients Then and Now

In the 100 years since the Children's first opened its doors as an orthopedic hospital, the hospital's staff have cared for nearly 1.3 million young patients, from infancy through adolescence. The nature of their ailments has changed greatly over the years, with orthopedic problems now only a small percentage of the hospital's cases, and many diseases that once claimed lives are now eliminated or treatable. The technologies and techniques used in diagnosis and treatment have come a long way, and the philosophy of patient care has altered significantly. But one thing has not changed. Whether they come for simple stitches or complicated surgery, children are the focus of the hospital's mission.

ONE SIZE DOES NOT FIT ALL

"No longer are young children treated medically as 'small adults'; their specific physiology and biochemistry have been studied and appreciated; their particular requirements for growth and development have been recognized."

DR. JESSIE BOYD SCRIVER, MCH PEDIATRICIAN,
The Montreal Children's Hospital,
Years of Growth, 1979

If a Montreal-area child was sick prior to 1904, he was seen by a general practitioner—if the family could afford to pay. Pediatrics as a specialty did not exist, and there was no publicly funded health care. If hospitalization was required, the child was admitted to an institution where the equipment and treat-ments were designed for adults, and where the medical staff rarely understood the extent to which the needs of their young patients differed from those of adults.

By the early 1900s, members of the medical community in Montreal and elsewhere began to acknowledge that children have special requirements. They understood that because children's bodies are developing, the causes, symptoms, and consequences of their ailments are often very different from those

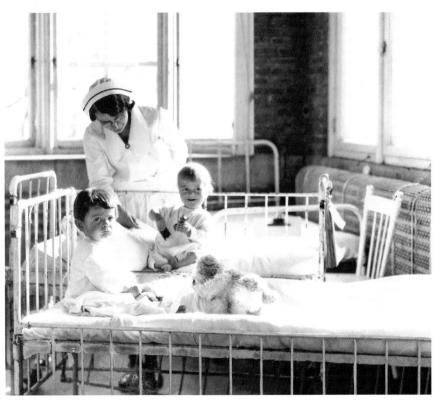

A nurse with patients at the Children's Memorial Hospital, 1939

of adults. Children may suffer from illnesses rarely found in the adult population, and treatments designed for older persons can have devastating effects on growing bones and organs. Specialized equipment is often needed, and staff must be trained to deal with children at different stages of development —from infants who cannot speak or understand what is happening to them, to adolescents who,

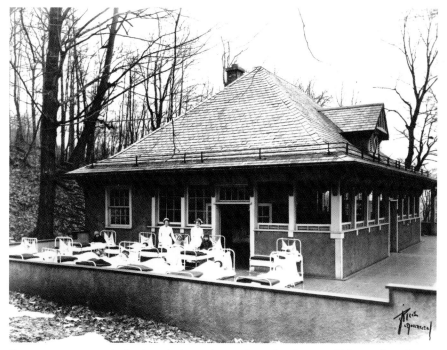

From 1909 to 1956, the hospital was located on the slopes of Mount Royal. This country-like setting enabled many children to take advantage of the sunshine and fresh air, considered vital to recovery from diseases such as tuberculosis. On the occasion of the hospital's 90th anniversary, nurse Dorothy Goulet shared her memories of Ward K (an orthopedic hut built in the 1920s) in Au Courant, the nursing newsletter:

"Ward K was built alongside the road that ran around Mount Royal ... which was patrolled by the Royal Canadian Mounted Police. They stopped in to see us frequently. We had a large verandah that could accommodate 10–15 beds side by side, which was used summer and winter almost daily. When they patrolled the road, they would come down the hill and tie their horses' reins to the wooden railing which surrounded the verandah. They allowed the children to pet the horses. Those who couldn't reach them rolled or crawled from one bed to the next until they were able to. If the children weren't outside, the RCMP would come in and talk with each child. They looked forward to it because some had been there for 13–15 years. They knew each other by name."

while they may be almost adults, are still undergoing major developmental changes.

Initially, the Children's Memorial Hospital was designed to deal exclusively with orthopedic cases— youngsters crippled by tuberculosis, congenital defects, and complications from a variety of illnesses. After 1913, however, when the first infants' ward opened at the CMH, full pediatric care was available, and children with medical conditions as diverse as rheumatic fever, rickets, appendicitis, and pneumonia finally had a place designed especially for them.

From the beginning, the CMH Board of Administration insisted on an open-door policy. There was no discrimination based on language, creed, or ethnicity, and no child was refused treatment because the parents or guardian could not pay. Treatment priority was based solely on medical need.

This meant that the number of children served by the hospital grew rapidly. The first patient was admitted on January 30, 1904, and by the end of the first week, five children were being treated—four inpatients and one non-resident. By May 20, 1905, care had been provided to 122 inpatients and 195 outpatients. The humble 10-bed facility on Guy Street was soon filled to overflowing, with 40 to 50 children spending the summer months in tents across the street and returning home for the winter. Over the years, each time new facilities were added, this story was repeated, with beds being almost immediately filled to capacity. Waiting lists in the 1940s rose as high as 1,500 children.

The following figures, based on the hospital's annual reports, give some idea of the progression:

Total	1915	1935	1954/55	1975	2002/03
Inpatients	394	3,198	5,300	12,213	6,779
Outpatient visits	998*	35,412	65,000	198,535	265,337

*It is not clear from hospital records of 1915 whether this is the number of outpatients or the number of outpatient visits.

TREATING THE WHOLE CHILD

"Just as the advances in medical knowledge increased our usefulness to the child population, so did the realization that the child is a person cause us to become acquainted with the behaviour and emotions of the child and the social forces which surround him."

DR. ALTON GOLDBLOOM,
PHYSICIAN-IN-CHIEF, 1946–1953
Small Patients, 1959

In the hospital's early days, patient care focused primarily on meeting the children's physical needs, with limited attention paid to their developmental, social, and emotional requirements. The educational needs of sick children, however, were met from the very beginning. Members of the Ladies' Committee were concerned about the lack of education for patients who often spent months and even years in the hospital. A regular teaching program, under the direction of Miss Sarah Tyndale, was established at the Guy Street facility and continued when the hospital moved to Cedar Avenue. Even today, school-aged patients who are hospitalized for more than two weeks, or who come in regularly for lengthy treatments at outpatient clinics, such as dialysis, can receive help with schoolwork from experienced teachers.

In the 1930s, the Children's became the first hospital in Canada to recognize the therapeutic value of play. As Dr. Jessie Boyd Scriver recounts in her history of the Children's, "the Department of Recreational Therapy was established under Miss Alice Burkhardt. This innovation was the first of its kind in Canada. It was her concept—in the pre-television days of medical care—that enjoyable pursuits could offset boredom and restlessness in the constrained patient. Long-term surgical and orthopaedic cases particularly benefited from the new ancillary service which contributed more than its share to the hospital's reputation for happiness among its children."

By the 1940s, psychiatry was becoming widely accepted as an important component of medical treatment, changing the way doctors and other health-care professionals viewed their patients. It became recognized that the most effective way to treat a medical condition was often to take social, emotional, and psychological factors into consideration.

At the Children's, Physician-in-Chief Alton Goldbloom recognized that many of his small patients suffered psychological distress not only from discomfort or pain, but also from anxiety and separation from their parents during hospitalization. He advocated the creation of a department of psychiatry at the hospital. Formally established in 1950 under the direction of Dr. Taylor Statten, it was the first such department in a Canadian pediatric setting. Its establishment ushered in a period of change in all aspects of patient care at the Children's—from the role of the family, to the relationship between children and staff, and the availability of psychosocial support services.

Since the 1940s, it has been recognized that sick children experience less anxiety and recover more quickly when their families take part in their hospital care. Today, children can be accompanied by family members not only in the waiting room, but also in most diagnostic and treatment areas.

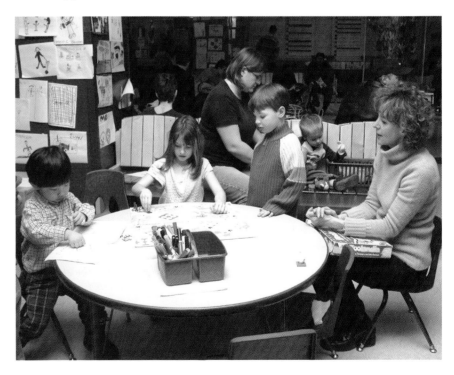

CHILDREN HAPPIEST WITH THEIR FAMILIES

One of the first major changes was the elimination of strict visiting hours for patients' families. Prior to the 1950s, hospitalized children rarely saw their parents, and visits from siblings and friends were prohibited. Dr. Statten and others realized that children tend to be more calm and cooperative if their parents are with them, and that a child's separation from the family during treatment, particularly when there are long-term or repeated hospitalizations, can have devastating, sometimes long-lasting, emotional effects.

Today, hospitalized children can spend time with their parents 24 hours a day and receive visits from siblings and other relatives and friends throughout the day. With family members there to feed, bathe, and play with them, and to bring toys, clothing, and treats from home, patients' daytime routines are kept as positive and as normal as possible. A child waking at night is often reassured by the sight of a parent sleeping on a cot beside him. With parents present during most diagnostic tests and participating in many treatment procedures, the child's anxiety is decreased and recovery sometimes accelerated.

Children's need to be with their families also led to the development, in the 1960s, of a home care program—now called Intensive Ambulatory Care Services—whereby children with chronic illnesses could be cared for at home with back-up from hospital staff. The program has expanded dramatically over the past 40 years, with new technology and training enabling parents—and sometimes the children themselves—to perform procedures that in the past had to take place in the hospital setting. The quality of life for most of these youngsters has improved dramatically.

Children with certain neuromuscular disorders, for instance, who previously would have been hospitalized for extended periods, and often died by the time they were teenagers, can now be connected to non-invasive, portable ventilators at home. They hook themselves up at night, get a good night's sleep, and function almost normally during the day. They may have physical restrictions—many are in wheelchairs, for instance—but they can go to school, to the movies, and to the park with family and friends.

Some children with chronic illnesses spend part of the day in hospital receiving treatments, then go home to sleep. Regular interventions for diseases such as leukemia, for instance, previously involved long hospital stays. Today these patients might come to the Children's in the morning for hydration, which requires connection to an intravenous line, then receive chemotherapy, have a lumbar puncture and any other necessary interventions, and return home at the end of the day.

Other children with chronic illnesses, such as juvenile diabetes or childhood arthritis, come to the hospital's outpatient clinics for periodic checkups and treatments, and otherwise lead relatively normal lives at home.

Day surgery has provided another way to avoid the psychological trauma of hospitalization. Since the 1970s, an increasing number of procedures such

Many children who would previously have been hospitalized can now live at home and receive regular outpatient treatments at the hospital. Anik comes to the Children's for dialysis three times a week.

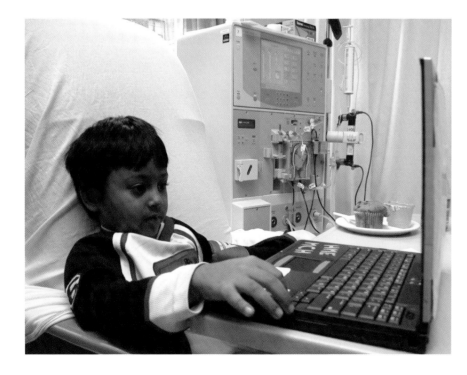

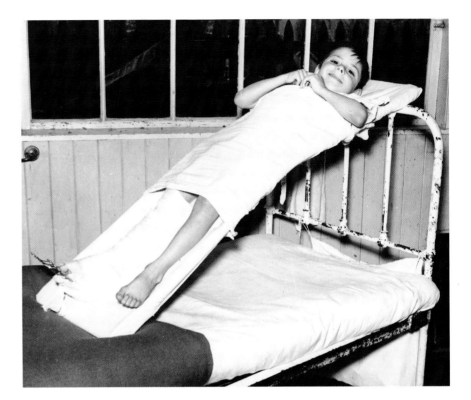

as orthopedic surgeries, hernia operations, dental work, and some ear, nose and throat operations can be performed on an outpatient basis.

Prior to the late 1970s, a child scheduled for a tonsillectomy would be admitted one day, have the operation the following day, and spend another night in hospital recuperating. Today, with new anesthetics and operating techniques, the child can go in for preoperative workup a few days prior to surgery, then come back for the operation and return home the same day. By 1985, 60% of surgeries were performed as day surgeries; today, the figure is more than 70%. Other operations that in the past might have involved many days of hospitalization now require only a single night's stay.

In 1915, the average patient was hospitalized for 50 days. For many, it was much longer. The Children's was often a place to recuperate from illness, with only a small percentage of the children acutely ill. By the early 1950s, with many previously long-term illnesses now treatable with antibiotics, the average stay was reduced to 12.5 days. By the early 1970s, with home care and outpatient clinics expanding, it was just over 7 days, and in 2002/03, it was 6.1 days. Only the most critically ill children are now hospitalized.

STAFF AND ENVIRONMENT REDUCE PATIENT STRESS

Another important development at the MCH in the 1970s was the way patient care was organized. Because the whole child was now the focus of treatment, teams of professionals from a variety of disciplines began working together to diagnose and treat each child. A youngster who had been in a car accident, for example, might be cared for by a multidisciplinary team made up of medical and surgical specialists, nurses, a social worker, a pharmacist, a physiotherapist, and any number of other healthcare professionals.

In addition to meeting medical needs, members of the multidisciplinary teams are trained to make each child feel as safe and comfortable as possible. They know that if a child is afraid and out of control, test results may be compromised. Stress can also affect the immune system and other systems, slowing recovery and even putting the child at risk.

Prior to the 1940s, children often spent months and even years in the hospital, suffering from diseases that have since been eliminated or greatly reduced in severity. This boy, suffering from tuberculosis of the spine and hip, was hospitalized for two years.

MCH doctors and other professionals are experts at explaining tests and procedures to children in age-appropriate language. Here, Dr. David McGillivray, Associate Director of Medical Emergency, sticks out his own tongue to show a young child how it's done.

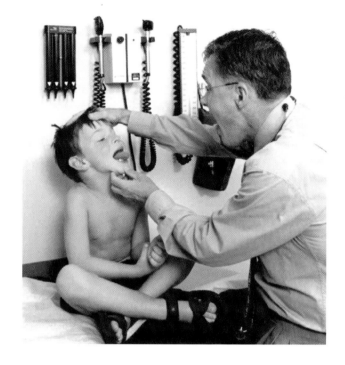

There is always a role for "low tech," especially in a hospital dedicated to caring for children. Here, young Tommy visits the 8th-floor outdoor play area with child life specialist Bertrand Dupuis. Tommy is able to get around by pulling along an IV pole attached to his little wagon. There are other low-tech conveniences, too: some small patients are encouraged to get themselves to the operating room under their own steam — by tricycle!

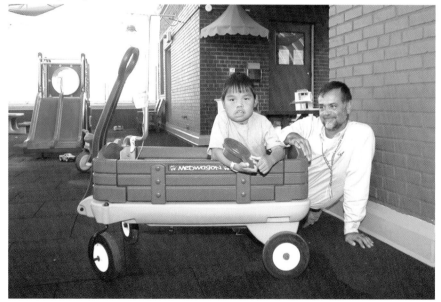

Surgery and tests can be scary experiences for children, so hospital staff try to make them as easy as possible. Masks to deliver anesthetics have familiar smells in them, such as raspberry, and the masks are clear so the children can look around. Many young patients are interested to see all the machines in the OR. Meanwhile, music helps relax children while they undergo tests like MRIs. They wear headphones so they can listen to music, and the technician can interrupt to give instructions.

Whenever possible, staff members take the time to show or explain to children, in developmentally appropriate terms, what specific tests and procedures will entail. For young children, they may use puppets and dolls, equipped with tubes, bandages, and masks, to explain what will happen during an operation or medical procedure. For older children, audiovisual materials have been developed. In the preoperative clinic, a video shows young patients what an operating room looks like, what staff members look like with their masks on, how the doctor or person who puts them to sleep will talk to them, why parents aren't allowed in the operating room, and so on.

The physical environment itself is also designed to reduce stress and make the hospital experience more pleasant for the young patients. There are bright play areas and colourful murals throughout the building. Toys, television sets, and video games are available to distract and entertain. And an outdoor terrace, renovated in 2004, is available for fresh air and play during the summer months.

The hospital can be especially scary and confusing if the child and his parents do not speak English or French and are newly arrived in Canada. Today, roughly one-third of patients at the MCH speak French as their mother tongue, one-third English, and the rest another language. Since 1986, the hospital's Multiculturalism Program has provided interpreters in roughly 40 languages and helped staff deal sensitively with children from different linguistic, religious, and cultural backgrounds.

In 1996, the Transcultural Child Psychiatry Clinic was launched to help children from other cultures deal with psychological problems. Since its inception, the clinic has seen children from more than 70 countries, the majority being newcomers to Quebec, many from countries that have recently experienced armed conflict.

No matter what the children's language or culture, the hospital's staff is concerned with their safety and the protection of their rights. An important part of the MCH's mission, in fact, is "to be an advocate for the rights of all children to reach their full potential." Within the hospital, issues related to the physical and psychological welfare of the children and their families are considered in every treatment plan. The Children's also has a history of supporting and mobilizing parents and community groups in developing programs, standards, and legislation that result in the improved health and welfare of children.

In the early 1960s, the hospital launched its Child Protection Team (later Committee), a multidisciplinary group designed to diagnose, treat, and provide help to children in need of protection and to their parents or guardians. It offers advice and clinical consultation, acting as a liaison with outside organizations in cases of suspected abuse or neglect.

FROM INFANCY TO ADOLESCENCE

The hospital's mandate is to treat children from birth to age 18. Today, the majority—roughly 63%—are under the age of six, as that is when common pediatric illnesses are most prevalent. Another 27% are between seven and 14, with the remaining 10% between 15 and 18 (2002/03 figures).

Tremendous changes have occurred in the care of all age groups since 1904, but perhaps the most dramatic is in the treatment of newborn babies. Although babies are not born at the Children's, newborns with medical problems have been transferred to the hospital since its first infants' ward opened in 1913.

THE AFTERMATH OF WAR

Some of the most challenging cases seen at the Children's are refugees who have lived terrifying experiences in their native countries before coming to Canada. Dr. Cécile Rousseau, who specializes in transcultural psychiatry, recalls one such child—13-year-old Marie (not her real name), adopted by a Canadian family after being rescued from her African homeland. During atrocities there, Marie's hands were cut off, and she had seen her own friends and family murdered.

The prostheses she used to replace her hands were a constant reminder to her teachers and fellow students of what she had been through. They expected her to speak about these horrors so they could sympathize and she could deal with the terrifying memories—our own culture's way of dealing with tragedies. However, Marie responded with silence, broken only by terrible rages that frightened them. She refused to speak her native language to the African member of her transcultural psychiatric team, and would give only her adopted name. "I'm Marie Tremblay," she would say.

The first breakthrough came when she received her immigration papers and felt safe enough to open up to the past. She began to ask for music from her native country, lullabies that she would hum to herself. Gradually, she then began opening up to childhood memories, such as well-known sayings, day-to-day activities, familiar smells—all the memories she had hidden away. The silences and the rages subsided. Marie's schoolmates are no longer afraid of her.

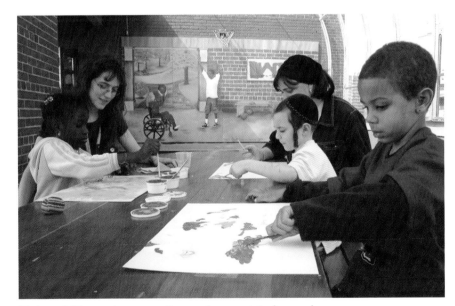

Today, children who are well enough may visit the newly renovated 8th-floor terrace, where fresh air and play provide a welcome change from the nursing unit.

The hospital's first neonatal intensive care unit (NICU) was established in 1957. As described by Dr. Eugene Outerbridge, then Director of the NICU, in the 1978/79 Annual Report, it was a primitive unit by today's standards:

"As a small 12 bed Unit, it had limited facilities; moreover it could not offer the intensive care for which it is known today. In fact, in the late '50s, there was very little awareness of the premature's sensitivity to temperature change and to taking proper precautions against infections or to proper food requirements. As a result, often babies born before term would not survive. Unfortunately, in the 1950s prematures were also too often the victims of an infant technology; for example, very little was done with incubators and infants were not given glucose and fluids intravenously. There were no respirators until the mid-1960s and intravenous feeding was not developed. There was no hospital policy fostering that initial parent–child contact which has since been found to be crucial."

NEW APPROACHES FOR NEWBORNS

By the 1970s, all that began to change. The Division of Neonatalogy was renamed the Division of Newborn Medicine in 1970 and was mandated to develop an active program of research into the causes of illnesses in newborn infants. A new 26-bed facility was created in the late 1970s, and a number of new programs encouraged parent–child contact and infant stimulation. Virtually every department was now involved with the care of newborns, from Physiotherapy and Dietetics to most of the hospital's laboratories.

The survival rate of premature babies increased dramatically in the late 1980s, as many health-care enterprises invested in research and development to produce new equipment and medications. Better incubators helped prevent heat loss in babies and more sophisticated ventilators supported tiny lungs.

In 1989, Dr. Robert Brouillette was invited to join the Children's with a view to expanding the staff and activities of the Division of Newborn Medicine. Since then, the medical staff has doubled, neonatal follow-up activities have grown considerably, and the division has brought in new techniques. Surfactant is now used for respiratory distress syndrome and the hospital has been the first in Quebec to work with high-frequency ventilation, nitric oxide, and ECMO for respiratory failure (see Chapter 9).

Today, the NICU provides specialized care to neonatal patients with surgical and cardiac conditions, as well as to those needing multidisciplinary care or with more common neonatal problems. Each year, 300 to 400 newborns are referred to the Children's from some 40 birthing centres in and around Montreal, brought to the hospital by its state-of-the-art neonatal transport team.

The development of intensive care was also a major advance in the treatment of other pediatric patients. While the NICU specializes in disorders of prematurity, the pediatric intensive care unit (PICU), established in 1969, deals primarily with older children. It is equipped to handle virtually any acute surgical or medical problem, including severe asthma (the most common). Some newborns who are not premature are also treated here, particularly those requiring the unit's cardiac specialists. The average stay today is three and a half days, after which patients are generally transferred to other nursing units.

ADOLESCENT SERVICES COME OF AGE

The care of adolescents, too, has changed a great deal over the years. In a 1948 lecture, Dr. Alton Goldbloom, then Physician-in-Chief, referred to "adolescence—that great unknown no man's land of medicine." Since then, the Children's has been a pioneer in the field.

Until the early 1950s, the hospital made little distinction between ages, except for newborns, and a nursing unit or clinic might include the whole spectrum. Older teens were often sent directly to adult hospitals. In 1961, recognizing the special needs of young people between the ages of 12 and 18, the hospital established the Adolescent Outpatient Clinic, the first of its kind in Canada. The clinic was designed to oversee all aspects of adolescent health care, providing medical services, counselling, and psychotherapy in an atmosphere of acceptance and confidentiality. This approach was important, as it still is today, because a large percentage of the teens treated for physical ailments also have emotional problems. They might be worried about sexually transmitted diseases, pregnancy, or family problems, or suffer from eating disorders, substance abuse, or depression.

During the 1970s, demands on the Adolescent Clinic, like other outpatient clinics, grew by leaps and bounds. By 1979, there were more than 3,500 visits to the clinic annually, about half for medical care and half for gynecological services.

A separate nursing unit for adolescents existed at the hospital until the late 1980s, housing boys and girls suffering from chronic illnesses that predominantly affect teenagers, such as cystic fibrosis, cere-

TEENS AND CONFIDENTIALITY

In the 1950s, Dr. John Elder was the first to insist that some of his adolescent patients should be seen without their parents. This was a revolutionary concept. Dr. Elder recognized that teens have unique emotional and psychological needs, and this sensitivity became part of the Division of Adolescent Medicine's approach to patient care. In 1981, adolescent services were moved to the Gilman Pavilion, separate from the main hospital, where teens could have a sense of privacy and independence.

Since the Quebec Public Health Protection Act of 1972, the right of teenagers aged 14 and over to make their own medical decisions has been entrenched in law. Although most adolescents continue to want their parents to be present during diagnosis and treatment, this is not always the case in matters of sexual counselling, eating disorders, and other sensitive areas.

BATTLING ANOREXIA

"People think that if you are anorexic you do not want food. In my case it was the opposite. I was so obsessed with food that it became my only thought. It consumed me until it hurt inside," says former patient Melissa in a 2001 edition of the MCH Foundation's publication *The Children's Own*.

Eating disorders such as anorexia nervosa have become increasingly prevalent among adolescents in recent years. In Melissa's case, the disease became literally a battle for life. At 5 feet 7 inches and 113 pounds, she decided to cut all fats from her diet in an attempt to lose weight. Before long, the weight loss was spiralling out of control, but still she wanted to lose more. Melissa's heart was affected and on the recommendation of Dr. Franziska Baltzer of the MCH Adolescent Medicine and Gynecology Clinic she was hospitalized twice.

Melissa realized that to prevent repeated hospitalization she would have to stop "cheating" and take control of her behaviour. She accepted the need for regular monitoring by the hospital and expressed the hope that, in time, she would become a peer counsellor for other adolescents battling anorexia.

bral palsy, muscular dystrophy, and eating disorders. Over time, these conditions have been increasingly managed without admission to hospital. In 1988, most MCH nursing units were reorganized to allow for more efficient treatment of patients with similar diseases and conditions, regardless of age. Adolescents requiring hospitalization are now admitted to these specialty-based units with children of all ages, while outpatient services are still provided in a variety of specialized adolescent clinics.

By the 1980s, the number of outpatient clinics for adolescents had expanded to include general medicine clinics, a sexually transmitted diseases clinic, a contraceptive clinic, and a teen discussion group. Today, sexually transmitted diseases and contraception are dealt with in the general clinics, while addi-

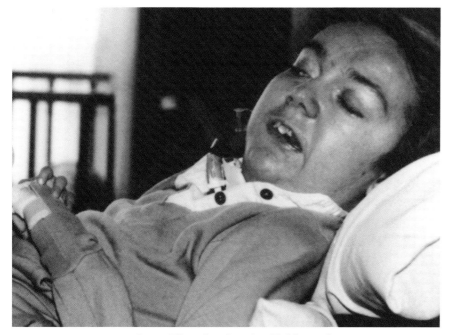

Joyce Elliott lived at the Children's for many years. Diagnosed at a young age with a neurodegenerative disorder, she was hospitalized in her teens, suffering paralysis and dependent on a respirator at night. The hospital's staff members were like family to her, taking her shopping and inviting her to their weddings. She joked that her role was to train new residents. "It's been a rough day," she'd say. "There was a whole new crop of residents who didn't know anything about my disease."

Joyce was very upbeat and determined, and knew what she wanted. In 1990, when she was in her late 20s, she had little movement left and knew it wouldn't be long before she couldn't even ask for help. She requested that her respirator be turned off, and people came from all over to say goodbye.

"She was very courageous," recalls nurse Brenda Wilson. "She died the way she lived — her way."

tional clinics have been set up for eating disorders, sexual abuse, complex menstrual disorders, teenage pregnancy and motherhood, and depression.

In 1993, Adolescent Medicine and Gynecology were merged. Since that time, despite limited medical staffing, the number of patients seen by the clinic has risen significantly. In 2003/04, staff responded to 5,300 patient visits. The clinic's patient population has also become increasingly more complex, often with multiple diagnoses.

In most cases, patients still requiring care when they turn 18 are transferred to adult hospitals, but there are exceptions. A patient who had a heart disorder treated as a child, for instance, may have problems lingering into adulthood that are best treated by pediatricians who understand the disorder. There are also home care programs based at the Children's for adults suffering from hemophilia and thalassemia, and in other programs patients might stay with the MCH into adulthood if they are receiving palliative care.

CHANGING ATTITUDES

Elisabeth Gibbon, Coordinator of Community Relations and Ombudsman, tells how attitudes towards Inuit children have changed since she started at the hospital in the late 1960s.

"When I first worked here, Inuit patients didn't have family names; there was a first name and a number. I remember working on the wards and being told that these kids don't laugh or smile, that it's a cultural thing. Of course it wasn't true. It was because they were in such a strange place—in a big city, away from home—and in those days they were very often brought down alone. Now, they usually bring a family member with the child."

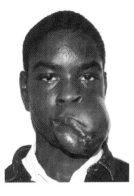

Ricardo came from Haiti in the fall of 2001 to have a massive vascular tumour on his face removed. The tumour was composed of very large arteries and veins that were present at birth and gradually enlarged, causing severe deformity. A special program at the Children's allows for surgical removal of such tumours by a team of plastic surgeons, cardiac surgeons, cardiologists, imaging specialists, anesthesiologists, and nurses, headed by Dr. Bruce Williams, plastic surgeon and Surgeon-in-Chief. So that the tumour could be removed with minimal bleeding, Ricardo had to undergo a cardiac bypass procedure.

The photos show Ricardo prior to surgery and in November 2003. Whereas before the operation Ricardo would not attend school due to his severe deformity, he is now doing well at school and participates in many sports.

CHILDREN FROM NEAR AND FAR

Most of the hospital's patients have traditionally come from Montreal and surrounding areas. Currently, 60% live in the Greater Montreal area, while the rest come from other regions of Quebec, elsewhere in Canada, and other countries.

Some children and their families have travelled great distances to seek specialized treatment at the Children's. In the 1930s, for instance, word of the remarkable work being done in correcting cleft palates brought cases from across the country and beyond. In the 1940s, '50s, and '60s, the volume of patients with cardiac problems referred from throughout North America increased steadily. Today, patients are brought from afar for treatments such as cardiovascular surgery and neurosurgery, kidney transplants, orthopedic procedures, and plastic surgery.

Since the 1960s, a number of native children from remote areas of northern Canada have also been flown to the Children's as part of its Northern and Native Child Health Program. These children require specialized care that cannot be provided locally.

TOUCHING OUR HEARTS

From the very beginning, the Montreal Children's Hospital had a definite personality. In 1913, a visitor remarked, "The children in this hospital seem like a big, happy family." Many of them, of course, were convalescing from long-term illnesses and did not feel all that sick, and knew the staff and other patients well. In contrast, the children who are hospitalized today spend much less time actually in the hospital, and at the same time, tend to be much sicker. Some are in pain, and a few will not respond to treatment. Yet there is still a sense of caring and hope throughout the building, and more laughter than one would expect.

Those who work at the hospital do so because of the children. Of the many patients who leave a lasting impression, there are some who stand out.

They are of different ages, backgrounds, and medical conditions, but have one thing in common: an indomitable spirit, an ability to smile through the pain and inspire those around them.

Elisabeth Gibbon remembers Kim, a young girl with cystic fibrosis who had lost a sister to the same disease. Kim received treatments at the Children's for many years, and was always incredibly positive and good-tempered. She died only a year after realizing her dream of having a heart and lung transplant.

"In spite of all her problems," says Gibbon, "she really lived life. I think the gene that passes on cystic fibrosis also passes on niceness."

Diane Borisov, Director of Nursing, recalls two Inuit children who were brought from the North at different times but with the same condition, intractable diarrhea. Both girls arrived unaccompanied by parents, and both were very sick. They were as malnourished as children from famine-plagued countries. Doctors couldn't find the root cause and normal treatments didn't work.

"Despite the needle pricks and other interventions," Borisov says, "they both had incredible smiles. They became very special to the staff due to their exceptional drive, personalities, and long stay on the unit. And despite the odds, both survived."

Franco Carnevale, Coordinator of Critical Care, remembers a five-year-old girl who was hospitalized for many months with kidney problems. The two became very close (she planned to marry him when she grew up!).

"I had the privilege of knowing her well for over a year. I had the opportunity to get inside the world of a child who was a patient, who still had lots of hopes, who could still play, who still had wishes, who responded to things being done to her. I was saddened when she got an infection and eventually died. But in her short life, I was important to her. That's quite a privilege."

Each staff member has stories such as these. Stories of children devastated by disease, who never lose hope and sometimes beat the odds; of children so weak they can barely care for themselves but unselfishly take care of other patients; of children who reassure their parents, and even give them permission to let go. Stories of children who recover and go on to do amazing things with their lives.

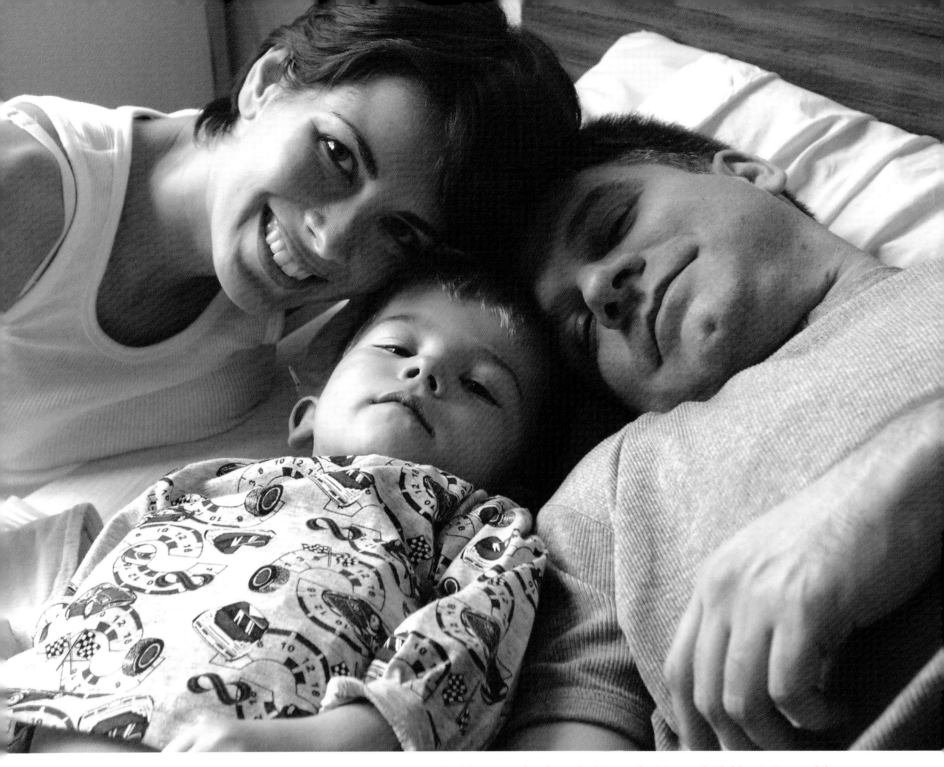

Alexis' parents first brought him to the Montreal Children's Hospital from Sherbrooke, Quebec, when he was just 10 days old. Alexis was born with only one functioning ventricle in his heart, a life-threatening malformation. From the beginning, Stéphanie and Nicolas, the boy's parents, had full confidence in their son's cardiologist, Dr. Luc Jutras, and cardiac surgeon, Dr. Christo Tchervenkov. Above, the family enjoys time together in Alexis' hospital room one week after the four-year-old's third and final open-heart surgery in 2004.

"A sustaining family network is critical to the care provided, whether ambulatory or hospitalized, and is vital to the successful integration of the child back into the community."

DR. HARVEY GUYDA, PHYSICIAN-IN-CHIEF

The Family Circle:
Caring for Kids and Their Parents

3

Families are an integral part of life at the Montreal Children's Hospital. Parents, siblings, and other family members keep children company in waiting rooms, reassure them during diagnostic and treatment procedures, and participate in their care on the nursing units. Whether a child is at the hospital for a few hours or for many months, the family's support and care are recognized as invaluable to the child's well-being.

This was not always the case. During the hospital's first half-century, families played a minor role in the child's hospital care and were sometimes viewed more as a hindrance than as a help.

FAMILY'S EARLY ROLE LIMITED

Prior to the late 1950s, parents were allowed only limited access to the hospital's clinics and wards. There were strictly enforced visiting hours, and parents could only stay overnight if the child was critically ill and might die. There were no cots or other facilities for them. Siblings were not allowed to visit in case they spread infections.

While parents were kept informed about their child's condition, they were usually told only as much as the physician felt they absolutely needed to know. Most parents relied unquestioningly on the doctor's expertise.

The child's family situation was usually only taken into consideration by hospital staff when it interfered directly with the child's medical treatment. In the 1916 Annual Report, for instance, the newly appointed social worker, Amy B. Hilton, reported:

"It has been found that a number of patients who were brought in here for malnutrition and whose condition was so improved by treatment in the Hospital that it was possible to discharge them as cured, were brought back again and again because of relapses and often in increasingly poor condition. This meant that the work of the Hospital was being wasted, and the care that ought to have been available for new cases was expended on those who had not profited wisely. Almost invariably the cause of the patients' return was bad home surroundings and ignorance on the part of the mothers. This was especially true of the infant patients, where generally the blame could be laid on careless feeding."

Main waiting room, circa 1946. When this photo was taken, the parents' role in their child's hospital care was usually confined to the waiting room and to strictly limited bedside visits.

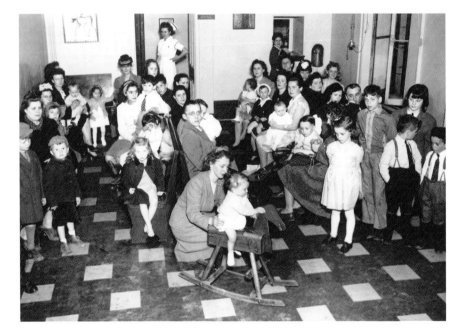

The following year she wrote, "Why do we need Social Service in Hospitals? The reply is because the sickness and suffering seen there is often due to bad housing, bad habits, ignorance, lack of sufficient income, domestic worries and many other non-medical, non-surgical causes which the doctor cannot investigate or remove."

To help reduce the effects of these conditions on children's health, CMH social workers and volunteers were trained to teach parents the importance of hygiene, fresh air, and nutrition, including the preparation of the complicated baby formulas of the day and the proper handling of food in warm weather. They even helped some parents find jobs and seek treatment for problems such as alcoholism.

Parents sometimes had to be reminded to take their children to the hospital for follow-up appointments, and transportation was arranged if necessary. Prior to the move to Tupper Street in 1956, even getting to the hospital was an ordeal for most families. With the sick child and often several other youngsters in tow, parents had to trudge half a mile uphill from the streetcar stop on Côte-des-Neiges Road to the hospital site above Cedar Avenue.

MANY TOO POOR TO PAY

Throughout much of the hospital's early history, the majority of families taking children to the CMH could not afford to pay all or even part of the modest hospital fee. (When the Children's first opened, the cost per patient day was 28 cents.) Records show that in 1938, for instance, only 3.8% of families paid the full cost of treatment. Until the Quebec government provided universal coverage for inpatient care under the Quebec Hospital Insurance Plan in 1961, and then expanded it to include outpatient care in the Health Insurance Act of 1970, parents often spent years paying off their child's treatment, and when even that was impossible, the bill was often simply cancelled.

Not knowing that the CMH accepted all patients regardless of the family's financial situation, many

parents in the early 1900s delayed taking children in until they were so sick that they died. This was one of the factors contributing to the high mortality rate at the time.

Beginning in the 1920s, a special fund was established by the CMH Social Services Department to provide families with emergency relief, sometimes paying for food, clothing, and medical equipment such as braces, crutches, and special boots. Parents usually repaid the cost of medical equipment on an instalment plan, but in some cases the equipment was given outright. Such assistance was in particular demand during the Depression, but it has continued to be part of the hospital's commitment to needy families ever since. Today, part of the hospital's Tiny Tim Fund goes to helping families with limited financial resources.

MEMBERS OF THE CARE TEAM

"The parents as part of [the] family constellation require no less understanding than the child. We speak so often of child psychiatry, when what we really mean is the sum total of interacting forces within the family group and their effect on its component parts."

DR. ALTON GOLDBLOOM,
PHYSICIAN-IN-CHIEF, 1946–1953
in a lecture at McGill University, 1948

In the 1940s, the hospital staff began to recognize that having a family member nearby and actively involved in the child's care could not only reduce the patient's anxiety but also speed recovery. By the early 1950s, families began to be included as part of certain outpatient treatment programs. A Saturday morning speech clinic for stutterers, for example, involved parents in a co-educational program, and a mothers' group for diabetic children was established and later expanded to include fathers. Individual and group education and therapy sessions were also begun with parents of children with chronic diseases and conditions such as cerebral palsy, cystic fibrosis, and mental handicaps.

By the late 1950s, the Children's had begun to relax visiting hours on the nursing units, abolishing them altogether by the early 1970s—the first pediatric hospital in Canada to do so. Hospital staff encouraged parents to spend as much time as possible with their hospitalized child. By the early 1980s, more than 25% of patients had at least one parent staying with them overnight. Today, it is more than half. There are almost as many parent cots as patient beds in some areas, while family lounges on each floor, a kitchen on the oncology unit, and some shower facilities make the family's stay more comfortable. Improved facilities for families are an important part of the plans for the Children's in the new McGill University Health Centre complex.

Some parents can be found at their child's bedside virtually around the clock for days, weeks, and sometimes even months. Friends and other family members, including young siblings, visit throughout the day. When family members are unable to be at the hospital due to distance, work, or other commitments, the hospital's staff and volunteers spend as much time as possible providing the child with personal care and support, staying in touch with the family through frequent telephone calls, e-mails, and faxes.

One of the last areas to encourage parent participation was the Neonatal Intensive Care Unit (NICU). Prior to the 1970s, the importance of early infant stimulation was not recognized, and glass panels, intended for infection control, limited the amount of contact parents could have with their babies. In the 1970s, numerous programs encouraging parent–child contact were established, and as Dr. Eugene Outerbridge, then Director of the Neonatal Unit, wrote in the 1978/79 Annual Report, "parents today can be seen touching, fondling and playing with their infants. As a result, today's premature babies are not only very much alive, they are indeed very lively, more mentally alert and better cared for."

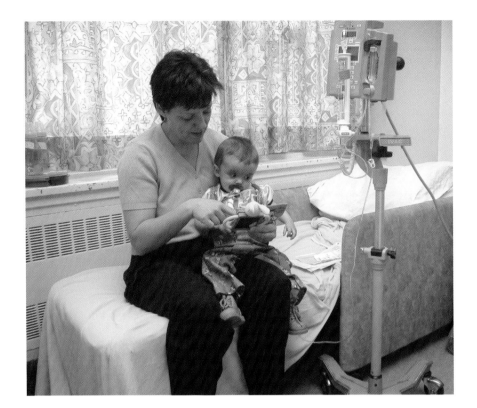

Families today also tend to play a more active role in the treatment process itself. On the inpatient units, nurses assess to what extent a family member is ready and able to assist with the child's care. A mother might learn to change a burn dressing, for instance. A father might be great at persuading the child to take medicine, or to get out of bed after surgery. An older brother or sister can assist with simple physiotherapy. It's comforting for the patient to be cared for at least in part by family members, and the families themselves often appreciate being able to contribute to the child's well-being.

Occasionally, family members can contribute to the child's health care in an even more substantial way, by donating blood, bone marrow, or even an organ for transplantation.

Families today can be involved in their child's hospital care around the clock, and cots are provided so parents can spend the night. Here, Manon Fortin entertains her son Gabriel Jacques.

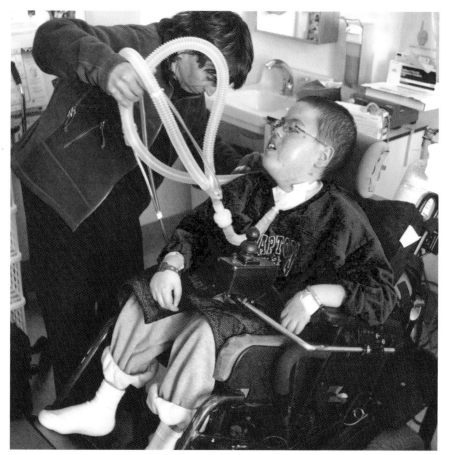

Lucy Cokay's son Erek lives at the hospital. She has been visiting him there for nearly 10 years, and has learned to perform many of the procedures on which his life depends. She suctions secretions from his windpipe and checks his feeding bag, which drips nutrients into a tube in his stomach. When Erek has to leave his room in his motorized chair, Lucy can detach the ventilator from the wall so it runs on batteries. She has even "bagged" him — that is, squeezed an ambulatory bag to give him air — when his ventilator failed on a field trip with the Mackay Centre School, where Erek attends classes.

Erek has a severe form of myotubular myopathy, a rare genetic disorder that causes muscle weakness and degeneration. He can no longer walk, speak, or swallow, and has limited use of only one arm. Lucy has been unable to care for him at home since he was a year old, and even taking him out of the hospital for brief periods is now difficult.

Lucy is a widow who lost another child at a young age, probably to the same disease, and has a healthy 13-year-old daughter. She is invariably cheerful and loving with her son, and sees how his face lights up when she enters the room. But she admits that helping care for a chronically ill, hospitalized child is extremely difficult. She is grateful to the staff members who have supported them both over the years, including nurses, doctors, social workers, the palliative care team, and Father Paul Geraghty, who visits Erek every day and has become a father figure to the boy.

Since the 1960s, many children who would previously have been admitted to the hospital have been cared for at home, thanks to training, medications, and equipment provided to their families by the Children's. Parents can now administer home antibiotic treatments, for instance, to children with illnesses such as pneumonia, who were once routinely hospitalized. Families can care for children with kidney disease or many forms of cancer, taking them to the hospital for daily or weekly dialysis or chemotherapy.

The Home Oxygen Therapy Program teaches parents of infants with chronic respiratory problems to operate oxygen machines at home. Until the early 1980s, these children stayed in the hospital, often for a very long time. Parents of children with some forms of sleep apnea are trained in CPR and provided with sleep apnea monitors in case their child stops breathing during the night. These are just a few of the home care programs supervised by the hospital's Intensive Ambulatory Care Services.

Another major change has been in the area of children's surgery. The combination of outpatient preoperative workups, modern anesthetics, and improved surgical techniques has contributed to a significant rise in day surgery, in which children can often go home just a few hours after their operation. There has also been an increase in same-day surgery, in which children are operated on the same day they are admitted, although they then stay one day or more in hospital for recovery.

Prior to the 1970s, children undergoing planned surgery were normally admitted at least a day ahead of time for preoperative tests and procedures. In the 1970s, Associate Director of Nursing Gwen Olivier —who was also instrumental in eliminating restricted visiting hours for families—introduced the concept of doing preoperative workups on an outpatient basis. Children are then only admitted on the actual day of surgery. Same-day surgery both reduces the amount of time children are in hospital and makes

HOME CARE PIONEER

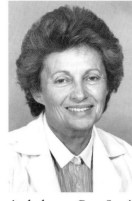

Dr. Hanna Strawczynski believed that children belong with their families and should spend as little time as possible at the hospital. Trained as a pediatrician in Poland and Canada, Dr. Strawczynski joined the MCH in 1964, doing home visits to sick children as part of the newly formed Home Care Program—now Intensive Ambulatory Care Services. It was the first such program in North America designed specifically to meet the needs of children and their families in their homes. Home care enabled children with chronic illnesses such as cerebral palsy—who previously spent years in hospital—to live dramatically improved lives at home. When founder Dr. Brian Wherrett left in 1969, Dr. Strawczynski took over the department, expanding services to include children suffering from conditions leading to frequent acute episodes such as hemophilia and thalassemia, who prior to this were admitted many times a year for short stays.

Today, Intensive Ambulatory Care helps parents provide care at home to children with severe progressive neuromuscular disorders, hemophilia, thalassemia, chronic lung disease, or HIV disease; those needing home ventilation, or with tracheotomies; those requiring home parenteral antibiotic therapy; liver and heart transplant patients; and children receiving palliative care at home.

better use of available beds. After surgery, children stay in the hospital for as long as their recovery requires. In day surgery, a child having a simple hernia operation might be discharged after only two hours in the recovery room, while a child over the age of three undergoing a routine tonsillectomy might stay for four hours. For both day surgery and same-day surgery, parents are provided, during the preoperative visit and before the child is released, with detailed instructions for follow-up care.

SUPPORT FOR FAMILIES

In many cases, the at-home treatment of a chronically ill child can be incorporated into the family's regular routine, with the child and other family members living virtually normal lives. When a child has juvenile diabetes, for instance, measuring blood sugar levels, administering insulin, and planning appropriate meals often become just part of the day's activities.

But sometimes the level of home care required is such that looking after the child becomes not only very time-consuming but also emotionally draining. In these cases, support from the hospital becomes extremely important.

Although home visits from staff have been rare since the 1960s, a 24-hour-a-day telephone service is available to most parents caring for chronically ill children at home. For most chronic illnesses, there's an identified nurse or clinical nurse specialist the family can contact in case of crisis. When the burden of taking care of the child around the clock becomes too much, the hospital will sometimes provide respite care. A home aid worker may go into the home, for instance, allowing parents to go shopping, get a haircut, or spend time with the other children.

Support is also available for families of hospitalized children and those attending outpatient clinics, when they need help dealing with the stress of their child's injury or illness. This is particularly vital in the case of frequent or lengthy hospitalizations, or the death of a child.

One of the hospital's most important support functions is providing families with as comprehensive information as possible about the child's condition, upcoming tests, and treatments. It is now recognized that being well-informed can alleviate some of the anxiety parents feel when bringing their child to the hospital, and can also help them prepare their child more calmly for hospitalization or outpatient treatments. While parents continue to rely primarily on the knowledge and expertise of the hospital's physicians and other health-care professionals, they

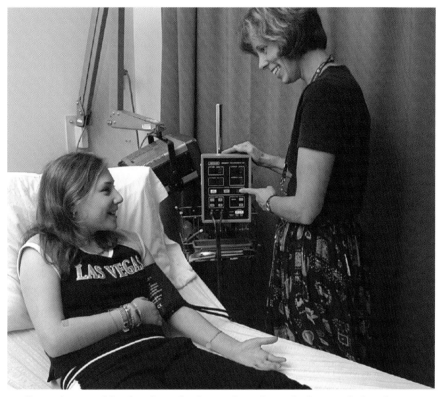

Malka Labow and husband Michael Hart have been dealing with daughter Hillary's illness at home since she was a baby. At three and a half months, Hillary was diagnosed with glycogen storage disease, a rare metabolic disorder caused by the absence of a liver enzyme that converts glycogen to glucose. For this reason, her blood sugar levels must be constantly monitored to prevent severe hypoglycemia.

The hospital staff taught Malka to test Hillary's glucose levels and to insert a tube through the child's nose into her stomach at bedtime. The tube was attached to a machine that provided continuous liquid formula to keep her blood sugar stable. Since Hillary was reluctant to suck on a bottle during the day, Malka would feed her daughter the special formula through a syringe. By age one, Hillary was drinking the formula from a spill-proof cup.

Today, Hillary's condition is controlled with a very restricted diet eliminating all sugars, and by having cornstarch with water at meal times to help sustain blood sugar levels. She still has to wake up once every night to drink cornstarch and water, but at age 14 she's able to take more responsibility for her own care. She's an active teen who dreams that research will one day discover how to replace the enzyme her body is missing, allowing her to have an entire ice cream cone instead of just an occasional lick.

Her mother brings Hillary for checkups at the hospital every nine to 12 months. (Above, Hillary's blood pressure is checked by nurse Lina Moisan.) "It's like a family, even though we're not related," says Malka. "We know the doctors and nurses in the CIU [Clinical Investigation Unit] and have a profound respect for one another. Treating Hillary is a partnership between us and the hospital staff. They have really made things easier for us."

also tend to ask more questions than in the past, and often do additional research so their decisions may be as informed as possible.

When a child is hospitalized unexpectedly, and when parents face difficult medical decisions, members of the multidisciplinary care team take great care to explain the child's condition, treatment options, and possible consequences as comprehensively and sensitively as possible. They know that in crisis situations parents may have difficulty absorbing information and need help to decide quickly among several options.

Sometimes a family member has difficulty accepting the child's condition. Occasionally, parents disagree about their child's treatment. Balancing the

The Family Resource Library is a place where families can find health information about children's medical conditions, parenting, and pain management. Filled with books, videos, pamphlets, and a computer station for parents, the library also houses a toy-lending library and a computer centre for children. Here, Kiraly Batist helps parent Mary-Lou Sims with some research.

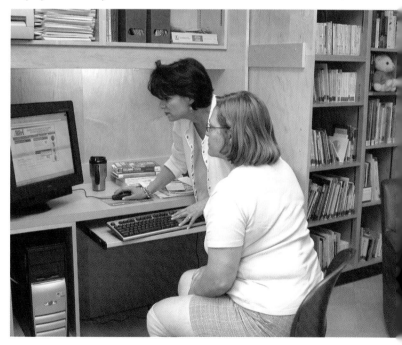

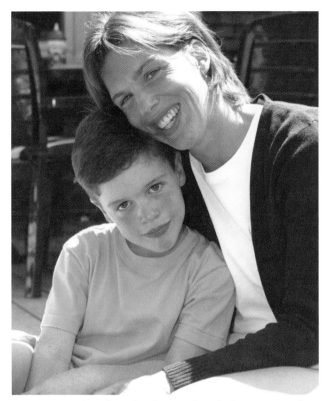

Sara Provencher thought the care her diabetic son Jack receives at the Children's was standard practice — until she spoke to mothers of diabetic children elsewhere.

When Jack was first diagnosed and briefly hospitalized at two and a half years old, Sara was taught how to control her son's diet, test his blood sugar, and give him insulin injections. She was also told about parent support groups. But it didn't end there. During the nine years since his diagnosis, Jack has received follow-up care at the hospital's endocrinology clinic every three months. He has blood tests and a checkup, including measuring his weight and examining his eyesight. Sara regularly discusses her son's condition with his doctor and dietitian.

After speaking with mothers in other settings, she says, "In most places, they pretty much diagnose you and throw you out on your behind. They say, 'Here's the medicine, here's the book, do it by yourself.' I was taking what we have here for granted. Now I'm really grateful."

care of a sick child with work and other family responsibilities can also be difficult, and siblings may experience anxiety or feel neglected. In each of these cases, individual or family counselling can be provided, and families can be put in touch with one of the many support groups based at the Children's. The hospital also provides important follow-up support so parents don't feel abandoned after the child is discharged.

GOING THAT EXTRA MILE

When a family comes to the Children's from out of town, the hospital's Social Services Department can help them find reasonably priced accommodation in a nearby hotel. Social workers can also connect parents with a wide array of other community services. They might help parents get a wheelchair for the child, for example, or assist them in applying for a grant to make their home wheelchair-accessible.

When a family has recently immigrated to Canada, the language, customs, and medical treatment options may be foreign to them. The hospital's Multiculturalism Program can provide interpreters to assist parents who are unable to speak English or French or whose comprehension of these languages

THANKS AND CHEERS

In the 1960s, Dr. Brian Wherrett, head of Home Care, would take a nurse, a social worker, and medical students with him on Fridays to visit ambulatory care patients and their families throughout the Montreal area. Many of the families were recent immigrants from Italy, Portugal, and Greece, and their way of saying thank you was to offer a glass of homemade wine. It was lucky the staff took a taxi, because it was hard to refuse!

"I even changed my itinerary so that I would go to the established French and English areas of Montreal first," he recalls, "so that the smell of alcohol was not on my breath when I came to see children from cultural backgrounds where this would have been inappropriate."

IN LOVING MEMORY

Several times a year, a memorial service is held for children who have died at the hospital during the past few months. The services were originally for staff members who couldn't attend the funerals and needed to say goodbye, but today they include a mix of families and staff. Although some parents find it too difficult, about 60% of them attend, often with the child's siblings and other family members.

The service is a moving tribute to the lives of these special children. Staff members read stories, poetry, and prayers in a variety of languages and sometimes dedicate special songs. A candle is lit for each child and every family receives a white carnation. It is a reminder that the child was important to the staff.

"We knew the staff cared," said one father. "But now we really know how much."

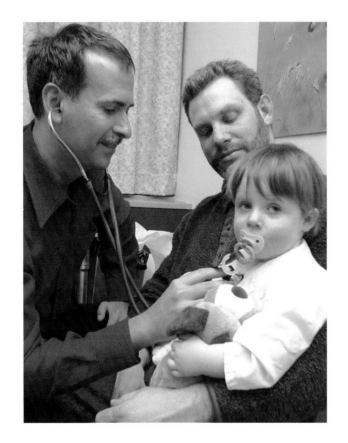

Sylvain Chapdelaine holds his son, two-year-old François, as Dr. Luc Jutras listens to the boy's heart. As a pediatric cardiologist, Dr. Jutras spends much of his time reassuring families and helping them sort out information about their child's condition.

is limited. Liaisons have also been developed with ethnocultural communities served by the MCH, to allow staff a better understanding of and respect for cultural values and practices and how they relate to the child's health care.

No matter what the family members' religion, they may receive spiritual support from the hospital's multifaith Pastoral Services Department. Since 1989, a chaplain has been assigned to each nursing unit and to the Emergency Department, with links to virtually every religious denomination in the area. Even if family members are not religious, the presence of a chaplain can be a real comfort as they live through the difficult experience of a child's illness.

The chaplains are also part of the hospital's Palliative Care Service. First established for hospitalized patients in 1991—the first such program in a Canadian pediatric hospital—the palliative care team supports children and families dealing with critical illness and helps family members cope with the loss of a child. They know that if the family receives good support at the time of a child's death, their grieving may be less complicated.

Virtually every member of the hospital's staff and dedicated team of volunteers contributes in some way to the support of families at the Children's, whether it's by reassuring anxious parents at the reception desk, or offering an exhausted family member a cup of tea.

Sometimes a small act of kindness can make a difficult situation more bearable. In one case, an Inuit mother who had to be away from her hospitalized baby for many months received a scrapbook of photos and comments created by the nurses, recording the child's development. Another mother, who visited her infant at the hospital every morning before work but was late one day, was touched to find a housekeeper singing to the baby until she arrived.

GIVING BACK

Throughout the MCH's century-long history, families have come to care deeply about the hospital and its patients, and have wanted to give something in return for the care and support they and their children have received.

Many parents take the time to send cards and photos to express their appreciation and show how well their children are doing. Even parents of children who didn't make it are often impressed enough with the hospital and its staff that they look for ways to turn their grief into something positive. Some parents donate their time—volunteering in the hospital, working with support groups, or raising funds. Some sit on the Family Advisory Forum, a parent group whose purpose is "to provide input and feedback on delivery of service for children and their families, establish channels of communication between families and staff, and represent parents on certain hospital committees."

Sometimes families generously donate items for the nursing units, waiting rooms, or library. Others turn their energies to the overall environment by raising funds to improve facilities, purchase equipment, or support a special program. And sometimes, by courageously allowing staff to try new medications and treatments when these offer the possibility of hope, parents and children contribute to the well-being of future patients.

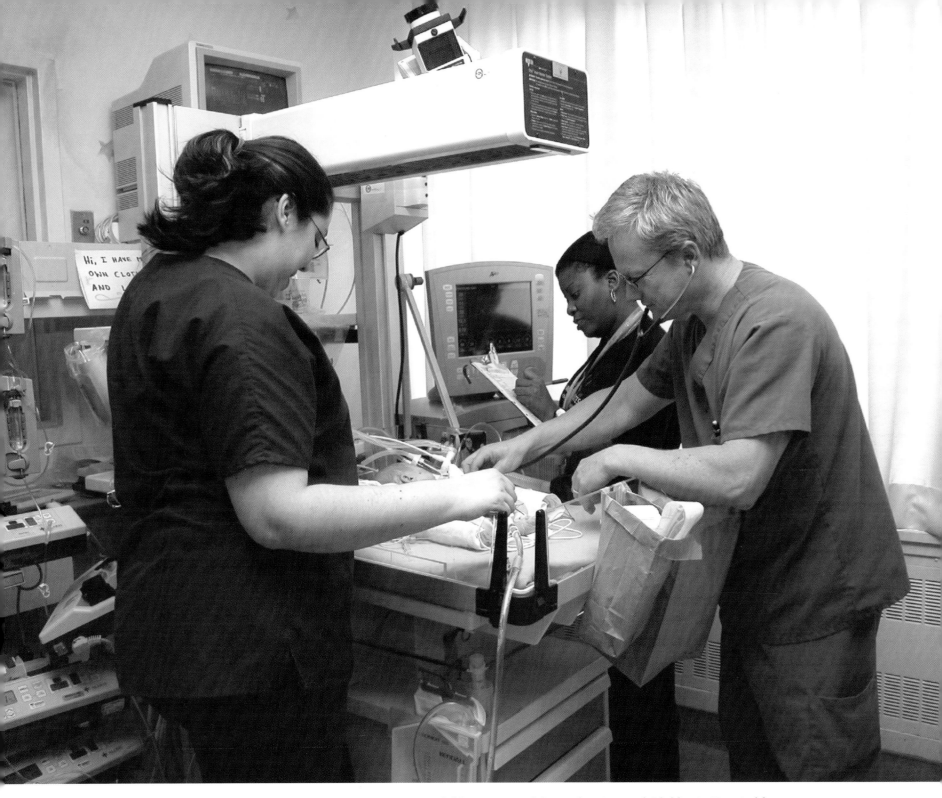

Children are cared for at the Montreal Children's Hospital by multidisciplinary teams of professionals. Here, nurses Beatrix Silva and Mario Bonenfant and inhalation therapist Stacey Broom (checking chart) examine a patient in the Neonatal Intensive Care Unit.

"In a children's hospital the staff must have very special
qualifications. Each member must be an expert of the highest
order in his own specialty and he must have a strong sense of
concern and devotion to the children he serves."

DR. DAVID R. MURPHY, SURGEON-IN-CHIEF, 1954–1974
1973 Annual Report

4

The Staff:
A Shared Spirit, a Shared Goal

If the hospital's founders were to walk through the halls of the Montreal Children's Hospital today, they would be astounded, not just at the number of individuals who work there, but also at the wide variety of specialized tasks they perform.

In 1904, the staff consisted of two part-time doctors, a head nurse, two assistant nurses, and a housekeeper. As patient numbers swelled, hospital facilities expanded, and public awareness of the importance of health care heightened, the number of staff members also grew. Today there are over 1,500 employees and more than 300 surgical and pediatric specialists and subspecialists.

Patients at the Children's are now cared for by a comprehensive team of physicians, surgeons, nurses, allied health professionals, technical and administrative personnel, and support staff. Whether it's a cardiac surgeon performing a delicate operation on a newborn, a nurse offering bedside care to a child on a respirator, a maintenance man modifying adult equipment to meet a child's needs, or a food services employee preparing child-friendly meals, each member of the MCH family plays a vital role in ensuring that all patients receive the most effective pediatric care possible.

A DOCTOR IN THE HOUSE

When the hospital first opened, there were only two part-time doctors on staff: Drs. Alexander Mackenzie Forbes and Harold B. Cushing.

Dr. Forbes (1874–1929) was an orthopedic surgeon working in the Outpatient Department of the Montreal General Hospital and in the clinic of the Montreal Dispensary when he became concerned about the number of crippled children in the streets of Montreal. Many were from poor families with little access to health care. To provide them with early treatment, he convinced a group of local physicians and community members to establish a small pediatric hospital specializing in orthopedics. By 1913, through his vision and that of his colleagues, the Children's had become a general hospital for infants, children, and adolescents.

Forbes' colleague, Dr. Cushing (1873–1947) had trained at McGill University's medical school and was working as Registrar of the Royal Victoria Hospital. Dr. Cushing was particularly interested in contagious diseases and the illnesses of children, and agreed to be associated with the new hospital even before it opened. In 1905, he was named Physician-in-Charge (responsible, at the time, for only one other physician), a position he held until his retire-

MEMBERS OF THE MCH FAMILY

In 2004, the employed staff of the Montreal Children's Hospital consisted of:
- 496 nurses
- 157 other professionals
- 371 technical and para-technical staff
- 452 support staff
- 67 managers

The MCH family also includes staff not on the hospital's payroll: more than 300 physicians and surgeons, and hundreds of volunteers.

A TALENT FOR DIAGNOSIS

Dr. Cushing had "a rare gift" for diagnosing patients, according to colleague Dr. Alton Goldbloom. In his book *Small Patients,* Dr. Goldbloom recalled the time Dr. Cushing was called in to see a sick child whose family lived behind a grocery story that sold aerated water.

"A tank of carbonic-acid gas connected to the water faucet by a flexible lead pipe dispensed the soda water at two cents a glass—three cents, if flavoured. Cushing walked through this little store to the back of the house where the child lay and having satisfied himself that the child showed no readily diagnosable symptoms, promptly made the diagnosis of lead poisoning. As he told it when the child was admitted to the hospital and his diagnosis corroborated, he had reasoned that the transient customer absorbed very little lead from occasionally drinking such aerated water, but that the child living as it did on the premises probably helped itself frequently and thus absorbed enough lead to cause poisoning."

ment in 1938. Dr. Cushing was instrumental in the acceptance of the Children's Memorial Hospital as a McGill teaching facility in 1920. He is remembered as a gentle man, a skilled physician, and an inspired diagnostician.

Dr. Alton Goldbloom was the first physician in Montreal trained to devote his entire attention to children and their illnesses. Educated at McGill University, with postgraduate work in Boston and New York, he joined the Children's Memorial Hospital staff in 1920, as one of a total medical staff of three, plus a surgical staff of two. In the 1952/53 Annual Report, on the occasion of his retirement, he described how he had been hired:

"Toward the end of 1919, when I was Resident Physician at the Babies' Hospital in New York, I received a letter signed by Dr. H.B. Cushing which said that at a meeting of the Committee of Management of the Children's Memorial Hospital, I had been appointed Assistant Physician. I had not applied to any hospital for an appointment, and this came as a welcome and pleasant surprise ... I subsequently learnt that a meeting of the Committee of Management consisted of Dr. Cushing, Dr. Forbes and Dr. Rhea (the hospital's Pathologist) meeting by chance on the Hospital grounds, seating themselves in the sun on a bench facing the Hospital and discussing hospital policy. Dr. Cushing had just been to New York, had made rounds with me at the Babies' Hospital and my appointment was the result of this visit."

In the 1920s, pediatrics was still in its infancy, not yet recognized as an official medical specialty. Dr. Goldbloom's work with children, like that of the other CMH pediatricians who followed shortly thereafter, was viewed with scepticism and resentment by many in the medical community, who did not recognize that the treatment of children was different from that of adults. Local obstetricians, for instance, felt they were quite capable of caring for newborns, and resented what they saw as interference by Dr. Goldbloom. He was only admitted to the newborn nursery of the local maternity hospital at the insistence of the mothers.

MONTREAL'S FIRST PEDIATRICIAN

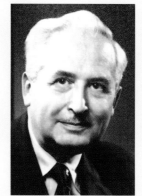

Dr. Alton Goldbloom (1890–1968) was Montreal's first trained pediatrician. He went on to hold many positions in the Montreal medical community, including Physician-in-Chief at the Children's and Professor of Pediatrics at McGill University from 1946 to 1953. Dr. Goldbloom contributed greatly to the hospital's development. It was during his term of office that the services of Cardiology, Hematology, and Human Genetics, as well as the Department of Psychiatry, were established and the Medical Library was founded.

A SPECIALTY IS BORN

As they watched pediatricians rapidly diagnose and treat obscure childhood conditions, however, many previously sceptical physicians began willingly to hand over care of their young patients to the doctors at the Children's. As CMH patient numbers swelled, the staff grew by leaps and bounds. By 1935, there were already more than 100 individuals listed among the hospital's medical staff, including consultants.

None of these doctors was based full-time at the Children's, and none was paid by the hospital or government to work there. Until Medicare took effect in 1970, physicians made their living in private offices and volunteered their time at the Children's, treating poorer children there in exchange for the privilege of admitting their private patients to the hospital. Still, the hours they spent there were often long. In the 1930s and '40s, for instance, it was not uncommon for a surgeon to operate all day on emergency cases, then work well into the night on elective surgeries, cleaning instruments in between. As there was no intensive care unit (this was only established in 1969), the surgeon would sometimes even sleep next to a child in case post-operative complications should arise.

"People today would be surprised to know that in the 1940s we didn't get paid anything—not one cent—and it was considered a great privilege to be on the staff of the hospital and to receive that kind of education, that kind of postgraduate training. And it absolutely was."

DR. VICTOR GOLDBLOOM, PEDIATRICIAN
who joined the staff of the Children's in 1950, and who, alongside a distinguished career in public service, has been associated with the hospital ever since

---

In the early 1950s, when planning the move to Tupper Street, the administration decided to provide office space for the Physician-in-Chief and his assis-tant, the Surgeon-in-Chief and his assistant, and certain other key staff members. In 1952, they appointed the first full-time physician, Dr. Ronald L. Denton. Director of Hematology since the end of World War II, Dr. Denton now divided his time between the Hematology Department and Pediatric Medical Services, supervising patients, staff, and intern training. This was the beginning of the concept of geographical full-time hospital appointments at the Children's.

Today, the majority of physicians working at the MCH are full-time, in contrast to most physicians treating adults, who generally have private practices outside their hospitals. Many community-based pediatricians also work at the hospital part-time. The full-time staff contribute to patient care, teaching, and research, in addition to assuming national and international responsibilities in professional societies and academic organizations.

INCREASING SPECIALIZATION

In the hospital's early days, its staff included few specialists. The 1905 Annual Report records the part-time services of one oculist, one anesthetist, and one pathologist/bacteriologist. A dentist was added shortly thereafter, and by the 1920s there were specialty clinics for dermatology, diseases of the eye, ear, nose and throat, and of the genitourinary tract. The rest of the physicians treated everything from broken bones and rheumatic fever to malnutrition and mental disorders.

By the 1940s, knowledge and technology in all areas of medicine, including pediatrics, were increasing so rapidly that it became impossible for one doctor to know everything about every disease and condition. Physicians and surgeons at the Children's and elsewhere began increasingly to specialize, becoming experts in new fields such as cardiology, neurology, endocrinology, and genetics, to name just a few.

Today, the Department of Pediatrics includes 17 divisions: Adolescent Medicine; Allergy and Immunology; Cardiology; Dermatology; Emergency Medicine; Endocrinology and Metabolism; Gastro-enterology and Nutrition; General Pediatrics; Medical Genetics; Hematology and Oncology; Infectious Diseases and Microbiology; Newborn Medicine; Nephrology; Neurology; Pediatric Critical Care; Respiratory Medicine; and Rheumatology.

FATHER OF PEDIATRIC EMERGENCY MEDICINE

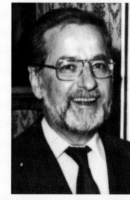

Emergency Medicine became a recognized field of medicine in this country in the late 1960s. Dr. Donald Clogg, who spearheaded the establishment of pediatric emergency medicine at the Canadian Pediatric Society, is known by many as the father of pediatric emergency medicine in Canada. Dr. Clogg was Director of Medical Emergency at the Children's from 1977 to 1980 and then Physician-in-Charge of the Pediatric Intensive Care Unit until 1983. He is also remembered for his organization of full-scale mock disasters, bringing in busloads of children and putting the entire hospital on alert.

In *A Fuzzy but Affectionate Look at the History of the Emergency Department* (1997), Dr. David McGillivray, then Director of the Medical Emergency Department, described Dr. Clogg's commitment to patient care:

"Like the captain of a ship, he took responsibility for every child who came through the 'room' ... His most famous case is the child of one of our esteemed hospital attending staff, who was critically ill with an illness that no one could understand. Don Clogg spent almost two solid weeks in the library and the ICU personally caring for this child. I don't think he slept for the two weeks. The story has a happy ending in that the patient made a full recovery. This was the most impressive commitment to a patient I have ever seen."

Closely linked to Pediatrics is the Department of Psychiatry, which treats both children and adolescents.

The Department of Pediatric Surgical Services has 10 divisions: Cardiovascular Surgery; Dentistry; General Pediatric Surgery; Gynecology; Neurosurgery; Ophthalmology; Orthopedic Surgery; Otolaryngology; Plastic Surgery; and Urology.

The Department of Anesthesiology provides anesthesia service to patients not only in the operating rooms, but also in diagnostic imaging, interventional radiology, cardiac catheterization, gastroenterology, hematology/oncology, and respirology.

Within each specialization, there are now sub-specializations. One ophthalmologist might focus on muscles in the eye, for instance, while another specializes in the retina or in eye tumours.

Over the years, MCH physicians and surgeons have become renowned experts in many of these specialized fields. Their programs and techniques have become models for other pediatric hospitals, and physicians are often called upon to share their expertise with colleagues worldwide.

As a result, the MCH has become a magnet, attracting expertise from around the world. The hospital also trains physicians and surgeons in various specialties who go on to practise at other centres worldwide, taking MCH expertise with them.

DID YOU KNOW?

MCH surgeons perform roughly 7,000 surgical procedures each year. The number has not risen dramatically over the past 40 years—the 1965 Annual Report, for instance, records 6,777 surgical procedures. What has changed is that surgical teams now perform increasingly complex operations, sometimes on babies who are only hours old, and that roughly 70% of the procedures are now done as day surgeries.

NEWBORN MEDICINE COMES OF AGE

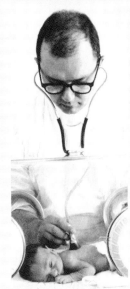

One of the pediatric subspecialties that has developed most dramatically over the past 40 years is neonatology. The Division of Neonatology opened at the MCH in 1961, with Dr. Leo Stern (left) as its director from 1961 to 1973. Now renamed the Newborn Medicine Division, it provides intensive care for premature and full-term newborns with genetic, neurological, cardiac, respiratory, and other serious disorders.

The division includes—in addition to the neonatal intensive care unit (NICU)—an extracorporeal membrane oxygenation (ECMO) program, a follow-up clinic, a transport service, and outreach programs. A multidisciplinary team made up of neonatologists, pediatricians, neonatal nurse practitioners, nurses, respiratory therapists, dietitians, pharmacists, and social workers cares for roughly 400 acutely ill newborns each year.

MULTIDISCIPLINARY TEAMS

For much of the hospital's history, each patient was the responsibility of a single doctor from admittance to discharge. Since the 1970s, however, doctors and other professionals at the Children's have worked in multidisciplinary teams to ensure that their patients receive the best care possible. A team might consist of any number of specialists—from doctors and nurses to biochemists, pathologists, dentists, and dietitians.

Clinical diagnosis, which was once based largely on a single doctor's observations, now often involves teams of skilled technicians and other professionals carrying out and analyzing multiple diagnostic tests. Treatment also improves with close collaboration among a wide array of clinical and laboratory colleagues. A cardiologist, for instance, might discuss a patient's case with other physicians, a cardiac surgeon, an anesthetist, nurses, laboratory technicians, and a social worker, to name a few. Modern communications technology also makes it possible to consult quickly with an extended team of specialists around the world.

Close liaison between specialties is critical as professionals treat increasingly complex cases. The repair of a complicated craniomaxillo-facial birth defect, for instance, might involve a variety of surgical specialists—neurosurgeon, plastic surgeon, orthodontist, dentist, otolaryngologist, and orthopedic surgeon—in addition to anesthetists, medical imaging specialists, and nurses.

THE NURSING TEAM

Many say the glue that holds the multidisciplinary team together is the nursing staff, as it is nurses who usually spend most time with the children and know them best. Nurses have always been at the forefront of patient care at the Children's, but their profession, like that of other health-care professionals, has seen great changes over the past century.

"Nursing has evolved," says the McGill School of Nursing Web site. "The typical hospital nurse as we sometimes picture her in a white uniform and cap, changing dressings, sheets and bedpans, exists only in old movies. The use of complicated equipment, rising demand for ambulatory care and home care, [a] population with more complex and long-term needs, and health needs of rural populations, have all led to a steep increase in demand for nurses with more skills, qualifications and experience."

When the Children's Memorial Hospital opened in 1904, nurses, like doctors, were not trained in pediatric care. As it was immediately recognized that the skills acquired in adult facilities and nursing schools were often not applicable to the treatment of children, the hospital opened its own training school for nurses in 1905. After the school closed in 1934, nursing students from other hospital-based schools came to the Children's for their pediatric experience.

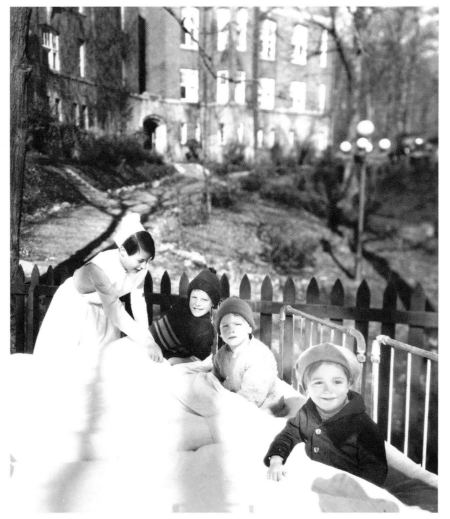

In the early 1900s, when fresh air and sunshine were considered vital to the recovery of many children, a nurse's job might include many hours spent outside, even in cold weather. Dr. Alexander Mackenzie Forbes once suggested that each nurse working in the hospital's outbuildings be provided with "a long sheep-skin lined cloak fashioned in duck ... [and] either overshoes or felt boots ... It is wrong to have them in their ordinary uniforms and clothes sitting and working down in God's fresh air."

Nurses no longer work outside, and their uniforms are very different from the one pictured here. Nurses' caps were eliminated with the advent of CEGEP and university training programs in the 1970s. According to some, they were too often left in lockers, where they collected bacteria and odours. Others say they were too hot, served no practical purpose, and scared the children. The polyester nurses' uniforms were eliminated in the 1990s because they were too hot. For a short time nurses wore street clothes, but since 2002 they have been supplied with light cotton uniforms.

JACKS AND JILLS OF ALL TRADES

Prior to the 1940s, the Children's, like other hospitals, isolated infectious patients from the rest of the world and hoped that natural forces would bring them back to health over time. Stays were long, families were hardly present, medicines were few, and most of the care provided was of a residential nature. Because doctors were only at the hospital part-time and the staff was small, nurses had to do virtually everything needed to run the institution. In addition to caring for patients' medical and health needs, they acted as administrators and assisted with cleaning and cooking—even stoking the coal stove to ensure patients were warm enough.

As the hospital increased in size and complexity, many of these tasks were taken over by other personnel. When the training of Quebec nurses moved from hospital-based schools to CEGEPs and universities in 1970, nurses were able to focus almost exclusively on the direct care of the children and their medical conditions.

Evelyn Malowany, Director of Nursing from 1976 to 1997, was an active proponent of the increasingly professional role of nurses at the MCH. Looking back on those days, she says she was confident in her cause, but also realistic about the challenges of bringing about change on an institutional level.

Mrs. Malowany promoted the training of nurses in the McGill Model of Nursing, a philosophy developed at McGill University under the leadership of Dr. Moyra Allen. The model emphasizes the importance not only of treating and preventing the child's illness, but also of focusing on the wellness of the whole child. It is a family-oriented approach that encourages the active participation of the child and the family in fostering health. To help develop this model as an integral part of MCH nursing practice, Margaret Hooton of the McGill Basic Nursing Program was contracted as consultant one day a week from 1981 to 1989.

The McGill Model of Nursing is still an important part of patient care at the Children's. As part of the family-centred approach, MCH nurses today offer ongoing support to parents and other family members—answering their questions, promoting prevention of injuries and illness, preparing them to care for children at home and connecting them with community services, as well as providing follow-up support.

NURSE–DOCTOR PARTNERSHIPS

Along with their enhanced professional approach, nurses began to take on more integrated management roles as well. During the 1990s, nurse–doctor management teams were established in MCH departments and services, such those of Dr. Ronald Gottesman and head nurse Franco Carnevale in the PICU, and Dr. David McGillivray and head nurse Carol Common in the ER. Their close communication and joint decision-making set the tone for a growing cooperative management model, giving a boost to the collaborative and innovative working atmosphere for which the Children's is known.

As nurses have become increasingly well-educated, many with baccalaureate and advanced degrees, their role in carrying out medical treatment plans has also expanded. Some tasks previously performed by physicians, such as connecting feeding tubes and starting intravenous lines, are now a routine part of the nurse's job. Others, such as administering chemotherapy treatments, are performed by specially certified nurses. Like doctors, many nurses now have specialized training enabling them to work with distinct groups of patients—psychiatric patients, for example, or newborns, or children in the pain management program.

As the caregivers who spend most time with the patients, nurses gain tremendous insight into the children and their families. With more scientific knowledge than ever, they are increasingly able to pick up subtle changes in patients and alert the rest

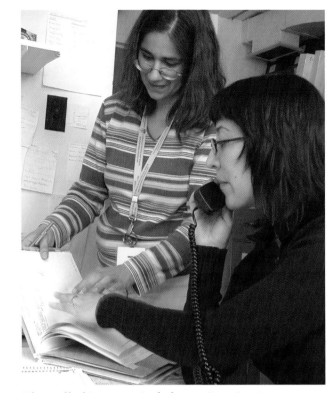

The staff of Intensive Ambulatory Care Services offers 24-hour-a-day consultation—no matter where the patient is. One night when nurse Tania Laflèche (above, right) was on duty, she received a call that a former heart transplant patient had come down with severe gastroenteritis on a family cruise in the Caribbean. Ms. Laflèche spent many hours on the telephone that night and the following day, speaking with the ship's doctor, the family, and physicians at the hospital in Nassau, where the girl was transferred, to ensure she got the treatment she needed. Because the child's system was immunosuppressed, doctors needed to act quickly to prevent deterioration of her condition.

After consulting with Dr. Geoffrey Dougherty, Director of Intensive Ambulatory Care Services, Ms. Laflèche was able to provide them with a treatment plan which may well have saved the child's life. The primary care nurse, Sylvie Canizares (above, left), followed up to ensure the child recovered fully. The parents were extremely grateful.

"This family knew they were not alone," said Ms. Laflèche. "The staff of the Children's made them feel secure, even if they were getting the actual treatment in an unfamiliar setting."

of the care team, leading to timely treatment and sometimes saving lives.

While nurses have for many years participated in research projects under the direction of other professions, in the past several decades, clinical and evaluative research has been directed by nurses themselves. As well, clinical innovations at the Children's have become increasingly nursing-driven. The beginning of this 21st century, for instance, has seen the development of a program of continuous insulin therapy for children and adolescents through infusion pumps, spearheaded by nurse Anne Bossy. She worked with physician colleagues on a proposal for the Children's to establish an insulin pump therapy centre for pediatrics, a first for Quebec, which opened early in 2005. In 2004, rheumatology nurse Gillian Taylor worked with the Quebec and Canadian arthritis associations to develop a one-week camp for children with arthritis. Nurses are also increasingly involved in outreach programs, sharing their expertise with colleagues at other hospitals and CLSCs (community clinics, or *centres locaux de services communautaires*).

Despite the changes, the philosophy behind the nursing profession—the best possible care for children—has not changed. Although they are extremely busy with patient and family care, administrative duties, teaching, and research responsibilities, they somehow manage, as one nurse put it, to be "every-

QUIET HERO

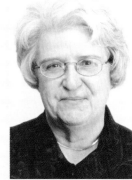

One of nursing's quiet heroes at the MCH, and the power behind a large number of innovations during the last quarter of the 20th century, was Associate Director of Nursing Gwen Olivier. Remembering her efficiency and creativity, Dr. Patricia Forbes recalls simply, "She kept this place going."

INFECTIONS AND DR. CRICKET

During the 29 years Susan Marshall has been a nurse at the Children's, there have been many exciting and challenging times. Once, for instance, there was an *E. coli* outbreak in a Northern community, and six Inuit babies arrived at the same time. "It was like the opening scene from [the TV show] M.A.S.H.," she recalls. "All six babies side by side across one stretcher, an IV pole with six IVs, nurses and doctors running down the hall ..."

There was also the bomb scare in the early 1970s. "Dr. Cricket was the code for bombs. When we heard it, everyone was evacuated to the park across the street, and there were IVs hanging from all the trees. Some nurses were assigned to check for bombs in the hospital bins."

Ms. Marshall has also seen many changes in nursing procedures and equipment since she began working at the Children's.

"When the kids had chest tubes, the tubes were attached to glass bottles. The bottles were taped to the floor so they wouldn't break and collapse the lung. We had to 'milk' the tube every hour, which meant that we took cream and rubbed it up and down the tubing to prevent clots from forming in the tubes.

"We also used glass thermometers. When one broke, housekeeping had to come with a special vacuum cleaner to vacuum up the mercury, which was poisonous. And nurses used to draw up chemotherapy drugs on the ward with no gloves; now the pharmacy does it, with special protection."

thing from entertainers and janitors to hairdressers." They rock babies while answering the telephone and organize impromptu birthday celebrations. Some write letters to schools to ensure that the children's needs are met once they leave the hospital, while others advocate for the children with providers of community health-care services.

In some outpatient clinics, nurses are aided by nursing assistants, who perform general nursing tasks such as receiving and preparing patients for tests, weighing them, taking vital signs, and so on.

There are fewer of these assistants than 20 years ago, however, as increasingly complex patient care now requires more education and scientific knowledge.

On the nursing units, some of the functions previously performed by nurses—such as feeding, changing, and bathing the children, cleaning and restocking equipment, and taking patients for tests—have been taken over by patient care attendants (PCAs). There are currently about 35 at the hospital, many working part-time.

ALLIED HEALTH PROFESSIONALS

In addition to physicians and nurses, today's multidisciplinary team is made up of a wide range of other health-care professionals, who not only treat medical conditions, but also support children's psychological, social, and emotional development. Many of these professions have long histories with the Children's.

Social workers

Social workers have been part of the hospital since 1916, when the first "head worker," Amy Hilton, assisted by volunteers, was appointed to perform home evaluations and help improve home conditions that might be detrimental to the patient's full recovery.

The 1919 Annual Report lists some of the social worker's duties at the time: instruction in hygiene; provision of massage treatments; supervision of tubercular patients in plaster casts; arrangement of summer outings; examination and treatment of families in which cases of venereal disease had been discovered; provision of special training for blind, deaf, or dumb children; investigation of cases when parents claimed inability to pay; purchase of special appliances for patients where applicable; and "disposition of children deserted at the hospital." Also listed are 3,325 phone calls, 1,382 letters, and 1,566 visits made by the head worker.

The Social Services Department's caseload continued to grow through the Depression years, with

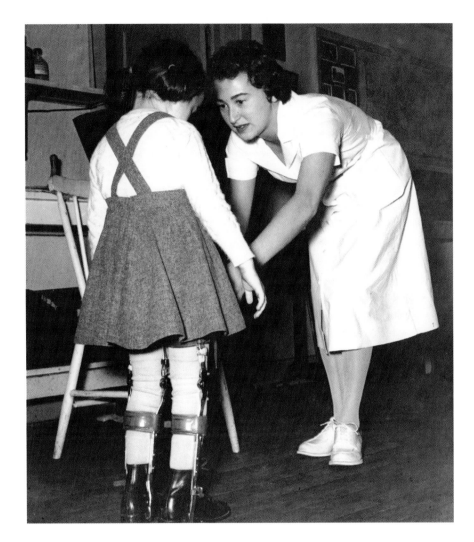

its three staff members seeing nearly 600 families per month—most being families of unemployed men, many with children suffering from malnutrition and tuberculosis. In the 1940s, the department was closed temporarily for financial and staffing reasons, but when it reopened in 1947, its staff continued to grow in size and function. Social workers reached their greatest numbers in the mid-1960s, before the years of serious government budget constraints, when the hospital had 43 social workers on staff, all with master's degrees.

In 1975, provincial government reforms made social workers part of the Ville-Marie Social Service

Physiotherapy has been an integral part of treatment at the Children's since the hospital's earliest days. This photo was taken circa 1950.

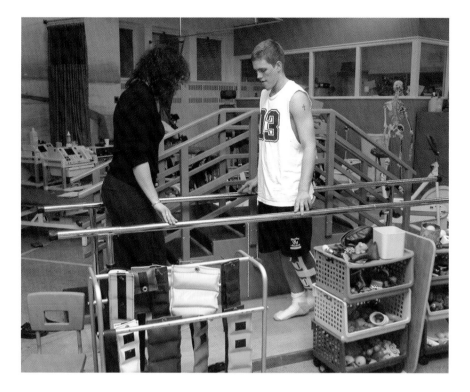

Andrew does his exercises in the hospital's well-equipped physiotherapy facilities. Physiotherapists follow children from birth through age 18 as inpatients and outpatients.

evolved over the years, and by the early 1950s, physiotherapists provided massage and remedial exercises, hydrotherapy, electrotherapy, and other treatments to patients with conditions as diverse as fractures and cerebral palsy, asthma, arthritis, skin grafts, and cardiac conditions.

Today, 10 physiotherapists (the equivalent of eight full-time positions) use modern techniques and equipment—some of it computerized—to help children with injuries, disabilities, and physical handicaps attain maximum mobility and strength. Their patients include many elite adolescent athletes who have had injuries and need help to resume their sport. There is also an active outpatient component, with physiotherapists participating in many clinics, including Orthopedics, Rheumatology, Pain Management, Neurology, Neurosurgery, Neonatal Follow-up, Spina Bifida, and the Spasticity Management Clinic. A physiotherapist is on staff in Intensive Ambulatory Care Services and in the Neuromuscular Clinic, and the department also participates in the Northern and Native Child Health Program.

In recent years, physiotherapists at the Children's have done less long-term rehabilitation of children with diseases such as cerebral palsy. Instead, they now offer assessment and short-term interventions,

Centre, providing services to the hospital on a contractual basis. Further reforms in 1993 brought them back into the hospital fold.

Today, a total of 26 social workers provide comprehensive psychosocial assistance to patients and their families throughout the hospital. This includes 24-hour-a-day service to the emergency room and to families in any crisis situation. Social workers arrange individual and group counselling, help parents gain access to hospital and community resources, and participate in shaping government policy and legislation to protect the rights of children.

Physiotherapists

The role of MCH physiotherapists, too, dates back to the hospital's earliest days, when members of the Department of Massage and Remedial Gymnastics, as it was called until the early 1930s, helped rehabilitate victims of "injuries, deformities, contractions, atrophies, diseases of the nervous system" and post-operative cases. Treatment techniques

TEACHING CHILDREN NEW SKILLS

Pediatric physiotherapy, says current department coordinator Eileen Kennedy, is very different from adult physiotherapy, particularly when dealing with infants. "With adults, when you're doing rehabilitation after an illness or an injury, you're giving them back motor skills they used to have. With children, we're sometimes teaching them skills they have not yet learned. A premature infant who has had brain damage at birth, for instance, has never learned any motor skills, so we're teaching him for the first time. We're also teaching the parents how to help the child develop the skills."

referring children to rehabilitation centres in the community for long-term treatment. Physiotherapy has also become more science-based, with MCH physiotherapists initiating and taking part in research to determine the effectiveness of various treatments and procedures.

Occupational therapists

Recognized as a separate profession in the 1930s, occupational therapy at the Children's has its roots in the volunteers of the 1920s who taught sewing, knitting, and basket-making to long-term patients as a way to pass the time and release pent-up energy. A Department of Occupational Therapy was established in 1936 with a view to helping children with disabilities, illness, or injuries become more functional and independent, able to complete daily activities such as dressing, grooming, eating, playing, and interacting with others.

Initially limited to the treatment of rheumatic diseases, the work of the occupational therapist soon expanded to children with pulmonary infections and to re-education after surgery. Today, the equivalent of seven full-time occupational therapists work in almost every nursing unit and outpatient clinic in the hospital, and provide services to children in the North.

Highly trained professionals, occupational therapists at the Children's today offer evaluation and therapy to help improve children's development in the areas of fine and gross motor skills, coordination, perception, and balance. They create customized splints for patients with acquired, traumatic, or congenital conditions. They also engage children with behavioural and psychiatric problems in therapeutic activities.

Child life specialists and teachers

Originally linked with the Occupational Therapy Department, the Department of Recreational Therapy was established in the late 1930s under Miss Alice Burkhardt to benefit children in long-

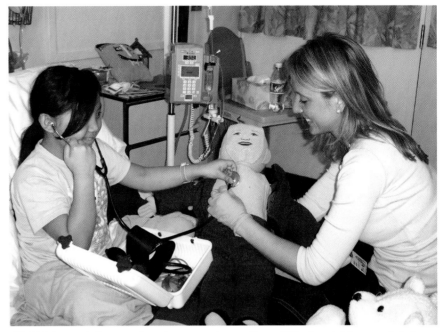

Child life specialists work to improve the quality of life for children and their families, using play, education, and self-expression to humanize the hospital experience. Through medical play—using puppets to demonstrate how blood tests are taken, for instance—they help children understand and cooperate with medical procedures. This is particularly important in cases where sedation cannot be used, either because of the type of test or treatment, or because of the child's medical condition. The child life specialist's assistance can not only reduce the anxiety of the child and family, but can also improve the chances that test results and treatments will not be compromised. Here, child life specialist Judy Edes shows young Kaycelyne how a physician listens to a child's heart.

term surgical and orthopedic care. The first of its kind in Canada, the department is now known as Child Life and School Services.

The precursors of today's child life specialists were the volunteer "play ladies" of the 1940s and 1950s, who used play as a therapeutic tool to relieve the stress and boredom of long hospital stays. Over time, child life specialists have become trained professionals, with backgrounds in psychology, education, and related fields. In addition to play, they use a variety of educational and creative techniques to help make the child's health-care experience understandable and as close to normal life as possible. They also assist families in dealing with their ques-

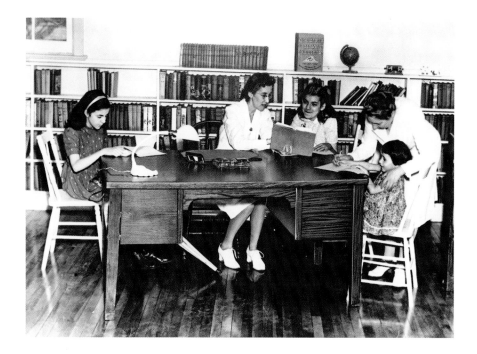

Since the hospital's inception, teachers have been available to help patients with their schoolwork. This photograph shows teachers working with ambulatory patients in the 1940s.

tions and concerns. Today, child life specialists work on all nursing units except psychiatry and in many outpatient areas.

Also part of Child Life Services is the hospital's school program. The importance of enabling children to keep up with their schooling has been recognized since the hospital's inception, when the Ladies' Committee established the first regular teaching program at the Guy Street hospital. In the days when patients spent months and even years at the hospital recuperating from illness, hospital teachers were often responsible for the child's entire educational program. Regular lessons would take place outdoors whenever possible, so patients could benefit from fresh air and sunshine at the same time.

With shorter hospital stays and an increase in outpatient care, teachers at the Children's now often focus on shorter lessons in specific areas of difficulty. Teachers provided by Montreal's English and French school boards tutor both elementary and secondary students—in the hospital classroom, at the bedside, or in the clinic, depending on the patient's condition and treatment schedule.

Clinical nutritionists

The links between nutrition and health have also been recognized since the hospital's earliest days, when malnutrition was at the root of many illnesses treated by the CMH, and nurses and social workers taught mothers about proper feeding and handling of food.

The first mention of a Dietetic Department in the hospital's annual reports is in the early 1930s. At that time, the department's staff was responsible for many of the same tasks as today's dietitians, including arranging for special patient diets, instructing parents, and teaching nursing students. They were also, however, in charge of the preparation of patient meals and the catering of special functions, along with care of kitchen equipment. The 1935 Annual Report, for instance, records that the department's staff "decided to replace the old enamel children's dishes by china dishes" and that "a coal range with blower control was installed in place of the old gas range."

Today, the 10 full-time and 15 part-time dietitians of the Clinical Nutrition Department are no longer involved in food preparation, but they do counsel patients and their families whenever a child's medical condition requires nutritional intervention. They are assisted by dietary technicians in fulfilling the needs of patients during their hospital stay. Each dietitian is assigned to a specific multidisciplinary team—such as the eating disorders team, the diabetes team, or the nephrology team.

"A dietitian evaluates the child's nutritional profile," explains the MCH pamphlet *Food for Thought*, "and makes recommendations on everything from menus and eating habits to feeding routines. Before a child leaves the hospital, the dietitian gives him and his parents advice to follow both at home and at school.

"Anorexia, bulimia, diabetes, cholesterol, severe burns, cancer, genetic diseases, cystic fibrosis, retarded growth and problems of the digestive tract or kidneys ... all are reasons for calling on the services of a dietitian. The dietitians have to adapt their recommendations to the specific needs of their patients taking into account the nutritional needs of children at different ages." They also take into consideration the children's cultural and religious backgrounds.

Speech-language pathologists and audiologists

Speech-language pathologists can trace the history of their profession at the Children's to Dr. Ernest Scarfe, a member of the otolaryngology staff in the 1930s who had a special interest in the speech problems of cleft palate patients. In 1933, he launched the MCH Speech Therapy Clinic, the first of its kind in a Canadian pediatric hospital. From the beginning, it was a comprehensive diagnostic and treatment facility, looking after not just the child's language, voice, or speech impairment, but also the accompanying learning difficulties, personal problems, and social development issues.

By the 1950s, speech-language pathologists were treating a wide variety of problems in the MCH's outpatient clinic, including stuttering, delayed language, voice problems, speech problems caused by hearing loss, and articulation problems. They treated children with cleft palate, cerebral palsy, and aphasia (the inability to use or understand words, usually caused by brain disease or injury), and did speech and language evaluation for other departments. They also, during this decade, established some of the hospital's first multidisciplinary teams in the Parent-Child Stuttering Clinic, the Cerebral Palsy Preschool, and the Cleft Palate Assessment Clinic.

The department offered services in both French and English as early as the 1940s, and today each therapist is fully bilingual. By the 1980s, when speech-language pathologist Dr. Ann Mary Stanton spearheaded a multiculturalism project in the hospital—which later grew into the Multiculturalism Program—services were offered in a variety of languages through interpreters.

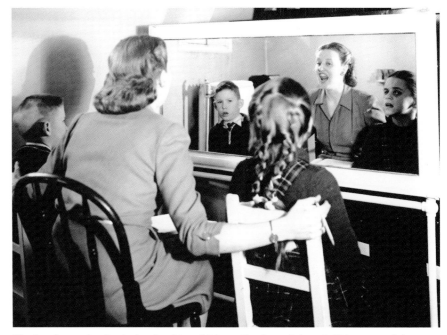

Under the enthusiastic leadership of Mary Cardozo (above), Director of the Speech Therapy Clinic from 1944 until 1991, the number of patients swelled and additional staff had to be hired. A summer speech camp was established in 1946 for out-of-town children with cleft palate who were unable to attend the hospital's clinic. In 1964, Mary Cardozo was a founding member of both the Corporation professionnelle des orthophonistes et audiologistes du Québec *and the Canadian Speech and Hearing Association.*

In 1995, the Speech and Language Pathology Department, in conjunction with the Division of Otolaryngology, established the first pediatric computerized voice lab in Canada. In 2003, they pioneered the use of telehealth (using communications technology such as a video camera, microphones, and screen) to provide speech therapy sessions to a patient in northern Quebec.

Today, MCH speech-language pathologists see children referred by professionals both inside and outside the hospital—about 1,500 patients a year, with many more on the waiting list.

Each child referred to the Speech and Language Pathology Department is also seen by an audiologist, to determine whether there is hearing loss or a related disorder. Audiologists also see patients from the Otolaryngology (or ENT: ear, nose, throat)

Division. While ENT looks at the medical causes of hearing problems, audiologists evaluate and treat the function of hearing.

Audiology at the Children's originated in the 1950s, when Mary Cardozo and ENT physician Dr. Hollie McHugh began evaluating children's

EARLY INTERVENTION

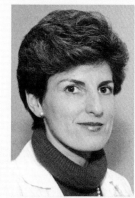

Louise Miller, who came to the Children's in 1968 as a student and has been Director of the Audiology Department since 1984, recently treated a 15-month-old boy who was diagnosed as profoundly deaf. His parents did not suspect he was deaf until they saw an MCH audiologist on television discussing hearing loss. They brought him for testing at the MCH, and the boy received a cochlear implant three months later.

"He is now just over two years old," says Ms. Miller. "He can turn to his name, has started to vocalize, and plays with his voice, which he never did before. The family is extremely happy with the progress and have promised to visit me. We do not usually see the children once they have started in the rehabilitation centre. It is so rewarding to be able to appreciate the results of our quick intervention."

MCH audiologists use a variety of technologies and screening measures to make a clinical assessment and come up with a treatment plan. When appropriate, they recommend hearing aids, rehabilitation, and even a special school. They also do counselling with the family, helping them adjust to the child's hearing loss or referring them to other specialists if the problem is something else, such as autism.

"The average age for determining deafness is over two years of age, which is still very late," says Ms. Miller. "However, we now have the tools to assess a baby a few hours old."

hearing and holding weekly "speech and hearing" conferences to discuss special cases. The Audiology Department was set up as a separate entity in 1973, going from one audiologist to six in the first year. It also moved from a tiny room near Dentistry—with cork walls supposedly making it soundproof, but with the noise of a constantly flushing toilet next door interfering with hearing tests—to the current department with three actual soundproof rooms.

Today, MCH audiologists see more than 3,600 patients a year, most under the age of five. While everyone in the department does standard testing and treatment, each staff member also has a subspecialty. One is on the head trauma team, another on the autism team, and several work with school-aged children having specific problems at school. Two are involved with the screening of hearing in newborns. All babies coming into the MCH Neonatal Intensive Care Unit are screened, but since 50% of hearing-impaired children don't have any risk factors (such as a family history of hearing impairment, congenital infection, or birth weight less than 1,500 grams, to name just a few), audiologists are advocating for standardized screening for all newborns in Quebec, as is already the case in several other provinces.

The audiology staff, in collaboration with ENT surgeons, are responsible for a number of "firsts" in the field, including the first cochlear implant in a child in Quebec (1986) and the first bone-anchored hearing device in a child in Canada (1990). They are also involved in a variety of research teams—evaluating the effects of specific eardrops and new implantable bone-conduction hearing devices, for instance, as well as looking at how chemotherapy affects hearing.

Psychologists

MCH psychologists have come a long way since the days when they were mostly administering and scoring IQ tests.

In the early 1950s, the hospital's first psychologist, Dr. Margie Golick, was appointed to use IQ and other tests to assess children with developmental delays. The relationship between medicine and psychology was established at this time, since these developmental delays were usually a result of illnesses such as meningitis, cerebral palsy, or polio. Since then, MCH psychologists have not only acquired more sophisticated diagnostic tools, but have also assumed a leading role in the treatment of children and their families.

The Psychology Department has consistently maintained a commitment to cutting-edge science and practice. In the 1970s, cognitive-behavioural therapy became an important part of treatment under Dr. Susan Campbell, and the psychologist's role became increasingly evidence-based under Dr. Anne Schlieper. The tenure of Dr. Philip Zelazo in the 1980s and 1990s saw the opening of a clinic to assess and treat developmental delays and autism, the Failure to Thrive/Feeding Disorders Clinic (under Dr. Maria Ramsay), the Eating Disorders Clinic (founded by Dr. Sam Burstein), and one of the first post-doctoral fellowships in pediatric psychology in North America. During that time, there was also a shift in emphasis from serving children in the community with no medical condition, to serving exclusively the sick children of the MCH.

There are currently 30 psychologists working at the MCH, representing a full-time equivalent of 18. Under the direction of Dr. Yves Beaulieu, they perform a variety of diagnostic procedures (e.g. neuropsychological, intellectual, and personality assessments) and evidence-based therapeutic interventions (e.g. individual therapy, group therapy, parental and family counselling). They also provide consultation and clinical services to nearly all departments and services.

Pastoral workers and chaplains

The provision of spiritual support for patients, families, and staff has also evolved over the years. In the hospital's early days, clergy were called to the hospital, either by staff or by families, when patients were dying. Eventually, a priest was assigned to the MCH by the Roman Catholic diocese, and a few years later, in 1987, a Department of Pastoral Services was created, based upon the standards of the Canadian Association for Pastoral Education.

As the profession of hospital chaplaincy evolved, the MCH moved away from offering services in only one denomination to a broad-based multi-denominational model that supports even those without religious affiliation or faith. Since 1989, when Reverend Donald Meloche became Director of Pastoral Services, a team of four chaplains has been available to provide spiritual support and guidance in all areas of the hospital, calling upon rabbis and representatives of virtually every religious denomination in the area, as needed.

Pastoral services team members are assigned to specific areas of the hospital—the Neonatal and Pediatric Intensive Care units, Hematology and Oncology, and Emergency—where they participate in the regular multidisciplinary meetings to discuss cases. Other areas of the hospital are divided among them, as well, but a chaplain will follow any child from one part of the hospital to another, if a bond has been established with the child or family.

Chaplains are often called upon when a family is in crisis, whether from sudden trauma, such as a car accident, or upon learning of a catastrophic illness. In these situations, they support the family emotionally and spiritually, and act as a link with the team treating the child. They are an important part of the palliative care team, as they are involved almost every time a child dies. They provide spiritual support and training to staff and hold teaching sessions with residents, medical and nursing students, and other trainees.

DIAGNOSTIC SERVICES

Laboratories

Some members of the MCH care team specialize in diagnostic procedures and assessments, working in the hospital's laboratories and test centre.

Prior to the 1940s and 1950s, much of the hospital's laboratory work was the responsibility of physicians and residents, sometimes with help from untrained assistants or medical students. Tests were often crude by today's standards, and processing was manual. While the hospital's facilities were adequate for routine tests, the Children's relied on other hospitals for more advanced testing and consultation.

Today, skilled professionals perform and analyze a variety of diagnostic tests and use a wide array of modern diagnostic equipment, much of it computerized. They collect and test specimens, such as blood, tissue, and body fluids, to assist in the diagnosis, treatment, and prevention of disease. They may work in specialized laboratories dealing with biochemistry, hematology, immunology, endocrinology, renal function, microbiology, genetics, or pathology. Some work in the hospital's Pediatric Test Centre, where blood procurement, urine collection, and swabs are performed and specialized diagnostic testing for cystic fibrosis is undertaken. The Test Centre serves the outpatient clinics and inpatient units.

The demand for laboratory technologists has increased continuously over the years, as patient numbers have risen, knowledge of diseases and conditions has expanded, and new specialized tests have been developed.

The growing role of clinical laboratories has demanded increasing expertise and vision, especially as labs combined their services with the other MUHC hospitals. Dr. Susan Tange, Director of Clinical Laboratories from 1988 to 2002, "brought a unique contribution to the MCH by having a vision of what clinical laboratories needed to become," says Dr. Claire Dupont, former Director of Biochemistry and later Director of Professional Services.

"She understood how integration of labs within the MUHC should look so that future excellence would be maintained. To her, this meant that the unique requirements of pediatric lab services had to be understood and preserved, while at the same time deriving all the benefits of coming together in a new structure."

Medical imaging

Pediatric radiologists have worked at the Children's since the Cedar Avenue days of the 1950s. Dr. Scott Dunbar, head of the Radiology Department until 1971, was "an icon of pediatric radiology,

ADVANCES IN IMAGING

Pediatric neuroradiology was a new subspecialty when Dr. Gus ÓGorman first trained as a resident at the Children's in the early 1970s. Neuroradiology provides images of the nervous system in the spine, spinal cord, brain, and other structures within the skull.

It was not an easy specialty in the early days, as many of the diagnostic procedures were invasive. Until the late 1970s, Dr. ÓGorman and his colleagues used angiography, or air studies, to look for tumours. They would do a lumbar puncture with the child in a sitting position, withdraw fluid, and inject air, which would rise and fill the cavities of the head. By seeing how structures were displaced, they could indirectly determine the location of tumours or other abnormalities.

"Air studies had to be done by tumbling children in a special chair," Dr. ÓGorman recalls, "turning them backwards and forwards to get air to go where you wanted it to go. It was difficult and painful for the patient compared to what we do now. Kids would get a headache and faint."

The procedure was the best the neuroradiologists had until the arrival of the CT scanner at the MCH in 1977, which enabled doctors to see brain structures in a painless way. With the arrival of the MRI in 1994, they were able to see the brain and other organs in much greater detail and in several planes.

and was a huge influence here at the Children's," says Dr. Gus ÓGorman, Director of Radiology from 1983 to 1999.

Radiology is now called Medical Imaging, and specialists in this field are trained not only in the use of X-ray equipment but also in administering and analyzing computerized tomography (CT), ultrasound, magnetic resonance imaging (MRI) scans, and other imaging technologies.

PHARMACY

There have been tremendous advances over the years, not only in terms of the number and variety of medications available, but also in the way they are prepared and distributed. Until the 1950s, nurses dispensed medications directly from a doctor's prescription, and medicine was kept on the nursing unit. Today, a pharmacist, with the help of a pharmacy technician, dispenses every prescription written for a hospitalized child. As treating hospitalized children has become more complex, the role of the hospital pharmacist has expanded to include preventing possible drug interactions and providing pharmaceutical care.

Each year, pharmacists and pharmacy technicians at the Children's prepare nearly 6,000 doses of total parenteral nutrition (for children receiving nutrition intravenously), more than 6,000 doses of chemotherapy, and 65,000 other medications of all types. Precision is essential. There are no standard doses at a children's hospital. Because of the variation in the sizes of patients, medications must be prescribed precisely according to each kilogram of weight.

The major challenge, says current director Jean-François Guévin, is the shortage of trained pharmacy staff in all hospitals. "Many choose to work in commercial pharmacies," he says, "as the salaries are much higher. They can earn right away what it takes 12 years to earn in a hospital." The department is currently short nearly three full-time-equivalent positions. Technicians play an increasing role, to free pharmacists for patient care.

SUPPORTING PATIENT CARE

Even MCH employees whose job descriptions do not directly involve the diagnosis and treatment of patients know that they are an important part of the care team, and that the special needs of children and their families must be taken into consideration when doing their jobs.

Creating supportive spaces

The hospital's architects, for instance, understand the importance of creating spaces that ensure the safety and security of MCH patients, families, and staff, and know how the environment affects the healing process. They design and implement projects to address basic needs, such as creating additional bathrooms and installing proper ventilation that provides complete air filtration. They are also responsible for installing state-of-the-art diagnostic technology. They have a special appreciation for colours, finishes, and different types of artwork that will create soothing, uplifting environments for patients and personnel alike, and carry out renovation projects using materials that are functional yet child-friendly.

Architectural Services was established at the Children's under Jean Dufresne in 1988, when the hospital had embarked on a capital campaign with a view to enlarging and adding to the hospital's buildings. Its mission, says current department manager Teresa Di Bartolo, is "to carry out projects that will bring added value to the patients, families, and staff by improving the functionality of the space, increasing efficiency, and creating environments that are safe, comforting, and healing." The department's staff also lends its expertise to various hospital committees such as the Space and Project Request Committee, the Task Force on Pediatric Design, the Committee for Quality of Life at Work, and the Infection Control Committee. Over the years, the department has built up a computerized databank of all the hospital spaces, ensuring that the locations of hidden services such as pipes, ducts, medical gases, sprinklers, and structural beams are known.

A responsive Architectural Services department like the one at the Children's makes it possible for the hospital to adapt rapidly, innovatively, and safely to changing clinical needs.

Invisible maintenance

Concerns for the health and safety of MCH patients, families, and staff are also the focus of the hospital's Maintenance Department. Whether they are painting a waiting area, replacing pipes, or creating a sterile area to store linens, maintenance employees must always be conscious of noise levels, dust, and other residue that might compromise healing or disturb the children and those around them.

"The ideal thing is to have the maintenance person be invisible," says Leonard Nixon, who has worked at the hospital since 1975 and was appointed Maintenance Manager in 2002. "Everything has to be done as quickly as possible, so as not to disturb the functioning of the hospital. In April 2004, we had to close the Emergency entrance to fix the expansion joint, and managed to do it in three days. The entrance was relocated to the old ambulance entrance beside the doctor's parking lot, off René-Lévesque Boulevard. But because of infection control, we can't cut corners. Sometimes a 15-minute job may take 10 hours because of the stringent criteria."

Keeping the hospital's buildings and grounds in good working order and looking respectable has always been a challenge. In the early days, much of the work was done by outside contractors. Today, the Maintenance Department's staff looks after all areas of the hospital—including the boilers, heating, and air conditioning systems, compressors for medical gases, electricity, plumbing, and refrigeration. They are constantly looking for ways to improve efficiency and reduce costs. Like many other MCH departments, they have begun to share certain responsibilities and tasks with other hospitals in the MUHC.

PLUMBING AND SURGERY

In the 1950s, the hospital's plumber did much more than look after the pipes. At the 90th anniversary celebration of the MCH, James Forsyth, who was responsible for plumbing and heating from 1957 to 1983, recalled his contributions to cardiac surgery.

"I used to go with every heart operation. A little baby would be lying on the table. I set up the machine. We had hot and cold water running through it. As they wanted the blood to be a little warmer or cooler, I used to work this machine right in the OR."

One of those tasks is the creation of signs. Because there are constant relocations, as well as new services and staff members, many new signs are needed each year. A full-time maintenance employee used to create each sign by hand. He would manually calculate the size of each sign and how far apart the letters had to be, then hand-engrave each one. Today, nearly 1,000 signs a year are computer-generated, and the sign-maker doubles as a locksmith.

Housekeepers essential in infection control

Whenever a construction or repair project is going on anywhere in the hospital, the housekeeping staff plays a vital role in keeping the area as clean and dust-free as possible. Housekeeping is also crucial in maintaining cleanliness and fighting the spread of infection throughout the hospital.

According to records from the 1920s, the MCH housekeeping staff included "kitchen help, waitresses, cleaners and helpers, housekeeper and maids, and seamstresses." Today, there are no waitresses, maids, or seamstresses, and the hospital's 60 housekeeping employees focus on cleaning and disinfecting, waxing floors, and moving furniture. They work in patient rooms, waiting rooms, diagnostic and treatment areas, and other areas such as kitchens, offices, and storage facilities.

The role of housekeepers in infection control is certainly not new. It has been recognized since "germs" were discovered in the 19th century that hospitals need to be hygienic. Infection control has always been a priority at the Children's, and took on increased importance during the typhoid, influenza, and polio epidemics that swept the Montreal area prior to the 1960s. Over the past 25 years, MCH infection control programs have become more structured, and housekeeping's role has become increasingly recognized.

With new viruses affecting hospitals today, and with better understanding of infectious diseases, the hospital is placing increased emphasis on infection control, which affects the workload of housekeepers. They now clean bathrooms at least three times a day instead of the previous two, for instance, and bathtubs at least twice.

They also take regular precautions to ensure children's safety. They don't leave their carts unattended in the hall, for instance, where children might play with the cleaning supplies. When moving carts or using large equipment, they continuously look to the front and back, to make sure they don't run into a small child.

Every employee in the hospital is involved in infection control in some way. There are all those with direct patient contact, of course, along with pharmacists, those who sterilize operating instruments, and laundry employees who provide sterile linens and gowns. The microbiology lab, medical records, information systems, and a variety of administrative and office staff help collect and collate data. The Infection Control Service develops standards and consults with departments throughout the institution regarding procedures and equipment.

Good food, prepared with care

Food Services is also involved in infection control. The employees in this department take great care in preparing, delivering, and storing food to prevent contamination by bacteria. They must maintain

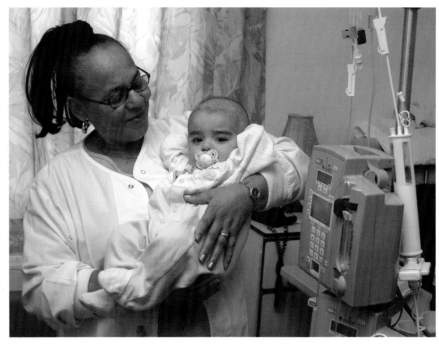

Housekeeping employees often get to know the children as well as do the nurses and doctors—sometimes better—and become an important constant in the lives of long-term and frequently hospitalized patients. As housekeeper Leonard Johnston says, "The kids are not afraid of the housekeeper. We're the friendly ones— we joke and have fun with them."

Ruby Wilson, seen here with Jordan, a patient on the Oncology Unit, often chats and laughs with patients as she cleans their rooms, and sometimes forms relationships with them that last even after the children's treatments have ended and they've gone home.

"I get courage from these kids," she says.

food at the proper temperature, avoiding unnecessary changes, and keep the handling of food to a minimum.

Today, a total of 50 Food Services employees, most working part-time, provide meals for patients, staff, and visitors. The largest number are "dietary helpers," who portion, prepare, and deliver food to the nursing units and cafeteria. Each day, they prepare between 300 and 325 meals for patients, including formula. In the cafeteria, they serve between 500 and 600 people a day.

Behind the scenes

The hospital's other employees also work—many behind the scenes—to ensure that all areas of the hospital function smoothly. They, too, know that their ultimate goal is to enable children and their families to be cared for as efficiently and comfortably as possible.

Staff in the Security Department, for example, know that by screening visitors and monitoring computer warning systems throughout the building—for everything from the level of oxygen reserves to the refrigeration system—they are keeping the patients, visitors, and staff secure, protecting the hospital's goods and preventing system breakdowns.

The Information Services Department ensures that the hospital's computer systems are kept as up-to-date as possible and functioning properly. They

KEEPING TRACK

About 35 people work in Medical Records—up to 42 during peak periods. They respond to hundreds of calls a day from the nursing units, Emergency Department, and clinics requesting patient files. Medical records employees are responsible for forwarding patient charts, tracking their whereabouts in the hospital, making necessary repairs to the charts from wear and tear, and, when the patient has been discharged, ensuring that all necessary paperwork has been completed, then filing the chart.

Each patient chart has a barcode, and is scanned—like at the grocery store—every time it leaves or returns to Medical Records. If a chart is transferred from one clinic to another, Medical Records is informed, and its new location is entered in the computer.

This means that the department's staff can locate each child's chart anywhere in the building at all times. There are only very rare exceptions. Once a resident, assuming the department closed at night (it doesn't), put a chart in his locker to protect it overnight, then forgot about it and left for Texas for three months. (Luckily, there were no serious consequences.)

SPECIAL GENES?

Dr. Harvey Guyda, Physician-in-Chief since 1996, thinks pediatricians are "genetically derived."

"I have no scientific basis for this," he says, "but I believe it. The environment will mould and shape the kind of pediatrician you become, but not every medical trainee can be a pediatrician, or work with kids."

assist individual departments in acquiring specific equipment and software to meet their needs, helping them to obtain from vendors whatever customized features are required to suit MCH-specific procedures.

Medical Multimedia Services contribute to a variety of clinical, legal, teaching, and research activities in the hospital. Technicians produce videos and photographs of patients and procedures and assist in telemedicine through the use of videoconferencing. They are involved in the rental and set-up of equipment for meetings and conferences, and the production of CDs, DVDs, videos, and publications aimed at patients, families, staff, and the community.

Public Relations and Communications is the hospital's link to the community. By keeping the general public, media, and other health-care professionals accurately informed about MCH developments and relevant health-care issues, they promote the public's interest in and support of the hospital's work.

And throughout the MCH, administrative and other office personnel coordinate a wide variety of activities involved in patient care, teaching, and research. They support front-line staff, develop office procedures, and organize committees. They make appointments, requisition supplies, process invoices, gather data, and plan special events.

A SPECIAL KIND OF PERSON

No matter what job they perform, there is something special about people who work at the Children's. It may be the kind of person who is hired, or the effect the children have on them. Most agree it's probably a bit of both.

Being able to explain circumstances and treatments in ways that are understandable to children of all ages—and empowering them to the greatest possible extent—requires flexibility and imagination on the part of the staff. Special skills and understanding are also required when dealing with the emotional reactions of children and their families to illness and hospitalization.

When families and patients are asked what makes MCH staff special, they use words like "caring," "patient," "open-minded," and "supportive." Many are impressed by how spontaneous and creative the staff can be, even when they're extremely busy. They tell of the maintenance workers, for instance, who when asked to repair a leak in the room of a dying child, repainted the entire room so the child could have a more pleasant place to spend his last days. They talk about the nurses who, while caring for Inuit children who couldn't eat the unfamiliar hospital food, arranged to have bannock bread and deer, moose, and whale meat shipped from the North.

> "The phone would ring and the nurse in PICU would tell me, 'A child has arrived who's been in a car accident. He's gone to the OR. He's not doing well and the parents are in shock. Could you come?' My knees would shake. They still shake, after 20 years. It's never easy."
>
> MICHÈLE VIAU-CHAGNON, COORDINATOR, PALLIATIVE CARE PROGRAM, 1995–2003

Working at the Montreal Children's Hospital has never been easy, of course. Watching children battle serious illness is extremely difficult. When long-term patients come of age and are transferred to adult facilities, it can be hard for both parties to say good-bye. And when a child can't be saved, it is not only the family that grieves, but also the staff. Support from the palliative care and pastoral services teams is invaluable at such times. The memorial services organized by Pastoral Services several times each year are an occasion for staff, family, and friends to grieve and celebrate together the lives of children who have passed away.

One effect of the movement toward keeping children's hospitalization to a minimum is that the workload is more intense and fast-paced than ever before. Twenty years ago, a third of the patients on any given nursing unit would be either waiting for elective surgery or on the road to recovery and requiring minimal care. Today, those children are at home, and it is generally only children who are critically ill or require complex care who are admitted, thereby increasing the overall service intensity.

Changes in medical knowledge and technology have always been part of the job, but today these advances are so rapid that keeping up is a constant challenge. To continue providing the highest level of care to their patients, staff must regularly take part in seminars, courses, and informal teaching sessions to upgrade their skills.

In 1936, the hospital was described as "an institution with little money but much faith," a statement that is still true today. The costs of equipment, facilities, and staff are higher than ever before, while funding, which comes from the public purse, is limited. Each member of the MCH staff has a role to play in the stewardship of the hospital. With modern information technology, employees can measure and keep track of their activities so they can make adjustments and ensure those resources are used to the best advantage.

Shortages of medical, nursing, and other health-care professionals are also a major challenge, and a great deal of time and resources are invested in recruiting and retaining staff.

THE REWARDS OF CARING

Luckily, the challenges faced by staff are usually far outweighed by the rewards. They see most children get better and return to their normal lives, including many who would not have made it just a

Leaders Set the Tone

What is it about the Children's that makes it such a special place to work? Jane Allan's response is "The staff: all of them. And good staff draw more good staff."

Jane's father was Dr. Alan Ross (1903–1998), who joined the Children's in 1931, and was Physician-in-Chief from 1953 until 1968. Dr. Ross had a gift for promoting team spirit and making staff feel appreciated. Jane remembers that when she was working at the hospital, she was stopped in the hallway many times by non-professional staff, to tell her how her father would talk to every employee, no matter what their position. "That summed up for me what kind of a man he was."

Dr. Ross created an atmosphere that attracted and retained energetic and versatile staff like Drs. Elizabeth and Donald Hillman, who in the 1950s were among the hospital's first full-time pediatricians. They remember that Alan Ross "established collaborative rather than boss-and-subordinate relationships. He gave you a sense of ownership of the hospital."

It was the Hillmans who encouraged Dr. John (Jack) Charters to take on the executive director-ship in 1970. Dr. Charters' administration reflected Alan Ross's collaborative, supportive approach. "Everything you wanted to try," recalls Liz Hillman, "he was willing. We had tremendous cooperation from administrators. We were all part of the family."

For Dr. Richard Hamilton, Physician-in-Chief and Chairman of the Department of Pediatrics from 1986 to 1996, "Jack handled things on a personal level. He had a real capacity to listen, patience in reaching decisions, and a forthright way of delivering decisions. He instilled a spirit of collaboration."

Dr. Nicolas Steinmetz, Executive Director from 1987 to 1995 and 2003 to 2004, remembers his predecessor as one who "managed to bring the hospital into the technological age without ever losing the human touch."

This spirit of collaboration and family atmosphere was not easy to maintain as the years went by. Specialization increased; professional boundaries changed and occasionally conflicted; hospital administration became more complex. Dr. Hamilton remembers his 10-year tenure as a time of "extraordinary evolution within the hospital." It was also a time of political and financial instability in Quebec, which posed a serious challenge to the Pediatrics Chairman, one of whose main responsibilities was to attract staff. According to Dr. Wendy MacDonald, who stood in for Dr. Hamilton briefly during that time, "Because of his international stature as a researcher and academic, Dr. Hamilton was able to attract people of high calibre despite the difficult time. He is a great judge of character and has great respect for people."

"The management teams and department heads have always been so talented and dedicated,"

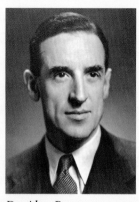 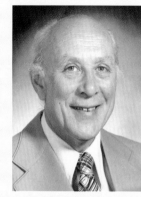 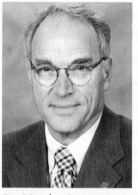

Dr. Alan Ross   *Dr. Jack Charters*   *Dr. Nicolas Steinmetz*

recalls Dr. Claire Dupont, who was Director of Professional Services from 1987 to 2001. "Our greatest challenges always seemed to relate to retaining and recruiting this kind of staff, especially in the challenging environments of government budget cuts, political pressures, and then the need to develop teams beyond our own 'MCH home and family,' such as within the integrated MUHC, and with Ste-Justine."

Dr. Steinmetz's mandate as Executive Director occurred during the same volatile period. Dr. Patricia Forbes describes Dr. Steinmetz's approach: "His clinical background and knowledge of health-care issues served him well as he guided the Children's into an era of more government control and the need to demonstrate innovation and excellence in care. He was open to new ideas, would discuss new projects, and was fully supportive of those that showed merit."

Despite the challenges of the times, the family feeling of the institution continued to flourish under Dr. Steinmetz's leadership. He maintained the tradition of entertaining personnel at his home. He was known for stopping in the corridors to speak to staff members of every rank. And he always made time to squat down in the hallway outside his office to chat with young children on their way to appointments.

few years ago. Most families are relieved of the stress they experienced when they first arrived at the hospital. Many families show their appreciation by sending cards and photographs, or making donations to the nursing unit or program. Some former patients come back years later to say thank you, and bring their own children for treatment.

Staff who have worked in other hospitals—even other children's hospitals—remark on the spirit of cooperation, understanding, and inclusion that characterize the way the Children's is run, from Board and senior administration through to individual work teams.

When asked why they stay at the Children's— many for their entire career—most staff members say it's because of the immeasurable rewards of caring for these special children, and because of the sense of camaraderie among the staff, even in sometimes difficult circumstances.

It's always been that way.

At the 90th anniversary of the hospital, a group of "old-timers" gathered to reminisce about "the good old days" of the 1950s, both before and after the hospital moved to Tupper Street. Many remembered picnics at Dr. Alan Ross's cottage and hockey games against the Montreal General Hospital. There were beer and oyster parties and dinner dances. Staff would gather around the ping-pong table—and the beer machine—in the lounge where the Human Resources Department is now.

Today the demands on staff are more complex and there isn't as much time to socialize, but the special feeling is still there. There's still a sense of commitment and of fun. There are still birthday celebrations and retirement parties. There are special cultural celebrations such as Greek Day, Black History Month, and the Hindu Festival of Lights. And there are annual Awards of Excellence recognizing staff at all levels.

There's also the sense that everyone is there for the same reason. Josefina Revuelta, a nurse on the

General Medicine inpatient unit, summed it up this way: "No matter what job they do, everyone on the staff works as part of a team; they are individuals first, and job descriptions second. They are all focused on the best interests of the children."

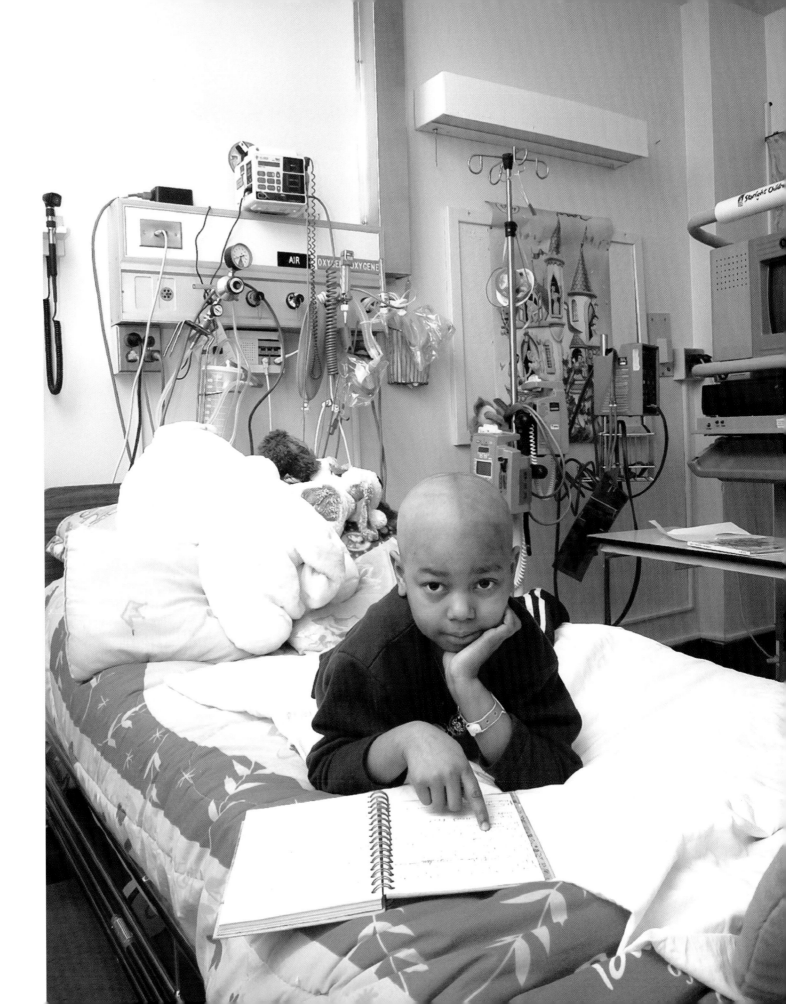

*Shilah, who
has leukemia,
has lost
her hair but
none of her
fighting spirit.*

"This Hospital will be, primarily, for crippled children, but if at any time, there should be unoccupied beds, those suffering from other surgical or medical affections may be admitted."

Press statement issued by the organizing committee for the proposed Children's Memorial Hospital, 1902

5

What Ails Kids:
Curing and Caring Then and Now

At the threshold of the 20th century, it had become abundantly clear that the children of Montreal needed a hospital to call their own. In 1902, a European visitor wrote, "I don't believe I ever saw so many people in one place deformed, or crippled, or with something the matter with their feet." A port city prone to epidemics, at that time Montreal had a higher infant mortality rate than most Third World countries today. In 1904, the rate stood at 375 per 1,000, with most infants dying from diarrhea. Contagious diseases such as diphtheria, scarlet fever, tuberculosis, measles, and whooping cough (pertussis) also claimed many children's lives. Between 1897 and 1911, one in three babies died before reaching the age of one.

In those days, children who fell ill were treated as if they were small adults, placed in overcrowded adult hospitals, with equipment and techniques designed for adults. There was a great need for additional beds, and for professional staff who could meet the special needs of sick youngsters. The community was quick to rally round the project, and all four local English-language newspapers publicized the hopes and aims of the new hospital.

The organizing committee, spearheaded by the visionary Dr. Alexander Mackenzie Forbes (the first Professor of Orthopedic Surgery at McGill University) and a group of public-spirited local citizens, further noted the need for children "to take advantage of the curative effects of the sun"—a radical concept at the time and precursor of the modern notion of the "healing environment." Soon after the Children's Memorial Hospital welcomed its first five patients on January 30, 1904, it was filled to capacity. Just five years later, the move to Cedar Avenue meant wide-open spaces, fresh air, and sunshine for the children.

MEETING VERY DIFFERENT NEEDS

Fast forward through a turbulent and eventful century, marked by major advances in medicine. Today, the healing environment of the Montreal Children's Hospital treats children with an enormous range of diseases and disorders, many of them fundamentally different from the health problems encountered in the early 1900s. In fact, the hospital's ever-broadening mandate has mirrored—and in many areas of medicine, led—the progress of pediatric medicine through the 20th century and into the 21st. While the hospital initially focused mainly on orthopedic cases and communicable diseases, the long list of problems treated today includes not only physical conditions, but also those with important societal, environmental, and psychological components, such as asthma and eating disorders.

The development of public health education, hygiene and prevention measures, and awareness of lifestyle factors have played prominent roles in preventing childhood illness and death, leading to a sea change in the kinds of diseases and disorders that are treated at the Children's today. Many illnesses that brought children to the hospital in the

- Department of Tuberculosis: separate pavilion added for contagious TB
- Department of Rheumatism: separate pavilion
- Department of Otolaryngology: tonsil ward
- Department of Congenital Syphilis: treating with arsenic compounds
- Department of Bacteriology: cultures, animal inoculation, production of antisera and vaccines
- Intensive studies of tuberculosis and rheumatic fever underway

"100 Years of Infectious Diseases—the Ongoing Battle between Microbes and Man," presentation by Dr. Dorothy Moore, Montreal Children's Hospital, June 2004

early days are now easily preventable. Vaccines have had a huge impact, rendering diseases such as polio virtually obsolete.

Antibiotics—introduced mid-century—have made many previously fatal diseases curable. Nevertheless, contagious conditions have not been completely eliminated. The use, and over-use, of antibiotics has created a new problem: major drug-resistant organisms. Over-reliance on over-the-counter remedies is another modern-day concern.

Many of the major shifts in disease patterns were reflected in the organization of the new facilities at 2300 Tupper Street, where the hospital moved in 1956. For instance, thanks to antibiotics, there were no more wards for rheumatic fever. There was no more polio ward, as the incidence had by that time decreased dramatically.

INFECTION AND POVERTY TAKE THEIR TOLL

A typhoid fever epidemic in the fall of 1909 that caused an acute shortage of hospital beds for both adults and children led to the first in the Children's Memorial Hospital's long series of expansions. An isolation ward was constructed in a separate building to prevent the spread of infection. Additional

isolation wards were built later for other infectious diseases as hospital staff dealt with successive waves of epidemics: the great influenza pandemic of 1918–1919; another typhoid epidemic in 1926; and polio outbreaks in 1931, 1932, 1946, 1949, 1954, and 1959.

The Great Depression of the 1930s exacerbated the effects of poverty: malnutrition, low resistance to illness, and slower convalescence. With low income

BED REST?

Rheumatic fever was one of the most common infectious diseases prior to the development of antibiotics. Treatment involved a long, strictly supervised convalescent period, thought to be best spent in hospital. Rows and rows of beds were occupied by children who no longer felt terribly sick but were required to rest in bed. Dr. Richard Goldbloom, who joined the staff in the 1950s, told the following anecdote about the rheumatic fever wards:

"Dr. [Arnold] Johnson [Chief of Cardiology] and the other cardiologists used to come around with the physiotherapist, and all the children used to be lying like statues under the covers, completely immobile. They would look over each child's chart and decide that Maryanne could perhaps increase from 10 steps to 15 steps today. This was to be overseen by the physiotherapist. They would finish their rounds and leave the building, and literally as the door closed, these kids would start leaping from one bed to the other. This idea of gradual mobilization and bed rest was a total illusion, but it had the cardiologists fooled for many years."

Or maybe not. In a 90th anniversary interview, Dr. Elizabeth Hillman recalled the time in the 1950s when she was on the ward with a new resident from the Dominican Republic.

"It was the first snowfall in Montreal, and she had never seen snow. She got all excited and ran outside and scooped up an armful for each child— each child supposedly on bed rest! Of course, you know what they did: they had a wonderful snow fight. Arn Johnson came in and found us ... and joined in the fight!"

and low morale, parents often found it difficult to help their children follow the advice and instructions of health-care providers. Before the advent of Medicare and government benefits, lengthy illness or unemployment, especially of the family breadwinner, could spell bankruptcy. What a blessed relief it must have been for such families to know that the hospital was equally "available to the children of the rich as well as the children of the poor."

TUBERCULOSIS AND SCARLET FEVER

Tuberculosis was another common infectious disease requiring long convalescence and its own ward. In the 1930s, sick children in Quebec were usually put into adult hospitals where they risked being exposed to advanced cases of TB in adults. Dr. H.P. Wright, who headed the tuberculosis ward at the time, insisted that the Children's accommodate as many infectious children as possible. Isolation cubicles were set up within the ward. The Royal Edward Laurentian Hospital (which later moved from Ste-Agathe-des-Monts to Montreal, became the Montreal Chest Institute, and subsequently merged with the Royal Victoria Hospital in the early 1990s) asked two staff members of the Children's to attend their children's clinic. Drs. Alan Ross and P.N. MacDermot answered the call, along with Dr. Ernest M. Worden, teaching generations of students and residents how to manage and prevent tuberculosis, which remains a problem in many areas of the world today.

Scarlet fever, another pre-antibiotic scourge, was contagious enough to require quarantine of the patient's home and could lead to rheumatic fever and consequent heart disease. The Children's did not see all these patients, as the most infectious cases were sent to other hospitals—the Hôpital Pasteur for French-speaking children and, for those who spoke English, the Alexandra Hospital in Pointe St. Charles. When these diseases became rare, the Alexandra was turned into a long-term care institution under the Children's direction and was ulti-

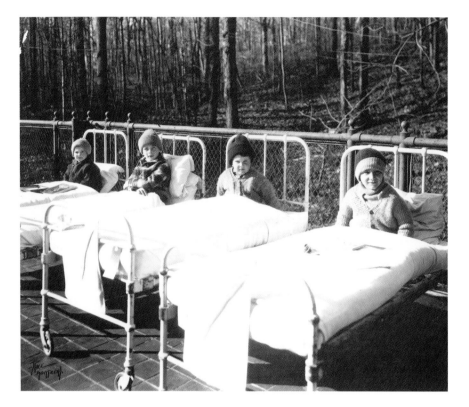

mately closed in 1988, after serving as a powerful learning resource for generations of residents as well as a centre of excellent care for these sick children.

ANTIBIOTICS AND VACCINES
CHANGE THE FACE OF INFECTIONS

Apart from improvements in socioeconomic conditions, the two major factors influencing the improvement of child health in the 20th century were antibiotics and vaccines. Infectious diseases lost ground very quickly once antibiotics became available—sulfa drugs in 1941, penicillin in 1944, and streptomycin after the end of World War II. Antibiotics have since saved countless lives and prevented many disabilities.

Although infections were now treatable, there was no overnight miracle. Insufficient supplies of penicillin at first left children vulnerable. While streptomycin controlled many forms of tuberculosis, it was not very effective in treating tuberculous men-

Four young boys enjoy the benefits of the "healing environment" from their beds, wheeled out onto a balcony at the Children's Memorial Hospital.

HIV-AIDS

The human immunodeficiency virus (HIV), unknown until 1981, has been the most devastating new infection to arrive in the last 50 years. Thousands had been infected, or had even developed full-blown acquired immune deficiency syndrome (AIDS), before there was any effective treatment for it—and in many cases, before HIV was recognized and understood. One of the ways in which children became vulnerable to the virus was through blood transfusions from infected donors.

Hemophiliacs were especially hard hit. Not only were they transfused many times, they received Factor VIII concentrate that came from "pools," or blood combined from thousands of donations. As a result, their chances of being infected were very high, and most transfused before blood testing was available contracted HIV. Children with thalassemia were another high-risk group.

Dr. Michael Whitehead, who headed the hospital's Hematology Division in those days, remembers those tragic consequences and how they broke the hearts of staff who cared for high-risk children, especially those in Home Care: "With advanced treatment methods, they had saved these children from a life of hospital confinement, only to see them fall victim to an even more serious threat."

In 1985, a reliable blood test became available in Canada and the Canadian Red Cross established a blood screening system. By the late 1980s, donated blood was no longer a risk.

However, by that time, there were still many former patients of both adult and children's hospitals who had been transfused a decade earlier and might not be aware of the importance of being tested for HIV. The Montreal Children's and Ste-Justine hospitals were among the institutions who made sustained efforts to track down all patients who had received transfusions between 1982 and November 1985—more than 1700 in the case of the MCH—and who had not already been advised by their doctors to have an HIV test.

In light of the widespread public attention to transfusion risks during the 1980s and '90s, it may come as a surprise that most children treated for HIV at the MCH over the years acquired it not from transfusions but from their mothers, before or at birth. In all, 39 such cases have been treated and followed at the Children's. (Four of these had acquired HIV due to other causes before coming to Canada.) Thirteen died, most of them early in the epidemic. Others moved on to adult centres as they got older. Of the 18 still being treated at the Children's in 2005, all but one were quite well, thanks to the powerful antiretroviral drugs now available. And transfer of infection to babies from their mothers is now quite rare, owing to the availability in Canada of screening and protective measures.

As Dr. Dorothy Moore of the Infectious Diseases Department notes: "The picture of pediatric HIV infection has changed dramatically over the years. In the early days, we only saw children who were quite ill in the first one or two years of life, and we could do nothing for them except keep them comfortable. Now, with early diagnosis and treatment, children are remaining healthy, never hospitalized, and living relatively normal lives."

ingitis, a common form of this disease in children. In time, antibiotics became more readily available and more effective drugs were produced. Over the last 50 years, antimicrobial treatments have been developed for a wide range of infections. Currently, the Montreal Children's Hospital's formulary contains more than 75 antimicrobial drugs.

Vaccines, an important preventive measure, also had a dramatic effect. Diphtheria, the major cause of childhood death from infection early in the century, became rare after widespread vaccination of children began in the 1930s. Polio, which once filled entire hospital wards, was virtually eliminated by the Salk and later the Sabin vaccines. The dreaded disease, then known as infantile paralysis, would cripple children by affecting the nerves and muscles, sometimes leading to death. Even once the disease was checked, the story was far from over. Children whose muscles had been affected needed physical therapy for years, and special clinics were established at the Children's to care for them. Unlike typhoid or rheumatic fever, polio taxed health-care facilities even long after the epidemic was over.

Other vaccines now routinely used in prevention include those for pertussis (whooping cough), tetanus, and *Haemophilus influenza B* (once the most common cause of meningitis in children), combined with diphtheria and polio vaccines in a single inoculation.

Another combination is the MMR vaccine, for measles, mumps, and rubella (German measles). Even before the 1960s, when these vaccines were not in wide use, only serious cases of these diseases were admitted to hospital. These children would have been admitted to the Alexandra Hospital or Hôpital Pasteur.

Today, children are routinely vaccinated against meningococcus and pneumococcus (which cause meningitis and other serious infections), as well as hepatitis B (which causes chronic liver disease). Many other vaccines are available for administration in special cases.

MALNUTRITION AND OBESITY

Despite great socioeconomic progress and increased public health education, the hospital still frequently sees health problems related to under- or over-nutrition. Obesity in children and adolescents has become a major problem as a result of limited physical activity and poor eating habits. Epidemic in the United States, the rate of obesity is also increasing in Canada—in fact, approximately 15% of Canadian children may meet current criteria for being overweight, according to a 2004 evidence report sponsored by the Institute of Nutrition, Metabolism and Diabetes that was co-chaired by Dr. Harvey Guyda, Physician-in-Chief of the MCH.

These days, the MCH's Weight Management Clinic is unable to accommodate all the referrals it receives. While obesity rarely results in hospital admissions on its own, it can lead to more serious conditions in the long term, such as Type II (adult-onset) diabetes, cardiovascular disease, hypertension, orthopedic problems, and sleep problems, not to mention the psychological problems that come from being teased, bullied, or rejected by other children.

GROWTH DISORDERS

Children with disorders of growth and puberty are frequently referred to endocrinologists at the Children's. Pediatric endocrinology, the medical discipline that deals with hormones and their influence on body metabolism and growth, treats illnesses caused by disorders of the endocrine glands, such as the pituitary, thyroid, and adrenal glands, as well as of the pancreas.

Dr. Frances McCall established the Division of Endocrinology and the Clinical Endocrine Laboratory in 1955. Two years later, Dr. Donald Hillman became the full-time Director of Endocrine Services, while Dr. Claude Giroux headed the lab and developed an active PhD training program in developmental endocrinology. The program started with Dr. Hillman in 1961 and ended in 1974 with Dr. Giroux's last PhD student, John Torday. The

REACHING HER FULL POTENTIAL

Maureen Smith and her brother were often mistaken for twins when they were very young, despite the fact that he was four years younger. Her short stature was a worry for her mother, who took her to four doctors—none of whom spotted her pituitary deficiency—before coming to the Children's in 1966. By that time, Maureen was eight years old and wearing size 4 clothes. At the MCH, she was enrolled in a new research program testing the use of human growth hormone. After starting the hormone treatments in January 1968, Maureen grew about an inch a month for a while. She spent a lot of time at the hospital, as her progress was checked regularly.

In 1976, when she reached five-foot-one, she chose to stop the treatments. "The waiting list for growth hormones was two years long in those days," she explains, "and I didn't feel I should be taking it from some other child who needed it more." Nowadays, the hormone can be created synthetically and is more easily available.

During Maureen's teen years, her faulty pituitary gland failed to make enough cortisone and she developed adrenal insufficiency, at one time lapsing into a coma. That meant spending more time in hospital. Not a great way to spend a childhood, you would think. And yet, for Maureen, there were happy memories.

"The MCH was just a place where you felt really loved. Jacqueline Rioux, head nurse on the Metabolism Unit, was always there for me."

There was inspiration, too. "I'd always wanted to be a teacher, although my mother warned me it might not happen. We came from a poor neighbourhood and kids from there didn't always get that kind of education. But the staff were really supportive. On my 15th birthday, just after I came out from that coma, Dr. Guyda gave me a chocolate apple and said, 'Here's an apple for the teacher.'"

Ms. Smith now has a master of education degree in educational psychology and is a member of two scientific committees on research. "I was motivated by the people at the Children's," she says. "They worked so hard for us. And being around educated people made you want to use your brain—I could see what it was possible to do."

Branchaud Lecture in Developmental Endocrinology is presented annually in memory of Dr. Charlotte Laplante Branchaud, an outstanding member of the endocrine research group at the Children's.

The approach to the diagnosis of endocrine disorders has changed enormously over the past 30 years. At one time, children would be admitted to hospital for up to 10 days of tests. Testing is now often completed in one day. Measurement of blood hormone levels is much more sophisticated and more readily available, and markedly improved imaging techniques have also led to more accurate diagnoses and more specific treatments.

IMPROVING LIFE FOR DIABETICS

Type I diabetes, diagnosed in childhood, is also known as insulin-dependent diabetes. The best-known "familial" disease, diabetes has been a special area of research focus at the Children's under Dr. Constantin Polychronakos for more than 20 years. The Diabetic Clinic set up by Drs. Mimi Belmonte, who joined the Children's in 1955 and taught at McGill for nearly 30 years, and Donald Hillman, has helped many diabetic children learn to live with their condition.

In the early 1900s, children with Type I diabetes did not generally survive beyond their teen years, as the daily insulin treatment they needed to live was not developed until the 1920s. Prior to the landmark discovery of insulin by Canadians Dr. Frederick Banting and Charles Best in 1922, those who were diagnosed with diabetes were put on extremely restrictive diets, causing some patients to die from under-nutrition rather from the disease itself.

Controlling diabetes at an early age has a positive cumulative effect, reducing long-term problems. Diabetics whose condition is not well treated live only two-thirds of the average lifespan. Once insulin became widely available, diabetic children and adults were administered life-saving treatment. New types of insulin and a variety of injection techniques, as well as simpler blood testing and treatment on an outpatient basis, allow children to control their diabetes at home, getting advice over the phone if necessary.

INNOVATIONS IN ORTHOPEDICS

Orthopedics has a long and proud history at the Children's, whose founder, Dr. Forbes, was an orthopedic surgeon. Until 1962, Orthopedics consisted solely of part-time doctors whose practice included both adults and children. Pediatric orthopedics, like most other fields of pediatric medicine, had yet to evolve as a separate subspecialty.

In 1962, Dr. J. Murray McIntyre left his adult practice to become the first staff surgeon to practise full-time at the Children's. Four years later, Dr. Robert Gledhill was the division's first clinical fellow in pediatric orthopedics, becoming Director of Orthopedics in 1973. The transition to a service consisting of full-time pediatric orthopedic surgeons was a gradual one. In the mid-1970s, Dr. Ken Brown, the first pediatric orthopedic oncologist at the MCH and probably the first in Montreal, introduced the operating microscope to the department and developed the division's skills in microvascular surgery. Microsurgical procedures for replantation of digits, free tissue transfers (transplanting non-essential donor tissue from one part of the body to another), and repairs were introduced in 1969–1970, making the Children's a world leader in this area.

Rehabilitation care has also been a major focus, notably through joint projects with the Mackay Rehabilitation Centre, where a Seating and Technical Aids Clinic was set up in the late 1980s that provides adapted strollers, wheelchairs, and positioning devices for disabled children. Residents in orthopedics frequently do rotations at the Shriners and Ste-Justine hospitals, establishing valuable links for training and clinical activities.

Multidisciplinary clinics bring together Children's staff from orthopedics, physiotherapy, and home care to look after children with rheumatoid arthritis and related disorders. Juvenile rheumatoid arthritis,

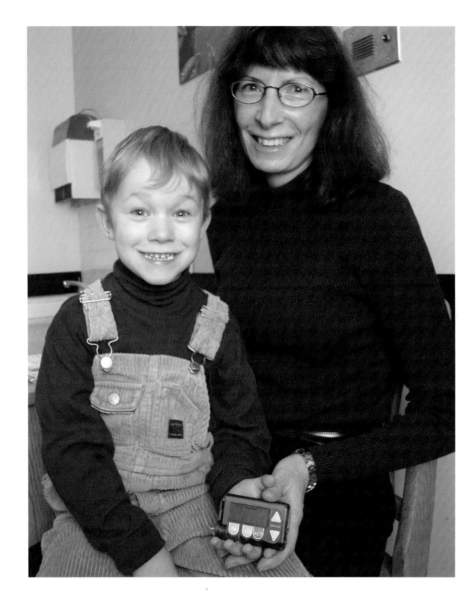

one of the most common childhood illnesses, affects an estimated one in 1,000 children under the age of 16. An unpredictable disease, it is marked by periods of remission between crises which can affect vision and growth, as well as cause deformities. "We try to make the joints as flexible as possible with the help of medication, exercise, prostheses, and sometimes surgery," explains division director Dr. Ciarán Duffy, who heads the multidisciplinary team that cares for children with chronic arthritis.

Nurse educator Anne Bossy of the Diabetes Clinic shows young Arnaud how to use an insulin pump. The pump, a pager-sized device, is changing the face of childhood diabetes.

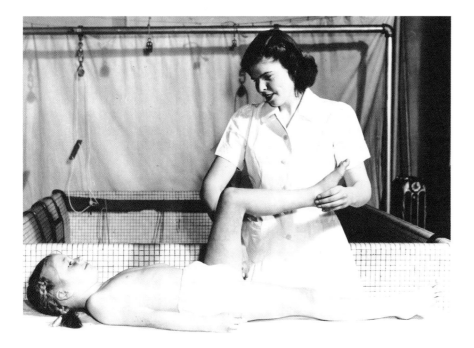

A physiotherapist helps a young girl increase her range of motion. This photo dates from the 1950s.

the MCH—quite an achievement, considering that the work was started before the era of the personal computer and all digitizing was done manually. Clinicians still use that algorithm today to evaluate various spinal deformities.

At the beginning of the 21st century, children with spinal abnormalities continue to come to the Children's from all over Quebec for innovative techniques that combine surgery with continual monitoring of spinal cord function.

MULTIDISCIPLINARY APPROACH REAPS BENEFITS FOR CHILDREN

Cerebral palsy is a disability caused by damage to the brain before, during, or in the early days after birth. In the first half of the 20th century, children with cerebral palsy were generally not treated until they reached school age, when their inability to walk became a more serious problem. Screening at younger ages, begun in the 1950s, made it possible to provide earlier treatment and alleviation of symptoms.

By the 1960s, children with cerebral palsy were benefiting from the combined expertise of orthopedics, neurology, and physiotherapy through the Cerebral Palsy Conference established by Drs. J. Murray McIntyre and Preston Robb. This multidisciplinary approach—teams from different disciplines working together to diagnose and treat the same patients—would become the wave of the future.

Yet another example of multidisciplinary teamwork is the Spina Bifida Clinic, organized in the mid-1970s by Dr. Patricia Forbes. Having patients see specialists in general pediatrics, neurosurgery, urology, and orthopedics, generally all on the same day, has proved to be an innovative approach, making it possible to synchronize treatment planning and to coordinate care, saving families many tiring hours of travel.

The Muscular Dystrophy Clinic established soon afterward through a grant from Muscular Dys-

Scoliosis, a deformity of the spine, frequently occurred as a result of polio, but it has many other causes as well. It can be a congenital abnormality, the result of other muscle paralysis, or associated with a multitude of diseases. The most common type by far is idiopathic scoliosis, which can occur in all age groups but most frequently arises during adolescence. If not treated early enough, it can cause severe physical deformity as well as impairment of lung and heart function. To foster early detection, which makes treatment easier and more effective, the Children's set up a school screening program for the City of Montreal in 1975, training school nurses in diagnostic techniques. Screening for scoliosis is now performed in most schools across North America.

The surgical treatment of scoliosis and other spinal abnormalities at the Children's has evolved considerably over the years (see Chapter 9). In the 1980s, a technique for radiographic three-dimensional analysis of the human spine was developed by Tom Szertes of the Department of Mechanical Engineering at McGill University and Dr. Gledhill of

trophy Canada (MDC) gradually evolved into a combined Neurology/Orthopedic Clinic, serving children with all neurological disabilities, including muscular dystrophy.

The Home Care Program, developed by Dr. Elizabeth Hillman, inaugurated in 1964 under Dr. Brian Wherrett, and continued under Dr. Hanna Strawczynski, was the first such program in North America specifically designed to meet the needs of children and their families, and to free up hospital beds previously occupied by chronic custodial-care patients. The program has grown rapidly and has been extended to include children with chronic illnesses or conditions such as hemophilia or thalassemia. Parents are taught how to deal with emergencies at home, helping them avoid midnight visits to the Children's.

KIDNEY DISEASE—EXTENDING AND IMPROVING LIVES

The most common cause of kidney failure in North America is complications from diabetes, or diabetic nephropathy. In the days before dialysis and transplants, kidney disease was an extremely serious diagnosis—frequently a death sentence, in fact.

Dr. Keith Drummond, Canada's first pediatric nephrologist and MCH Physician-in-Chief from 1974 to 1986, set up a research laboratory and clinical division for kidney disease at the Children's in 1964. He was a pioneer in evaluating glomerulonephritis (inflammation of the internal kidney structures), using biopsy results to determine the most effective treatment with different types of drugs. Dr. Bernard Kaplan, who chaired the division, led an active research program in nephrology, and Dr. Patricia Forbes taught children with kidney disease how to manage their condition. A major milestone occurred in 1989, when Dr. Lorraine Bell started the Kidney Transplant and Dialysis Program at the Children's.

The challenges associated with treating children with kidney disease are many, starting with the fact that their blood vessels are so small. Today, kidney transplantation in infants has become the standard of care, with extremely encouraging results. With better immunosuppression, advances in techniques, and the contributions of the intensive-care team caring for small patients, many hurdles have been overcome. Kidney failure can now be postponed or even prevented.

In 1991, the Children's set up Quebec's first living-donor pediatric kidney transplant program. Living-donor transplants have become easier to plan and easier on the donor (usually a parent or sibling), thanks to laparoscopic surgery. They have also achieved a high rate of success. A child who receives a kidney from a living donor at the Children's today can expect to enjoy 25 more years of healthy life.

Dialysis is a procedure that removes toxic substances from the blood when the kidneys are unable to do so. Hemodialysis, in which blood is cleaned through a machine with a special filter that removes wastes and extra fluids, imposes a rigid schedule that requires frequent hospital visits, up to five times a week for babies and three times a week for older children. The trend is to slower, more continuous therapy through daily hospital visits or home hemodialysis.

Peritoneal dialysis is a less restrictive process in which a catheter is used to fill the abdomen with a cleansing liquid and the peritoneum, a membrane lining the walls of the abdominal cavity, lets waste products and extra fluid pass from the blood into the dialysis solution, which is then drained out. Children on peritoneal dialysis can follow a less restricted diet and go to school, coming to the Children's for dialysis two afternoons a week and Saturdays so that family life and schooling continue with fewer disruptions. During their treatment sessions, they can catch up on schoolwork with the help of the teachers working in the Dialysis Unit.

POOLING EXPERTISE TO HELP CHILDREN WITH CANCER

One of the most frightening diseases, and the most common cancer in children, leukemia has seen a spectacular turnaround in recovery rate. As recently as the 1960s, a diagnosis of leukemia was virtually a death sentence. However, by the 1990s, the survival rate had climbed to 85%, mainly thanks to the development of better chemotherapy drugs, notably

Dr. Sarah Campillo examines young outpatient Vancleef-Emmanuel at the Children's.

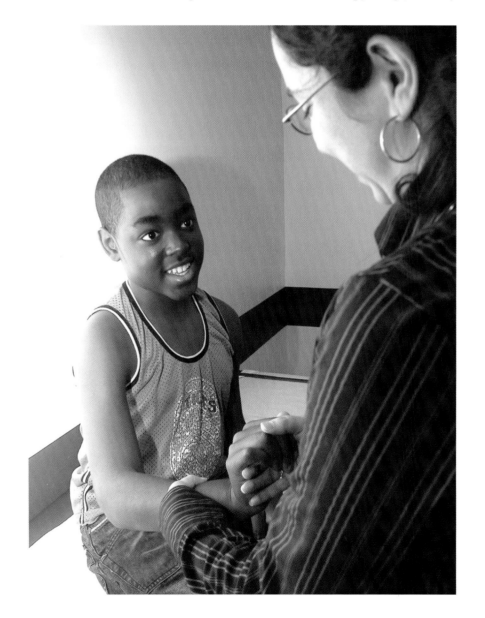

methotrexate. Children no longer routinely spend months in hospital with little hope of getting out. Today, they come to the clinic for chemotherapy, going home between treatments.

Cancer specialists at the MCH have been at the forefront of research into and treatment of leukemia and other childhood cancers since the mid-20th century, soon after the development of the first chemotherapy drugs. In the 1950s, several pediatric hospitals came together in cooperative groups to pool information and data. The MCH is a founding member of the Pediatric Oncology Group (POG), a network of more than 90 major and smaller institutions that share research findings and develop innovative treatments. The hospital's participation in this group, spearheaded by Dr. Michael Whitehead, led to its carrying out the first bone marrow transplant in a pediatric setting in Canada.

The first bone marrow transplants on MCH patients were carried out at the Montreal General Hospital, but in 1981, Dr. Penelope Koch arrived to set up a program at the Children's. She headed up the highly successful MCH Bone Marrow Transplant Program until her retirement in 1998.

While chemotherapy has made a huge difference in recovery rates of children with leukemia, it does not necessarily make that recovery much more pleasant. Over the years, however, drugs to control nausea have made some difference, as have implantable lines, through which medication can be administered without a new injection, making chemotherapy much less invasive and painful.

In cases where doctors arrive at the reluctant conclusion that nothing further can be done for a patient, the time has come for palliative care. Depending on their condition, some children will die in the hospital, where staff do their utmost to control the pain and make their final days as peaceful as possible, with the support of the hospital's palliative care program. This service has been available to hospitalized patients since 1991, and in 1994, the

Children's set up an award-winning program that combines the resources of intensive ambulatory care and palliative services to help parents care for their dying child at home. Nurses in the program play a liaison role, facilitating care and the family's interaction with the hospital.

OUTPATIENT CARE AND DAY SURGERY

As the 20th century turned to the 21st, most of the patients being cared for by the Montreal Children's Hospital had conditions that its founders would not have been able to treat 100 years earlier. In fact, the founders would be astounded at the number of children treated outside the hospital setting. The majority of the hospital's young patients are looked after by hospital staff during clinic visits, and by their families at home. Most of those who have surgery are sent home within 24 hours, receiving post-operative treatment at outpatient clinics or at home, in a comforting and familiar setting.

Day surgery, developed at the Children's by Dr. Herbert Owen, was yet another Canadian first. It is now commonplace for many straightforward procedures, such as tonsillectomies, to be done without admitting the patient to hospital. Developments in anesthesia over the years have gone a long way towards making day surgery, and surgery on smaller and smaller babies, possible.

Anesthesia has been an important part of the surgical department since the days when Dr. Morton Digby Leigh, hailed as the father of pediatric anesthesia in Canada, worked at the Children's Memorial, from 1939 to 1947. Fifty years ago, anesthetized children were monitored with a stethoscope and the anesthesiologist's finger on the pulse. Techniques developed by leaps and bounds in the 1950s under Drs. H.T. (Tony) Davenport and José Rosales. Today, sophisticated monitors measure the child's oxygen level non-invasively and check breathing and circulation. Anesthetists are key members of the surgical team, meeting with the children before surgery to allay their fears about being "put to sleep."

INTENSIVE CARE FOR TINY INFANTS

Today, premature infants born at extremely low birth weights, who in previous decades would have died, are routinely saved and live to be healthy children and adults. The backdrop for many such success stories is the Neonatal Intensive Care Unit (NICU), established in 1957. Dr. Mary Ellen Avery, a renowned neonatologist, discovered and established the use of surfactant (a complex and essential fluid formed late in fetal life without which premature infants may die) in small premature infants with respiratory distress syndrome. Dr. Avery, Physician-in-Chief and Chair of the Department of Pediatrics from 1969 to 1974, played a key role in the development of the NICU. Dr. Eugene Outerbridge, Director of the NICU from 1976 to 1988, established the first Neonatal Nurse Practitioner training program in Quebec in 1994. Nurse practitioners started to practise two years later.

"If you look at surgery 25 years ago and now, what has made the most significant impact is the relationship between basic laboratory investigations and their transposition into clinical surgery. At that time, surgery was less complex. Today, due to important improved surgical techniques and advancements in anesthesia, it is possible to perform many more difficult procedures with improved outcomes."

DR. BRUCE WILLIAMS,
SURGEON-IN-CHIEF

HEALING CHILDREN'S HEARTS

Since before World War II, children with congenital heart defects have been coming to the Children's for surgery from across the country and beyond. Pioneering heart surgery has been performed at the Children's since the late 1930s, when Dr. Dudley Ross perfected some groundbreaking techniques. The Division of Cardiology was founded in 1947. Ten years later, when the first pediatric open-heart surgery in Quebec was performed at the Children's, the heart-lung bypass machine was an integral part of the procedure. That event not only opened the door to life-saving surgery for young patients, but also drew attention to the fact that they could be helped and started the surgical world on the path to increasingly daring interventions.

Dr. David R. Murphy, Surgeon-in-Chief from 1954 to 1974, and Dr. Anthony Dobell, who suc-

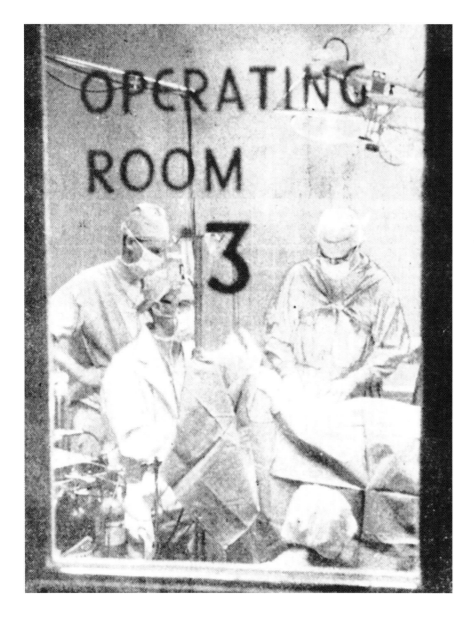

ceeded him, presided over an era of stellar achievement in heart surgery at the Children's, along with Dr. Arnold Johnson, who performed the first pediatric heart catheterization in Canada in 1946, and Dr. Maurice McGregor, Dean of Medicine at McGill University from 1967 to 1972, who took a special interest in pediatric cardiology.

The first operations using the heart-lung bypass machine were performed in 1957. Initially, surgeries on heart defects were palliative, prolonging children's lives, but not always to adulthood. However, each year of life gained provided more hope and opportunity for further treatment. Due to the challenges of operating on a very small heart, surgery was often performed in stages, with repeated operations every few years, each step making the next one possible. Prior to 1984, less than 20% of open-heart surgery at the MCH was done on children under one year old; by 1991, that figure had risen to 70%, with 25% of operations performed on newborns less than a month old. Most importantly, the risks for these babies have proven to be the same as or lower than for heart surgery in older children.

In 1987, Dr. Christo Tchervenkov returned to the Children's after studying under Dr. Aldo Castaneda in Boston, where he witnessed the early development of neonatal and infant cardiac surgery. The MCH's Neonatal and Infant Corrective Cardiac Surgery Program combined Dr. Dobell's extensive experience and Dr. Tchervenkov's newly acquired surgical techniques at a time when very few such programs existed in the world. In 1988, the team performed Canada's first heart transplant in a baby.

The process of developing operative procedures for a wider range of complex malformations has continued, and virtually any malformation can now be repaired. By the 1990s, surgeons at the Children's were able to correct even major congenital heart defects with a single operation on the infant's tiny heart just days after birth. These babies grow up and develop normally, avoiding the multiple palliative operations that used to be the norm.

Cardiac surgery at the MCH has been a remarkable success story, largely due to a strong, dedicated team that includes doctors, nurses, technicians, perfusionists, intensive-care staff, and other hospital personnel.

DEVELOPMENTS IN PEDIATRIC NEUROLOGY AND NEUROSURGERY

A child's brain presents special difficulties because it is still in the delicate process of developing. Before World War II, children with neurological problems were generally referred to the Montreal Neurological Institute. In 1946, after extensive training in the United States, Dr. Preston Robb returned to the Children's Memorial Hospital to work as a pediatric neurologist. The Division of Neurosurgery was formed in 1961, with Dr. John Blundell as Director.

The hospital was busy in those post-war, baby-boom days, and the outpatient clinics saw many children who had, as a result of tuberculous meningitis, suffered brain damage that could have been prevented by early treatment. The clinics were also seeing increasing numbers of patients with epilepsy, familial diseases such as Tay-Sachs or cystic fibrosis, mental retardation, and various types of cerebral palsy. A multidisciplinary group started the Cerebral Palsy Conferences, in which parents were actively involved as part of the health-care team—an innovative concept at that time.

TREATING LESS COMMON CONDITIONS

Children with hemophilia, a rare disorder, used to have to go to hospital when their bleeding became uncontrollable. Thanks to more effective blood clotting factors, which help to prevent blood loss, they are now better able to manage their disease. By the 1960s, thanks to the development of a model home care program, yet another Canadian first for the MCH, most children with hemophilia were receiving care mainly on an outpatient basis. By the 1970s,

THE "EXIT" PROCEDURE

On December 21, 2000, a team of surgeons, anesthetists, nurses, and other specialists and technicians from the Royal Victoria Hospital and the Children's achieved another Quebec first. At 18 weeks' gestation, a fetus was found to have a large neck mass—a partly solid, partly cystic teratoma (a form of cancer) that was three times the size of the head, preventing the fetus from swallowing. The mother decided to proceed with the pregnancy, despite the high risk of respiratory distress at birth. The team planned for a procedure called ex-utero intrapartum treatment, or EXIT—a Cesarean delivery under deep maternal anesthesia to relax the uterus and maintain placenta–fetal circulation while the airway was secured. At the time of surgery, the fetus was less than 33 weeks' gestation, but doctors determined that its lungs were sufficiently mature to proceed.

The mother was brought to the Alternative Care Module (ACM) at the Children's and taken into the operating room. The extremely complex procedure involved more than 20 people inside the operating theatre and a great deal of specialized equipment, some of which was specially imported. Thirty-seven minutes after the head was out of the uterus, the maternal anesthesia was modified to allow uterine contraction; two minutes later, the cord was clamped and divided and the baby—a girl—was born. The mass had to be lifted off her chest to allow adequate ventilation. Three hours after birth, excision of the rare tumour was started, under general anesthesia. The weight of the tumour and the fluid removed at the beginning of the EXIT procedure came to 1.4 kilograms; after removal of the mass, the baby weighed 1.6 kilograms. The procedure was considered a major success for both mother and baby, and a triumph of teamwork for everyone involved.

they were not admitted to hospital unless they had a major injury.

Muscular dystrophy (MD) is another group of diseases that now brings fewer children into hospital. Until recently, because most types of MD eventually affect breathing, children would have regular bouts of hospitalization. Thanks to newer treatments, they now have far fewer respiratory crises. Because they live longer, they require care for a longer period but can receive most of it while living in the community into their adult years. One example of this is the specially designed apartment for young men living with Duchenne muscular dystrophy, which the Children's was instrumental in setting up in the 1980s.

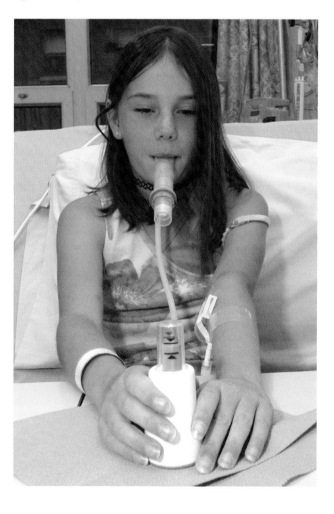

Stephanie, who has cystic fibrosis, has learned how to monitor her functioning thanks to the team at the Children's.

PEDIATRIC CONJOINT LIVER TRANSPLANT PROGRAM

In December 1985, MCH surgeons Drs. Frank Guttman, Luong T. Nguyen, and Jean-Martin Laberge performed a pioneering liver transplant on a 13-month-old infant with Crigler-Najjar Syndrome, an inherited disorder that causes jaundice and organ malfunctions. The operation was part of a highly successful ongoing collaboration with physicians from three other city hospitals: Notre-Dame, St-Luc, and Ste-Justine.

Cystic fibrosis (CF) was not even recognized as a disease until the late 1930s, and then usually only after a child had died from complications such as malnutrition or pneumonia. By the early 1960s, people were learning how to cope with the severe respiratory and digestive effects of the disease and physiotherapy was bringing some comfort and improvement, though the average lifespan of children with CF was still less than four years. However, as we enter the 21st century, research and treatment have advanced so much that patients are living into their mid-30s and beyond. Today, while many still have to cope with respiratory crises, young adults with CF are using genetic counselling services to plan families of their own.

DETECTING AND TREATING GENETIC CONDITIONS

Unlike the infectious diseases that filled hospital wards in the early years of the Children's, diabetes, hemophilia, muscular dystrophy, and cystic fibrosis are all diseases with genetic causes. This illustrates another major shift in the types of conditions leading to hospitalization among children, and reflects the overwhelming impact of heredity on childhood disease. These diseases and disorders existed, of course, when the Children's was founded, but were either unrecognized or impossible to treat. By the turn of the 21st century, however, genetic factors were contributing to 30% to 50% of admissions to pediatric hospitals in North America.

Fortunately for its young patients, the MCH's expertise in screening, diagnosing, and treating genetic conditions has a long history. In 1949, the Children's Memorial (as it still was then) established a Genetics Department—one of the first on the continent. The work of the team, starting with Drs. Clarke Fraser, Julius Metrakos, and Katherine Metrakos, earned a worldwide reputation. Much of Dr. Fraser's work focused on the genetic causes of birth defects, such as cleft palate. Dr. Charles Scriver, who founded the DeBelle Laboratory for Biochemical Genetics at the Children's in 1961, achieved widespread recognition for his stellar work in the study of basic and applied aspects of human biochemical genetics, as well as his discovery of hereditary forms of rickets in children.

MEETING NEW CHALLENGES

In the year 2000, the 10 most frequent conditions leading to hospitalization at the Children's were asthma, respiratory infections, urinary and kidney infections, seizures, epilepsy and related conditions, appendicitis, head injuries, chemotherapy, broken

"BACK TO SLEEP"

The Jeremy Rill Centre for Sudden Infant Death Syndrome and Respiratory Control Disorders was inaugurated in 1986 in memory of Jeremy Rill, a seemingly healthy baby who died of sudden infant death syndrome (SIDS), also known as "crib death." SIDS is the major cause of infant death between one and 12 months of age, with peak incidence occurring between two and four months. An estimated 6,000 babies die annually of this devastating syndrome in North America. The Centre provides bereavement counselling and support for families, as well as education programs. SIDS prevention programs have made a real difference through a simple change: placing infants under six months of age on their backs instead of their stomachs to sleep.

arms and legs, and gastroenteritis—a huge array of conditions requiring an enormous range of treatments.

THE ROLE OF THE ENVIRONMENT

Unlike conditions caused by improper sanitation or poor maternity care, which decreased over the years, asthma increased in prevalence throughout the 1980s and '90s. In part, this was a result of more accurate diagnosis; in part, some doctors believe, environmental pollution is to blame. Certainly, that is the current view of many respiratory allergies.

Allergens are even more mysterious in relation to food reactions, which are also turning up more often. An example of this is peanut allergy, which has increased in prevalence in developed countries. One reason for this may be increased consumption by either children themselves or breast-feeding mothers, as many prepared foods contain peanut products. The "hygiene hypothesis" posits that with the reduction in infections due to improved hygiene and vaccination, the human immune system no longer has to overcome the amount of infection it is designed to fight, so it turns on itself and creates allergies. This hypothesis seems to be supported by the fact that there are fewer allergies in farm families and in developing countries.

Peanut allergy has gained a high public profile, partly because it is so threatening. If epinephrine is not injected within an hour, a serious attack can be fatal. Exposure to peanut products is common and almost always inadvertent, and there is no way to predict the seriousness of an attack. Many parents fear sending their children to camp or on sleepovers. While some children outgrow it, 80% will have it for life.

The search is on for both treatments and preventive measures. As this book is being written, the Children's is preparing to take part in a study to determine the effectiveness of a medication that blocks the antibody that causes the reaction. In some

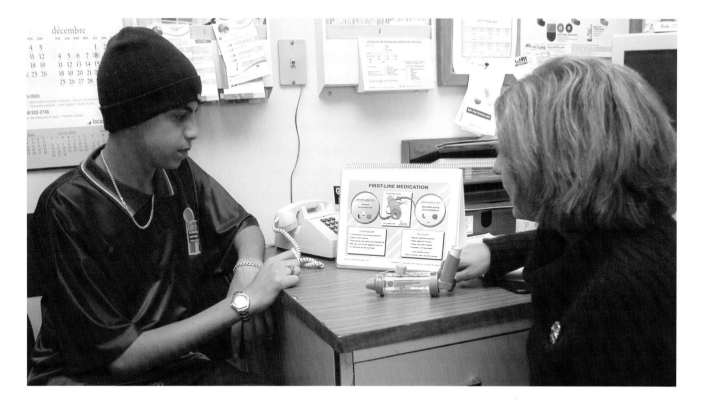

Inhalation therapist Georgia Kotsirilos helps Adam learn how to manage his asthma using pulmonary function testing.

COPING WITH ASTHMA

Asthma, the leading problem seen today at the Children's, is partly a phenomenon of our changing environment. The hospital's multidisciplinary Asthma Centre, which opened in October 1990, calls on a skilled team of specialists, including pediatricians, allergists, immunologists, respirologists, epidemiologists, nurses, psychologists, and social workers.

In 1999, an Angus Reid survey found that poor asthma control was responsible for 85% of hospital admissions in Canada and 78% of emergency room visits, and that one in two Canadian asthma patients had required urgent care for their asthma. While effective controls are available, they are still poorly understood by parents. The Children's has developed a simple and attractive tool, the Asthma Quiz for Kids, to help families cope. A follow-up clinical study will determine whether using the quiz can help school-aged children become more aware of coping strategies and lessen asthma's impact on their lives.

children, the medication may wipe out the allergy; in others, it may reduce severity, making life easier.

One pollutant that has increasingly been linked not only to allergies, but to respiratory conditions of all kinds, is cigarette smoke. As recently as a generation ago, families and employees—even doctors—thought nothing of lighting up in hallways, waiting rooms, and consulting rooms. Today, as society acknowledges the terrible risks of second-hand smoke, hospitals have become smoke-free zones, letting patients and staff alike breathe easier, and parents are encouraged not to smoke at home or during pregnancy.

CHALLENGING NEW INFECTIONS

Antibiotics, of course, have not turned out to be the panacea they were once thought to be. Some bacteria stay ahead by mutating and developing resistance to the drugs used. Resistance to antibiotics and over-use of antibiotics are of growing concern.

Many strains of influenza, pneumonia, and other infections are caused by viruses rather than bacteria, and while new medications are helping to combat some viruses, there are as yet no specific treatments for most. There are still outbreaks of influenza, with new strains developing all the time. Meningitis, both bacterial and viral, is much rarer than it used to be, but still brings between 12 and 20 patients to the MCH every year.

Today, infections in children can be caused not only by microbes that mutate, but also by microbes that have new opportunities to spread. Daycare and playgroups for the very young bring greater numbers of children into close contact at an earlier age. True, sharing infections has always been a feature of early school days. But younger children and babies tend to get even closer to one another than their older sisters and brothers: they put their hands into one another's mouths and chew on the same toys. Of course, many are still in diapers—a situation whose infection potential needs no further description! As a result, children are acquiring common infections at an earlier age.

Dr. Brenda Moroz, Director of the Dermatology Division since 1975, reports that skin infections such as athlete's foot, warts, and scalp fungus are increasing in children under five, likely because of close contact in daycare centres. "Small children go around in bare feet, and touch other children a lot."

Gastroenterology, the medical specialty concerned with the digestive system and its diseases, brings the MCH about 3,400 visits a year, with 1,200 new consultations and many patients followed on a continuing basis for inflammatory bowel diseases (IBDs), such as Crohn's disease, ulcerative colitis, and colitis of unknown origin. There may be a genetic predisposition to these conditions, as well as environmental influences. We do know that the incidence of IBDs is particularly high in Quebec and that they are more common in northern countries. Since there is no cure, the objective is to help patients to live as normally as possible—in most cases with drugs, but

sometimes with surgery. The MCH Gastrointestinal Motility Centre is an advanced facility that uses new technology to pinpoint the causes of intestinal ailments. Diagnosis can usually be made through a combination of laboratory tests and endoscopic and radiological exams. Diagnostic procedures are largely painless, except for mild discomfort caused by the presence of the probe, and the resulting measurements can be transferred to the computer for use in treatment, increasing the chances of success.

SPEECH, HEARING, AND LANGUAGE

The importance of normal speech development was recognized early at the MCH, which set up the first speech therapy clinic in a Canadian pediatric hospital in 1933. In those days, most children referred for delayed speech and language were at the preschool and school-aged levels, while today referral is likely to take place at an earlier age.

Speech therapy, essential for children who have speech delays or difficulties speaking, or who have conditions that lead to indistinct speech, has gone from simple beginnings to complex treatments, resulting in a body of valuable research and a heightened understanding of speech pathology. The multidisciplinary approach throughout the hospital has led to very close collaboration between specialists in the closely related fields of speech and audiology.

The Children's set up a pioneering voice lab for the school-aged group, enabling speech therapists and ENT specialists to conduct detailed investiga-

EVERYTHING BUT THE KITCHEN SINK

In a 1951 report, Dr. Hollie McHugh, head of the ENT Clinic, described, among other activities, the successful removal of various foreign bodies from the lungs of infants during the year: three carrots, seven peanuts, one chestnut, one eraser, and one nutshell. ENT remains one of the busiest clinics in the hospital today, handling 12,000 outpatient visits and more than 2,000 surgical procedures every year.

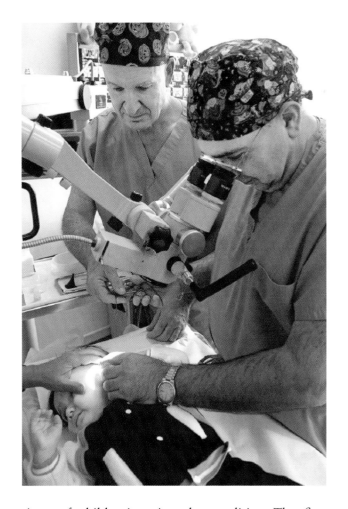

Drs. John Manoukian (front) and Melvin Schloss examine one-year-old Mustafa in the Ear, Nose and Throat Clinic.

tions of children's voice abnormalities. The first pediatric voice and speech laboratory in Canada was established at the Children's in 1995, with specialties including cleft palate, learning disabilities, dysphasic children, and those with physical handicaps, voice disorders, and stuttering. In fact, one of the earliest multidisciplinary teams for the treatment of children with cleft lip and palate deformities was formed at the Children's in 1960.

Middle-ear infections are much more common than they were a generation ago. Many of these can be controlled with antibiotics, but some recur so frequently that they require surgical intervention. Tubes are placed in the eardrums to facilitate drainage. While there is some controversy as to the long-term effectiveness of this procedure in some children, in others it has made an important difference. Small eardrums may perforate if the pressure of the infection is not relieved. In addition, children just developing language benefit from improved hearing, allowing normal speech development to take place.

Over the past 20 to 30 years, the Children's has made outstanding contributions to the field of otolaryngology. These include screening for hearing loss in infants, as well as the use of implantable devices for hearing loss, such as cochlear implants for children with profound bilateral hearing loss, and bone-anchored hearing aids for children with craniofacial abnormalities and hearing loss. Dr. Sam Daniel's research on deafness and middle-ear anatomy has made a major contribution to the development of this field. Sinus surgery and adenotonsillectomies are now performed with minimally invasive procedures that shorten hospital stays and reduce the risk of complications. And children with sleep apnea are now treated by a multidisciplinary team that includes otolaryngologists, anesthetists, and sleep researchers.

Plastic surgeons at the Children's have developed craniomaxillary surgical procedures designed to correct severe hereditary and post-traumatic facial deformities. The recent development of distraction osteogenesis, a surgical process for the reconstruction of skeletal deformities, is yet another advance that offers great promise for the treatment of small patients.

A VISION FOR EYE CARE

When it comes to the eyes, education and the use of protective devices to prevent injuries and illness have had a huge impact. Babies whose mothers caught German measles (rubella) when they were pregnant often developed cataracts; widespread immunization against this communicable disease led to a big drop in their incidence. The Children's has developed special expertise in the treatment of cataracts, as described in Chapter 9.

Sports-related eye injuries have also declined, although they still occur. Prior to 1977 there were always one or two children in the hospital at any one time in the winter with eye injuries caused by hockey sticks or pucks. Then the organization that oversaw amateur hockey in Canada made full visors and shields mandatory, and hockey eye injuries in children—when playing in supervised conditions—virtually disappeared.

TRAUMA CARE

Over the past decade, trauma care has become a vital part of the hospital's mission. The Trauma Program plays an important leadership role at the regional and provincial levels, serving the special needs of Quebec children and adolescents.

Today, trauma is the leading cause of death and disability in children and adolescents—a far cry from the days of the hospital's founding, when injuries didn't even figure in the top 10 causes of death. There are, of course, many more motor vehicle accidents, along with new risks from sports and recreational activities our great-grandparents could never have imagined. Over the past few decades, awareness of risks has grown greatly, with encouraging results. Between 1962 and 1996, fatalities from drowning fell by 44%; from poisoning, 47%; and from cycling injuries, 40%. Injury trends and data are tracked through the Canadian Hospitals Injury Reporting and Prevention Program (CHIRPP), set up in 1990, which currently contains about 1.5 million cases in its database.

The Children's is a provincially designated and accredited trauma centre and a centre of expertise in neurotrauma. Children up to the age of 18 are treated for various types and severities of trauma. These include neurotrauma (the first neurotrauma program in Quebec, developed in 1989 under the leadership of Dr. José Luis Montes and Debbie Friedman, now Trauma Program Head, evolved into the present-day Pediatric and Adolescent Trauma Program) and burns (the first pediatric burn unit in Canada was

DENTISTRY AND ORAL HYGIENE

Dentistry is another field in which research and knowledge have progressed by leaps and bounds over the years. Specialists in pediatric dental care (pedodontics) must possess infinite patience and gentleness to overcome the apprehension or downright fear most children feel approaching the dental chair. Dental surgeons at the Children's are known for their skill in treating complicated oral problems for children with multiple handicaps, following in the footsteps of Dr. George Brabant, a leader in providing free dental care for children with disabilities, who worked at the Children's from 1951 to 1995.

When the hospital moved in 1956, Dentistry had only three dental chairs and was split between the main building on Tupper Street and the Gilman Pavilion (then known as the Red Feather Building). Today, entirely in Gilman, the Children's has the largest pediatric dental clinic in North America, with 20 chairs and the latest technical instrumentation. It handles 16,000 appointments a year, providing free care—an important consideration given that 27% of the children seen by the Children's dental clinic are from families that live below the poverty line.

There are a number of specialty clinics for children with rare or severe problems. Some have such extensive decay that they need to have a general anesthetic during treatment, while others require hospitalization and intravenous antibiotics to control tooth infections. Some children have anomalies such as missing baby or adult teeth, while others lose teeth in accidents. The MCH's dentists provide them with a variety of appliances so they can smile, talk, and eat without embarrassment or discomfort.

The MCH's orthodontic team follows about 350 cleft palate cases a year and carries out reconstructive surgery in collaboration with the Plastic Surgery division.

THE BENEFITS OF FLUORIDE

In the 1940s, dentists discovered that fluoride could help prevent cavities, and manufacturers began adding fluoride to toothpaste in the 1950s. By the 1970s, dentists regularly sealed the pits and fissures of their young patients' back teeth with fluoride to prevent bacteria from penetrating the tooth and causing cavities. Many cities add fluoride to the municipal water supply so that everyone, even those who are not educated about oral health, can benefit. This is not yet the case in Montreal—despite the urging of senior staff from the Children's over many years.

established at the MCH in 1971 under Drs. Bruce Williams and David R. Murphy). Musculoskeletal trauma, chest, abdominal, and pelvic trauma, eye injuries, dental trauma, and poisoning complete the list. Common causes of trauma include motor vehicle accidents, falls, sports and recreational activities, attempted suicide, intentional injuries, violence and assault, and injuries sustained from swallowing harmful substances.

The Poison Control Centre at the Children's was a Canadian first, established by Drs. Elizabeth Hillman and Ronald Denton and expanded by Dr. Norman Eade, who was instrumental in persuading pharmacists to use child-proof caps on prescription medications.

The ER treats about 13,000 trauma patients every year. Of these, more than 700 sustain injuries that require hospitalization and the intensive involvement of the Trauma Program. An additional 200 patients are referred as outpatients for consultation, education, and interventions. This comprehensive interdisciplinary program includes medical and surgical specialties, as well as nursing, rehabilitation, psychosocial, and pastoral services. The goal is to go beyond physical care to address patients' psychosocial, academic, and spiritual needs as well—all in age-appropriate ways that include the family.

EXPLORING THE DEVELOPING MIND

Among the areas that have evolved at the Children's from informal practice to academically recognized specialties is the field of developmental and behavioural pediatrics. Until the 1970s, pediatricians and family doctors dealt with child develop-

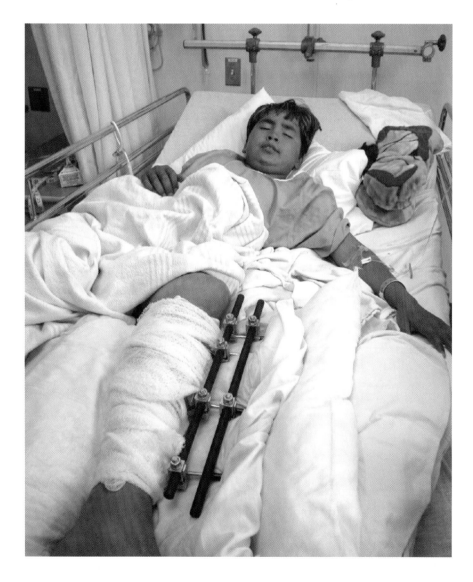

Qiiva's broken leg was treated by members of the trauma team at the MCH.

INTENSIVE AMBULATORY CARE

Intensive Ambulatory Care Services, described in earlier chapters of this book, give parents the knowledge and skills to provide their children with quite sophisticated care in their own homes. But they often go further than that. When the children go back to school, nurses will involve their teachers in meeting any special needs and, for those who need to do daily exercises, coordinate the setting up of an exercise program that includes their classmates, so the recovering child doesn't feel "different." Similarly, the Trauma Program helps injured children re-integrate into school. If a youngster has a head injury, for instance, trauma staff will let teachers know what kind of learning and memory abilities they can expect as the child recovers.

ment and behavioural issues in their everyday practice, but the specialty did not exist as such.

Then, in the 1970s, various clinics were set up at the MCH to see children with behavioural and developmental difficulties: a clinic in learning progress for children between the ages of six and 13; another in developmental progress for children from birth to five; and specialized clinics, such as the Failure to Thrive/Feeding Disorders Clinic headed by Dr. Maria Ramsay. Specialists from Occupational Therapy, Physiotherapy, Audiology, and Psychology were called upon as needed. In 2000, the team was consolidated into a single structure, the Developmental and Behavioural Pediatrics Service.

Even now, the borders of the program are far from clear-cut. It is inherently multidisciplinary, engaging the expertise of pediatricians and child developmental psychologists who understand how cognitive, emotional, and motor processes evolve over time. Other fields of specialization, such as psychobiology, child neurology, and child psychiatry, also contribute to knowledge in this field.

MENTAL HEALTH

The Children's has long recognized that the body cannot be treated in isolation, without consideration of psychological concerns. While Dr. Alton Goldbloom was Physician-in-Chief in the late 1940s, he recognized that many of his patients were suffering psychological distress—whether caused by illness or disability, or simply by being separated from their families while they were in the hospital.

The MCH was the first pediatric hospital in Canada to set up a psychiatry department (1950), and the first in the country with a centre for children's learning disorders. Dr. Taylor Statten was recruited to head the Department of Child Psychiatry. He ran a children's camp every summer and recruited several psychiatrists-in-training and social workers to join the team. He was instrumental in abolishing rigid visiting hours, encouraging parents to visit whenever they could and stay as long as they liked. A preschool nursery for autistic children was started, and a research program for hyperactive children began in 1960, with funding from the National Institutes of Mental Health (see Chapter 6).

Play therapy and family therapy have remained strong throughout the department's history. Under Dr. Klaus Minde's leadership (1989–2000), particular attention was paid to mother–infant relationships, especially in connection with premature infants. An innovative Adolescent Day Treatment Program uses music and art therapy, and new aspects of child and adolescent mental health and development are continually being explored. The department provides full services and introduces new ones to meet emerging needs, such as the increasing incidence of depression, transcultural issues, and eating disorders.

AUTISM—A GROWING CHALLENGE

One emerging need that presents a major challenge for diagnosis, treatment, and research is autism, a complex developmental disability that typically appears during the first three years of life and affects the normal development of social interaction and communication skills. Children with autism typically have abnormalities in language development, communications, and social skills, as well as repetitive behaviours.

In the decade leading up to the Children's centennial, the number of children diagnosed with this disorder increased tenfold. It now affects an estimated six in 1,000 people. It has been shown, though, that early intervention in teaching language and social skills can bring about great improvement.

Dr. Eric Fombonne, Director of Psychiatry and internationally recognized specialist in autism, oversaw the establishment in 2003 of the hospital's Autism Spectrum Disorders Program and its associated clinic. (The word "spectrum" is used because there is a range of disabilities associated with autism and related problems.) At the clinic, children of all ages with suspected autism spectrum disorders

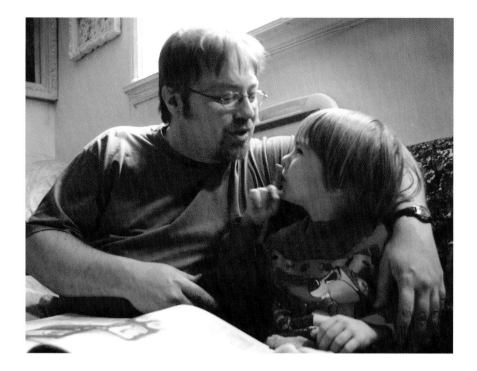

In 2004, Larry Hasting used techniques learned through the Children's Autism Spectrum Disorders Program to work with his four-year-old son Jacob at home. Here, they share a book and a song, "The Wheels on the Bus."

are diagnosed and treated by a multidisciplinary team that includes psychiatrists and pediatricians, as well as a nurse, a speech therapist, an occupational therapist, an audiologist, a psychologist, and a social worker.

"These children and their families have been faced with a chronic lack of services in the past," says Dr. Fombonne, "and we at the MCH intend to remedy this problem."

Dr. Fombonne also conducted a study into the incidence of autism in children who have received the MMR vaccine, which protects children against measles, mumps, and rubella (German measles). These three potentially serious childhood diseases can cause long-term complications or even death. Despite this, concern over a possible connection between the vaccine and autism has caused some parents to refuse the vaccination for their children. As a result, there have been outbreaks in the past several years of measles, a disease which had declined dramatically after the vaccine was introduced. Dr. Fombonne's study concluded MMR

vaccination is not associated with increased risk of autism.

THE LEGACY OF DR. SAM

Dr. Samuel Rabinovitch, hired as director of the new Psychology Department in 1950, set up the McGill–Montreal Children's Hospital Learning Centre in 1959. Affectionately known as "Dr. Sam," he was considered one of the world's leading authorities on specific learning disabilities (SLD), a condition that affects more than 10% of Canada's school-aged population. He and his colleagues explored the causes of learning disabilities and reading problems and probed a wide range of theories, using a smorgasbord of sometimes unorthodox tools, from playing cards to trampolines.

Reading disorders like dyslexia were poorly understood at the time, and a prevailing theory was that perceptual motor problems could be responsible. To test the hypothesis, Dr. Sam acquired balance boards, trampolines, skipping ropes, and bouncing balls for the 12th-floor Learning Centre.

Dr. Richard Goldbloom worked one floor below this treatment space. One afternoon, a loud thumping noise disturbed his work. Perplexed, he asked Dr. Herbert Owen about the infernal racket. His colleague explained, "Oh, that's just Sam teaching kids how to read."

Dr. Sam played a critical role in developing awareness of the needs of children with learning disabilities. In 1969, he hosted an acclaimed CBC television series on the subject that was used in schools across North America.

The Centre eventually outgrew its quarters in the hospital and moved to a building near McGill University on Mountain Street. Under Dr. Rabinovitch's leadership, and with staff from both the Children's and McGill, the Centre achieved international recognition for its work on assessing and teaching kids with learning disabilities and for training social workers and medical and psychiatry residents.

After Dr. Rabinovitch died in 1977, his colleagues continued his work. In the late 1980s, the hospital was forced to close the Centre due to a shortage of funds. The committed staff of the Centre opened a private, not-for-profit clinic called Learning Associates of Montreal, which is still operating with some of the original staff members.

ADOLESCENT MEDICINE

"On socially sensitive issues such as sexual behaviour, and the use of alcohol and drugs, adolescents are less likely than adults to seek care and, if they do, it may already be too late. In addition, our systems of health care are rarely designed to deal specifically with adolescents who are no longer comfortable with children's units and yet are not quite ready for adult treatment. Adolescents especially fear that health workers will be unsympathetic to their needs."

CANADIAN INSTITUTE OF CHILD HEALTH
*The Health of Canada's Children:
A CICH Profile, 1989*

As children grow up, the nature of the problems that bring them to the hospital changes. In adolescent medicine at the MCH, the clientele is mainly female—80% to 90%—reflecting the fact that the service began by offering gynecology consultations. When the adolescent medicine clinics were started at the MCH in the 1970s, the main problem facing these teens was recreational drugs, followed by sexual abuse and teenage pregnancy, with their attendant concerns. Eating disorders such as anorexia nervosa and bulimia, which have multiplied tenfold over the past decade, also require regular monitoring and, in some cases, hospitalization.

The Division of Pediatric Adolescent Gynecology, founded in 1968 by Dr. Robert Kinch, was yet another Canadian first, providing consultation services for medical or surgical gynecological conditions to both inpatients and outpatients. The prenatal clinic for pregnant teenagers is the only one of its kind in Canada, and the division runs a Well Baby Clinic for the offspring of teenaged mothers followed at the prenatal clinic. Contraception counselling has been an important focus right from the start, under Dr. Elsa Quiros. In 1993, Adolescent Medicine and Gynecology were merged under one director, Dr. Franziska Baltzer.

The prevalence of child abuse led to the establishment of a Child Abuse Team in the mid-1960s under Drs. Elizabeth Hillman, Herbert Owen, and Nicolas Steinmetz, and Margaret Ann Smith of Social Services—a Canadian first that was, sadly, much needed. Today, a team from the amalgamated services provides medico-forensic examination of children who have been sexually abused.

Adolescence is a turbulent time for many children, with effects that can last for many years, even a lifetime. Illicit drug use that starts in early adolescence, for example, can affect cognitive development for life. The long-term effects of teenage pregnancy, on both mothers and babies, are not known.

The Children's mandate, in this area as in so many others, is to intervene where needed and foster the healing process so that children can grow up with health and hope.

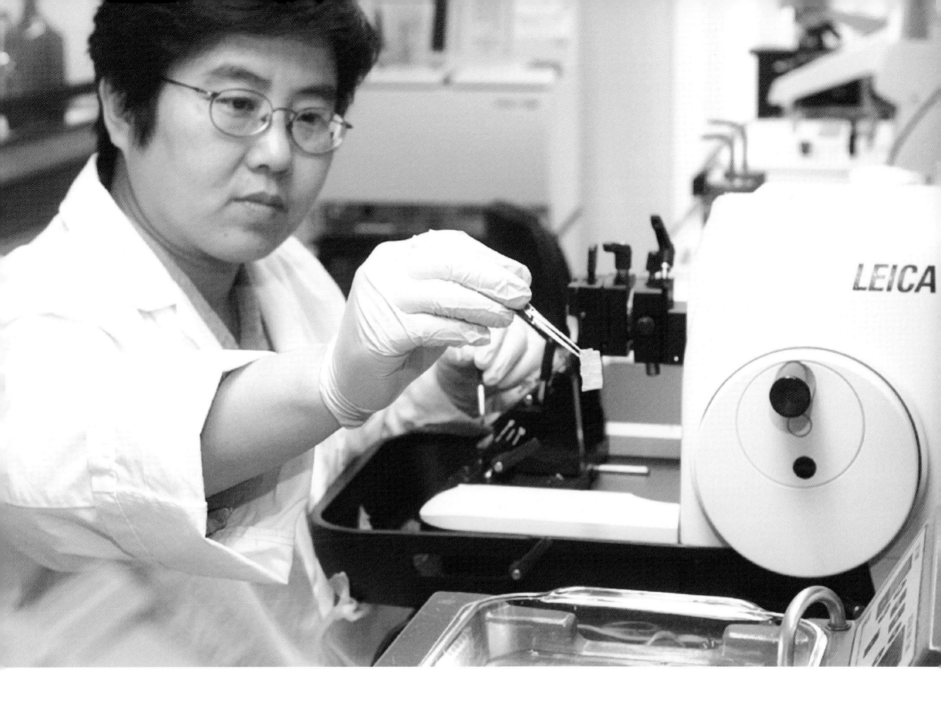

State-of-the-art research requires not only experienced researchers, but highly skilled technical and support staff, as well as a wide array of technology. Here, Dr. Xinying He, Coordinator of the Histology Service at the Research Institute, uses a microtome to cut tissue into very thin sections and transfers them to a floating bath, in preparation for staining and microscopy analysis. The Histology Service provides technical support to all the Research Institute's laboratories.

"The study of disease seems to go hand in hand with the relief of disease."

GEORGE H. SMITHERS, PRESIDENT, CMH, 1917–1933
1920/21 Annual Report

6

The Promise of Research: A Healthier Future

Research that focuses on adults or on children may ask the same questions, but these disciplines are not interchangeable. Some diseases affect children only, and others affect children differently from adults. Still others may be present in children, but not show themselves until adulthood.

Research, teaching, and clinical care at the MCH are inextricably linked. Ultimately, the children benefit from this dynamic interaction.

In 1928, George H. Smithers, President of the Children's Memorial Hospital, issued a "call to arms" to the hospital's Board of Directors. "We must not only combat disease, but we must exterminate disease," he proclaimed. "This can only be done through the study of the cause and the nature of morbid conditions. This study must be carried on in two ways. First, by observation at the bedside, and second, by investigation in the laboratory."

This bench-and-bedside approach to medical research remains a basic philosophy of the Montreal Children's Hospital. It defines the attitudes, values, and beliefs of the MCH scientists who are committed to finding new ways to better the lives of children of all ages.

THE EARLY DAYS: INDOMITABLE SPIRIT

One of the first mentions of clinical research at the Children's Memorial Hospital appears in the 1925 Annual Report. Amy B. Hilton, Director of the Social Services Department, surveyed patients to determine if they had received adequate treatment or needed more follow-up visits to complete their therapy. The study concluded that only 47% of patients were discharged from the medical clinic "creditably" and found "definite evidence, judging from complaints and medical diagnoses, that the other 53 per cent needed further treatment." Her work represents the earliest example of quality-assurance evaluations of hospital services that continue today.

From 1927 to 1934, expansion of facilities and staff in the Pathology, Biochemistry, and Bacteriology departments fostered the growth of research into childhood diseases. Many physicians at the CMH were affiliated with McGill University's Faculty of Medicine as teachers and researchers. Most experimental studies were clinical in nature, as the hospital lacked the laboratory facilities for basic research.

The academic medical environment in the 1930s was a world apart from what we know today—a world without computers and the Internet. Most articles in medical journals consisted of case reports, clinical discussions, and review articles. Literature searches were performed manually and familiarity with German, French, and other languages was a prerequisite for clinical research. Multicentre clinical trials did not yet exist, as coordination was next to impossible.

Despite the limitations, CMH researchers contributed significantly to fledgling medical journals, such as the *Canadian Medical Association Journal* and the *Journal of Pediatrics*. During his career, Dr. Alton Goldbloom, Physician-in-Chief and Chairman of Pediatrics from 1946 to 1953, published 53 articles in national and international medical journals.

"Adult medicine attempts to mend the errors of the past. Paediatrics should attempt to prevent the errors of the future; if this is its aim, its scope is limitless."

DR. ALTON GOLDBLOOM,
PHYSICIAN-IN-CHIEF, 1946–1953
first H.B. Cushing Memorial Lecture, 1945

The hospital's unique pavilion structure, which isolated children with particularly common chronic diseases at different sites outside the main hospital building, encouraged the study of children with tuberculosis, rheumatic fever, and polio.

Shortly after World War II, MCH surgeons took on the challenge of helping children with severe birth defects, particularly cleft lip and palate. Advances in research by Dr. Fred Woolhouse and, later, by Dr. Howard Oliver, a dental surgeon, earned the hospital an international reputation for excellence in this domain. In the 1960s, progress continued in infants with esophageal defects (Dr. Herbert Owen), in orthopedic surgery (Dr. Harry Farfan) and in children with cerebral palsy (Dr. David Forbes).

Research in endocrinology and metabolism, then in its infancy, began at the MCH in the mid-1930s, establishing a solid base for significant advances in later years. In 1955, Dr. Claude Giroux founded the Endocrine Research Laboratory, which investigated the function of endocrine glands and their hormones. Until his death in 1978, Dr. Giroux collaborated with Drs. Donald Hillman, Charlotte Branchaud, Eleanor Colle, Harvey Guyda, and Cynthia Goodyer to further medical knowledge of the function of the human placenta and fetal endocrine glands.

An explosion of scientific knowledge in the 1960s fundamentally changed pediatrics. New diagnostic techniques and therapies emerged in fluid and electrolyte imbalances, genetics, neonatology, cardiology, endocrinology, and congenital defects. The Montreal Children's Hospital was at the forefront of much of this research in Canada.

By this time, the practice of research in all departments was burgeoning but spatial limitations began to interfere with this progress. In 1963, Physician-in-Chief Dr. Alan Ross wrote, "The matter of space available for research laboratories is another of our real concerns. Lack of it has actually now brought the expansion of our program to a standstill."

RESEARCH IS NEVER DULL

In the early 1950s, Dr. Richard Goldbloom was studying a puzzling presentation among infants with skin rashes. When brought to Emergency, crying in pain, they bore a characteristic inflamed, red rash from head to toe. The emergency-room staff dubbed these infants "lobster babies."

Dr. Goldbloom traced the cause of the red rashes to boric acid, found in a popular brand of baby powder. With his father, Dr. Alton Goldbloom, he published a series of case studies in 1953 that deterred mothers from using boric acid powders on their infants.

One day, Dr. Elizabeth Hillman, Director of Emergency, and a few other practical jokers called Dr. Goldbloom to Emergency "on the double," proclaiming that a "lobster baby" had just arrived. Dr. Goldbloom interrupted his work and rushed to a room where a tightly swaddled bundle awaited examination. He drew back the coverings to discover ... a giant red lobster!

THE McGILL UNIVERSITY–MONTREAL CHILDREN'S HOSPITAL RESEARCH INSTITUTE

On January 8, 1964, Dr. Wilder Penfield, of McGill University's Faculty of Medicine, chaired a newly formed 14-member committee that recommended the development of a children's research institute. Two years later, on January 21, 1966, the McGill University–Montreal Children's Hospital Research Institute was born when the two parent institutions signed a memorandum of understanding to "stimulate, direct, supervise and coordinate, in cooperation with the hospital, all research work carried out under the aegis of the hospital."

The Board of Administrators' first meeting was held on May 25, 1966, when Mr. John H. Molson was elected as the first Chairman and Dr. Richard Goldbloom was appointed as the first Research Committee Chairman. The institute had 15 project directors, who worked in 600 square metres of space within the Montreal Children's Hospital.

By 2004, the Research Institute had 70 clinical and basic research scientists with at least 48 grants from major funding agencies, such as the Medical Research Council of Canada (MRC), the *Fonds de la recherche en santé du Québec* (FRSQ), the U.S. National Institutes of Health (NIH), the International Juvenile Diabetes Research Foundation, the Canadian Cystic Fibrosis Association, and other agencies. Over 80 research assistants and 107 graduate students and fellows now work with MCH scientists in 3,600 square metres of space spread over the hospital's main campus and two satellite buildings a block away.

Today, the Research Institute's major strengths lie in the fields of genetics; growth and development; preventive medicine; public health; psychosocial problems; cardiorespiratory health; neuroscience; and endocrine, renal, and musculoskeletal disorders.

The Institute has contributed to advancements that have helped to shape our understanding of the biological development of healthy children. "We have attacked the mechanisms of disease and claimed victories on many fronts, yet children still die in infancy and childhood. They succumb to the complications of prematurity, genetic disease, infection and injury," proclaimed Dr. Roy Gravel, then Scientific Director, in 1995. "We remain humble at the task before us and work unceasingly towards its fulfillment."

A NEW ERA OF DISCOVERY

Medicine is a science that advances not only through discovery but collaboration. MCH scientists participate in multicentre research on the provincial, national, and international fronts, frequently taking the leadership role.

Under the leadership of Dr. Charles Scriver, who succeeded Dr. Goldbloom as Scientific Director from 1968 to 1976, physicians, research assistants, students, and fellows worked as a team in the fight against pediatric disorders and diseases. "In our opinion, no one person is any more important than the next ...," wrote Dr. Scriver in 1970. "It is this combined effort that produces research."

The McGill University partnership enabled MCH researchers to extend their research on a much broader scale. In 1996, the research institutes of the Montreal Children's, Montreal General and Royal Victoria hospitals joined the Meakins-Christie Laboratories to form the McGill University Health Centre (MUHC) Research Institute. That year, the McGill University–Montreal Children's Hospital Research Institute finished the year on a high note with 74 clinical and basic scientists in pediatric research, 47 having received a record $5.9 million in competitive research funds.

Before the merger, Drs. Harvey Guyda, Roy Gravel, Rima Rozen, and others lobbied for a strong pediatric presence within the MUHC Research Institute, rather than a separate pediatric research institute. In 2004, Dr. Rozen, MCH Research Institute Scientific Director, also assumed the role of Deputy Scientific Director of the MUHC Research Institute. Today, pediatric research occurs within

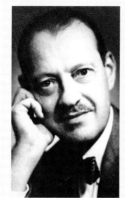

"IN PROUD AND THANKFUL MEMORY"

In the late 1940s, Dr. Alton Goldbloom, Chief of Pediatrics, negotiated with Dr. Wally Boyes, a McGill professor of genetics, and Dr. John deBelle, the hospital's Executive Director, to establish one of the first departments of medical genetics in North America.

Dr. John deBelle

In 1961, just after Dr. deBelle's death, the hospital's new biochemical genetics laboratory was named for him, as a tribute to his prescient support of medical genetics.

many of the 11 research axes of the MUHC Research Institute, touching on all areas of children's health, ranging from investigations of the fetus's genetic map to evaluations of a teenager's ability to cope with a psychiatric disorder.

OUR GENETIC HERITAGE

Genes play a determining role in childhood health and disease, with genetic factors accounting for 30% to 50% of admissions to pediatric hospitals. Congenital abnormalities, such as birth defects, present unique challenges to pediatric researchers. Malfunctioning genes can threaten survival during the transition from fetus to newborn, impede normal growth and learning, and cause serious childhood diseases and disorders.

In 1951, Dr. F. Clarke Fraser formally inaugurated, on a trial basis, the first hospital-based clinic in Canada for patients with medical genetics disorders. Dr. Fraser was the first of a long, prestigious line of genetic specialists at the Montreal Children's Hospital, which has been at the forefront of research in this field for more than a half-century.

Dr. Louis Dallaire, a PhD student under Dr. Fraser, was first to show that screening of sibling pairs with congenital malformations and their parents was a good way to find translocations, the displacement of genetic material to a different chromosomal location. He organized the first genetic amniocentesis laboratory in Quebec and, in 1964, founded a cytogenetics service laboratory for the MCH at the Douglas Hospital.

Dr. Leonard Pinsky, who trained as a summer student in the department's "mouse room," set up a laboratory of cell genetics at the Jewish General Hospital in 1967 and became the first director of the McGill Centre for Human Genetics in 1979.

Dr. Charles Scriver developed an interest in applying genetics to preventive medicine. During his residency, he set up the Biochemical Genetics Laboratory at the MCH.

Dr. Scriver also pioneered the establishment of screening programs to detect inborn errors of metabolism in all Quebec newborns and carriers in high-risk communities. The identification of a screening test for phenylketonuria (PKU), a cause of mental retardation in newborns, was "the paradigm for changing the thinking about genetics," said Dr. Scriver, "because once you identify PKU, you can treat it. It's no longer destiny." The laboratory's pilot studies screened the blood and urine of thousands of Quebec newborns for inborn errors of metabolism. In the 1980s, the mass screenings were woven into the Quebec Network of Applied Genetic Medicine.

Dr. Scriver and Carol Clow (see Chapter 7) were the first to introduce screening programs into Quebec high schools for Tay-Sachs disease, a fatal metabolic brain disorder afflicting children of Montreal's immigrant Jewish families, and thalassemia, a hereditary form of anemia usually afflicting children of Mediterranean descent.

Thalassemia is the most common inherited single-gene disorder in the world. Research into the detection of this blood disorder at the MCH meant that early treatment was possible, changing thalassemia from a fatal childhood disease to a treatable condition.

In 1972, the symbiotic nature of research in bio-chemical and medical genetics led to the formation of the Medical Research Council's (MRC, now the Canadian Institutes of Health Research, or CIHR) Medical Genetics Group, with Dr. Fraser as director and Dr. Scriver as co-director. At 33 years, it is the longest-running CIHR-funded research program in Canada. The group united researchers from the Children's, Royal Victoria, and Montreal General hospitals long before the advent of the MUHC. It has achieved many important firsts and contributed significantly to our understanding of diseases that progress well beyond childhood into adult life.

Early detection is the key to successful treatment of many life-threatening diseases in children. In the field of oncology, for instance, Dr. Mark Bernstein was instrumental in adding province-wide screening for neuroblastoma to Quebec's detection program for genetic diseases in the late 1980s. Neuroblastoma, a rare childhood cancer that arises from embryonic nerve cells, usually develops in the adrenal gland, then spreads throughout the body. The Quebec Neuroblastoma Screening Project ran from 1989 to 1994, and continued to follow up patients until 2001. Dr. Bernstein's research (now continuing at Hôpital Ste-Justine) has improved the lives of many children with this disease.

One in 500 children is born with an abnormally small kidney. In a child with two small kidneys, the mismatch between body size and functional kidney tissue grows with the child, who eventually develops renal insufficiency. Drs. Paul Goodyer's and Indra Gupta's laboratories combine experimental studies of cell cultures and mutant mouse models with clinical evidence from DNA studies in children to investigate genetic factors that influence kidney development in fetal life.

The mineral phosphate is essential for normal skeletal growth and development. Dr. H. Susie Tenenhouse, of the Department of Human Genetics, has studied inherited bone and kidney wasting disorders that may arise from disruptions in phosphate transport within the kidneys.

Birth defects may occur in a child whose father is exposed to certain drugs or environmental toxins. Dr. Jacquetta Trasler, of the Department of Human Genetics, investigates how exposure to chemicals interferes with the development and functioning of sperm cells. In collaboration with other researchers, she is developing ways to monitor and prevent drug damage to the sperm or egg cells of cancer patients in chemotherapy.

Dr. Roy Gravel and colleagues cloned the genes and identified the genetic mutations that are responsible for Tay-Sachs disease and another inherited disorder of vitamin B12 metabolism that causes severe metabolic acidosis in infancy.

Retinitis pigmentosa (RP) is the most common cause of inherited blindness, affecting over 1.5 mil-

WHY SCREEN FOR GENES?

The Tay-Sachs screening program grew out of the compassionate concerns of Peter Bronfman, then Chairman of the Research Institute's board. In the late 1960s, he came to Dr. Scriver with a request. "He told me that a colleague had a child with Tay-Sachs disease and asked me what I could do about it, and I said, 'nothing'." Bronfman challenged Scriver to find a way to prevent or help parents to avoid the inherited disease, which causes progressive mental and physical degeneration and death by age four in children of Ashkenazic and Sephardic Jews.

In the early 1970s, Dr. Scriver's team invented an automated test to detect the Tay-Sachs enzyme, then developed a screening program that has served as a blueprint for genetic screening programs around the world.

Groundbreaking work on Tay-Sachs has continued at the MCH. The seminal research of Drs. Peter Hechtman and Feige Kaplan into the defective gene responsible for Tay-Sachs has contributed to a significant decline in this lethal neurological disease.

"CHARLEMAGNE"

Dr. Charles Scriver's achievements as a pioneer in biochemical genetics are an outstanding legacy to Canadian medical research. At just 31 years of age, he was Canada's first faculty-appointed biochemical geneticist. One of his early discoveries was a method for testing the blood of newborns for devastating but treatable inborn errors of metabolism, such as phenylketonuria (PKU). Today, Quebec newborns are screened for more than 30 genetic diseases.

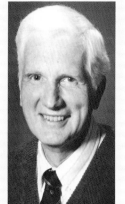

Dr. Scriver directed the McGill University–MCH Research Institute for 10 years, and in 2000, the DeBelle Laboratory was renamed the Charles R. Scriver Biochemical Genetics Unit–DeBelle Laboratory in his honour.

As a leader, he encouraged excellence and was a strong believer in the importance of cross-disciplinary research. He often invited fellow researchers to formal "soirées" at his Montreal West home, where they were expected to act, dress, and discourse with great intelligence. Yet this formality all but disappeared at annual staff celebrations, where younger researchers hosted talent shows, in which he was often the subject of much good-natured hazing. They dubbed him "Charlemagne"—the emperor of biochemical genetics—a title he bore with good humour.

lion people worldwide. There is no cure, but treatment may be a step closer, thanks to the work of Dr. Robert Koenekoop, Director of Pediatric Ophthalmology, who in 2003 identified two important gene mutations in French-Canadians that lead to severe RP and, in some cases, hearing loss. This finding may lead to the development of new diagnostic and screening tests for RP.

Dr. Serge Melançon, Director of the Division of Medical Genetics and the Biochemical Genetics Laboratory, was part of a team that identified the gene responsible for autosomal recessive spastic aplasia of Charlevoix-Saguenay (ARSACS), a rare neuromuscular disorder most often found in northeastern Quebec.

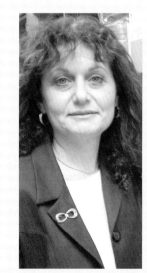

FRUSTRATION AND REWARD

With her team, Dr. Rima Rozen, Deputy Director of the MUHC Research Institute and Scientific Director of the MCH Research Institute, studies the role of folic acid, a type of vitamin B, in birth defects, cancer, and heart disease.

Their path to discovery was not an easy one. In the late 1980s, after almost two years of diligent work, Dr. Rozen's team succeeded in cloning a gene—only to discover that it was the wrong one. A U.S. collaborator had mistakenly sent them the wrong starting material. They began the painstaking work over again, eventually cloning the gene for methylenetetrahydrofolate reductase (MTHFR). Mutations of this gene are carried by about 10% of North Americans, putting them at a higher risk of spina bifida and heart disease. Consumption of folic acid during pregnancy wards off spina bifida and may decrease the risk of other disorders.

Although proud of these accomplishments, one of Dr. Rozen's most rewarding moments came in 1985, when she set up and became Director of the Molecular Genetics Diagnostic Service. This MCH laboratory offers prenatal diagnosis and carrier detection for genetic disorders. "It translates our experience in molecular genetics into a routine activity for the benefit of our patients and their families."

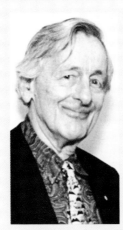

A PIONEER IN MEDICAL GENETICS

In the 1950s, Dr. F. Clarke Fraser was instrumental in establishing medical genetics as a focal area of research at the Montreal Children's Hospital. He founded a distinct discipline known as teratogenetics, which is the study of environmental agents or factors that cause genetic malformations resulting in birth defects.

He modestly attributes his success to lucky circumstance. "I was certainly lucky in the beginning of my career, just at the time when both medical genetics and teratology were about to take off, so I was able to get in on the ground floor.

"This may be why I was the youngest president of both the American Society of Human Genetics (ASHG) and the Teratology Society."

THE NEWBORN PERIOD

A century ago, children under two years of age were not generally admitted to hospital. Even a half-century ago, medical research into newborn development and diseases was still in its infancy.

Over the years, MCH researchers in the divisions of Newborn Medicine and Respiratory Medicine have explored the causes of respiratory problems that may lead to death or disability, as in the case of respiratory distress syndrome (RDS) or sudden infant death syndrome (SIDS).

In the late 1960s, under the leadership of Drs. Leo Stern and Pierre Beaudry, the Montreal Children's Hospital pioneered studies in the use of mechanical ventilators to help premature infants with undeveloped lungs to breathe.

In 1974, Dr. Mary Ellen Avery established the McGill University Neonatal–Perinatal Medicine Program, which combined the three neonatal programs at McGill teaching hospitals—the Children's,

Royal Victoria, and Jewish General hospitals—and fostered international-calibre neonatal research. Dr. Avery undertook experimental studies on the developing lungs of rabbits and lambs to better understand the underdeveloped lungs of premature newborns, which lack surfactants, the natural biochemicals that prevent the collapse of alveoli (tiny lung sacs that control oxygen exchange in the circulatory system). Her early work at McGill's McIntyre laboratories, which investigated the use of artificial lung surfactants, established the MCH as a leader in the field of respiratory medicine in newborns. Dr. Avery's work has been widely recognized with a number of prestigious awards, most recently (2005) an honorary doctorate in science from Harvard University.

Dr. Aurore Côté has identified the death of brain neurons as a pathological factor in SIDS. She directs the Infant Apnea and SIDS Group of the provincial research network in respiratory medicine.

Dr. Immanuela Moss, also in respiratory medicine, has studied neurochemicals as well as drugs, such as cocaine, that regulate the breathing process in the fetus.

Dr. Thérèse Perreault, a neonatologist, has studied the structural and functional changes that occur in the newborn's heart and lungs to enable the blood to absorb oxygen as it passes through the lungs. In primary pulmonary hypertension of the newborn, these changes are delayed or fail to occur.

Drs. Hélène Flageole and Jean-Martin Laberge, surgeons, have studied how surgical intervention *in utero* can help fetal lung growth to normalize before birth. In a multidisciplinary collaboration, Drs. Dominique Shum-Tim, Ronald Gottesman, Michael Davis, and Charles Rohlicek have studied how the heart-lung bypass machine, mechanical ventilation, and periods of low oxygen in newborns affect brain, lung, and heart development.

In the 1980s, Drs. Bernard Rosenblatt and Annette Majnemer, working in the Clinical Neurophysiology Laboratory, established the usefulness of evoked potentials testing, an electroencephalography (EEG) technique, in predicting the neurodevelopmental outcome of high-risk newborns deprived of oxygen shortly after birth. In the early 1990s, Dr. Majnemer, an occupational therapist who was at that time a graduate student in neuroscience, used the results of evoked potentials tests in high-risk newborns, such as premature babies, as predictors of later neurological problems. She followed these chil-

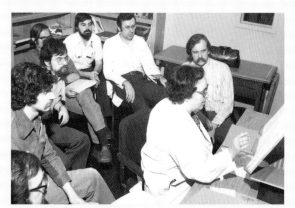

Dr. Kay Metrakos with MCH residents and students

THE BRAIN

Electroencephalography (EEG) can identify the function of brain neurons. In the late 1950s, two MCH neurologists, married couple Drs. Katherine (Kay) and Julius Metrakos, pioneered studies in the genetics of juvenile epilepsy in family members of children with idiopathic generalized epilepsy (petit mal seizures) using EEG studies of brain waves. They found that children under three years of age do not have seizures, while adolescents tend to outgrow them. In 1961, they published a seminal paper in Neurology, still quoted today, entitled "Genetics of compulsive disorders II: genetic and electroencephalographic studies in centrencephalic epilepsy." Dr. Kay Metrakos later directed the hospital's Convulsive Disorders Clinic.

In November 1991, the neurophysiology laboratory was officially dedicated as The Katherine Metrakos Clinical Neurophysiology Laboratory, in her honour.

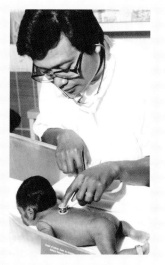

EARLY APNEA RESEARCH

In 1977, Dr. Jack Aranda pioneered the use of caffeine to treat apnea, the temporary suspension or absence of breathing, in premature infants. These unpredictable episodes rob the newborn's brain and vital organs of oxygen, threatening the development of higher brain functions.

dren for 10 years and found that newborns whose evoked potentials demonstrated abnormalities tended to develop motor problems or learning difficulties later on. Identifying children at risk of developing neurological problems opens up the possibility of being able to step in and help them earlier.

MCH researchers have also investigated the development of safe, effective drug therapy in newborns and infants. These studies have looked at the use of antibiotics, diuretics, respiratory stimulants, bronchodilators (drugs that open the lungs), and painkillers such as ibuprofen.

Dr. Hema Patel, of the MCH's Intensive Ambulatory Care Service, is carrying out studies to find the most effective treatment for acute viral bronchiolitis, one of the most common serious illnesses in infants.

During his career of several decades at the MCH, Dr. Ronald Barr (now at the University of British Columbia), investigated natural ways to lessen an infant's response to pain. His studies of crying in young infants have suggested that colic may be a normal phase of newborn development rather than a response to abdominal pain.

GROWTH AND DEVELOPMENT

Growth is a continuous, dynamic process. Because the bodies of infants, children, and teenagers are constantly evolving, they cannot be treated as if they were simply smaller versions of adult bodies. Research into normal growth and development is essential for our understanding of how children, at specific stages of their lives, will react to different genetic, environmental, physical, and psychological stresses.

MCH researchers in endocrinology and metabolism have achieved international recognition for their basic research in the study of human endocrine glands and growth hormone (GH).

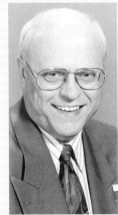

UNDERSTANDING GROWTH

For over four decades, Dr. Harvey Guyda has played a significant role in answering the question of what constitutes normal size in children. His basic and clinical research on GH and related growth factors has furthered understanding of the biochemical processes that stimulate or inhibit growth. This work has contributed to better treatments for children with GH deficiencies and genetic disorders, such as Turner and Down syndromes.

In collaboration with Dr. Gloria Tannenbaum, he developed a test to accurately identify which children with short stature are likely to respond to growth hormone therapy. This test was a direct outgrowth of Dr. Tannenbaum's studies of the hypothalamic regulation of GH secretion in rats.

Dr. Guyda's early work focused on basic research in pituitary function, and he helped to develop a blood test that was instrumental in detecting the presence of pituitary tumours in adults who secrete prolactin, a hormone that stimulates the production of human breast milk.

The fetal adrenal gland is remarkably large before birth and adrenal weight drops precipitously after birth. In the late 1980s, Dr. Charlotte Branchaud studied the growth and development of this gland, which controls the production of vital steroid hormones.

After birth, growth depends on the intricate interplay of a number of hormones, the most important of which is GH. Since the 1980s, Dr. Cynthia Goodyer has been studying how the fetal pituitary gland secretes its many hormones, and especially GH. She seeks to define the exact time around birth and the cellular mechanisms by which this hormone begins to influence growth in the neonate and infant.

Dr. Michael Kramer is exploring why some infants are born too soon or too small for their age. He is particularly interested in why low-income women are more likely to have low birth weight or premature newborns. As a leading specialist in infant nutrition, Dr. Kramer has studied the short- and long-term effects of breast-feeding versus formula feeding on infant, child, and adult health since the 1970s. A consultant for the World Health Organization, his work has established him as an international expert in breast-feeding.

Dr. Maria Ramsay, an MCH psychologist, has explored the physical and psychological basis of eating disorders and contrived creative ways to overcome feeding difficulties in infants and children.

The research of Dr. Richard Hamilton, gastroenterologist and former Physician-in-Chief, has focused on experimental and clinical studies that elucidated one cause of diarrheal disease in children. This research has made an important contribution to the management of diarrhea, particularly in Third World countries.

In children with severe kidney disease, normal growth and development may be compromised. Drs. Lorraine Bell and Atul Sharma have examined how a program of special nutrition and intensive dialysis, combined with GH injections, can improve the growth of these children.

Dr. Paul Goodyer has investigated the drug treatment of kidney failure due to hemolytic uremia syndrome, often called hamburger disease, which is caused by eating poorly cooked hamburger infected with *E. coli*.

Dr. Celia Rodd's research has focused on calcium and bone metabolism and thyroid function. She has studied osteoporosis in children with chronic diseases to discover new ways to reduce their risk of fractures. She has also studied genetic factors that enable Inuit children to adapt to low intakes of dietary calcium.

In the late 1990s, Dr. Reggie Hamdy, of the Department of Orthopedics, focused on how GH affects the formation and lengthening of children's bones.

The body's organ functions develop at their own speed, according to a pre-programmed schedule. Dr. Immanuela Moss has investigated the order of postnatal growth and development in the cardiovascular and respiratory systems and the sleep–wake cycle.

Sometimes neurological problems, triggered by illness, disease or injury, can delay a child's normal process of growth and development. Dr. Annette Majnemer is studying how sleep and awake positioning affects the development of early motor milestones in young children. She and Dr. Michael Shevell have studied the growth and development of premature infants and how cerebral palsy affects child development.

THE CHILDHOOD YEARS

Not all diseases and disorders appear in infancy. Some only become evident in preschool or school-aged children. A few examples are cancer, asthma and allergies, diabetes, cystic fibrosis, developmental delays, and learning disorders. Another common cause of hospitalization during childhood is preventable injury.

Cancer

Dr. Michael Whitehead's research focused on the development of effective treatments for childhood leukemia that saw mortality for this disease diminish from 75% to less than 25% in the last quarter of the 20th century.

In the late 1950s, there was no infrastructure for the management of clinical trial data. Dr. Louise Chevalier pursued this work with the California-based Children's Cancer Group, later known as the Cancer and Acute Leukemia Group B, which began the first international cooperative clinical studies of childhood leukemia. She extended the life expectancy of her young patients, while preserving their quality of life through a hospital-supported, at-home treatment program. She founded the Clinic for Leukemic Children and later became Director of the Oncology Clinic. At Dr. Chevalier's urging, the MCH became a founding member of the Pediatric Oncology Group (POG), a North American collaboration of oncology researchers in childhood cancer, in the mid-1970s.

Cancer in childhood is devastating to both patient and family. When therapy is unsuccessful, Dr. Stephen Liben, in palliative care, studies the respite needs of children with life-limiting illnesses.

INVALUABLE RESEARCH ASSISTANCE

Mary Jane Vuchich worked in the Penny Cole Laboratory with Dr. Michael Whitehead for 25 years, researching the best way to treat childhood leukemia with the powerful anti-cancer drug methotrexate. Dr. Whitehead would plan the experiments, then Ms. Vuchich and her staff would carry them out. "Theirs were the capable hands without which our research could not have been accomplished," says Dr. Whitehead. Ms. Vuchich was one of the many dedicated research assistants who have worked with MCH investigators on groundbreaking discoveries.

Asthma and allergies

Allergies are orchestrated by the body's immune system, which identifies and reacts to different allergens, such as ragweed or tree pollen. The body produces allergen-specific antibodies called IgE. These antibodies migrate to mast cells lining the nose, eyes, and lungs that release many chemicals that irritate and inflame the membranes lining the respiratory tract, producing the symptoms of an allergic reaction.

In 1933, Dr. Harry L. Bacal founded a clinic for children with allergic diseases in the Outdoor Department of the Children's Memorial Hospital. He and his successors, Drs. A.H. Eisen, Elena Reece and Jack Fong, helped to establish the MCH as an internationally renowned centre for the study of allergy, clinical immunology, and immunodeficiency diseases.

Dr. Rhoda Kagan, pediatric allergist and immunologist, has participated in studies that improve our understanding of how peanut allergy, a potentially fatal illness, affects the lives of afflicted children and their families.

Asthma is a chronic disease that stems from inflammation and muscle constriction in the lung airways. At the MUHC Meakins-Christie Laboratories, Dr. Bruce Mazer and his colleagues are studying cells that are responsible for allergy and asthma, defining cellular factors that trigger inflammation and finding ways to modify them.

Dr. Charles Larson's research is both far-reaching and far-flung. He has studied childhood asthma in Chelyabinsk, Russia, with an international team of health professionals. Since 1999, this project has surveyed over 20,000 Russian adolescents for asthma and other allergic diseases in hopes of learning what triggers asthma attacks and what factors can predict asthma severity.

KATHARINE

In August 1990, Katharine's mother noticed that her two-year-old daughter was limping. She had lost her appetite and developed flu-like symptoms. Her mother asked a physician at her local hospital in the Laurentians for a referral to the MCH. "We were in Emergency the next morning. With one X-ray, they knew there was something there." Katharine was diagnosed with neuroblastoma, a cancerous tumour, in her hip joint. She was placed on chemotherapy but, by spring 1991, doctors at the MCH knew she needed more aggressive treatment. They extracted her bone marrow, which was sent to the University of Florida for special treatment, then re-transplanted in Katharine. On her fifth birthday, Katharine was back on her bike and playing with her brother Jason.

The MCH is a pioneer in the treatment of neuroblastoma, one of the most common solid tumours in children less than five years of age. In the 1990s, it was the only Montreal hospital to perform bone marrow transplants for this disease.

The breath of life

Regular breathing, so essential for life, is affected by many childhood disorders, ranging from prematurity to sleep apnea.

Since the 1990s, Dr. Robert Brouillette's research has focused on sleeping and breathing patterns of normal infants and those with obstructive sleep apnea or birth defects, such as spina bifida. He has developed innovative ways of recording children's sleep and breathing patterns in their own homes, reducing the need for extensive hospitalization.

Dr. Larry Lands, Director of the Respiratory Medicine Service, has elucidated the need for better nutrition and skeletal muscle function in children and adults with chronic lung diseases, such as cystic fibrosis and asthma, to improve quality of life.

Community-based research

At the MCH, clinical research within the community has always enjoyed high priority and high visibility. Founded in 1976 under Dr. Barry Pless, the Division of Community, Developmental and Epidemiologic Research (CDE) has been one of the largest, best-funded aggregations of child health researchers in North America. As part of this division, Dr. Charles Larson established a program to evaluate ways to smooth the progress of mother–child bonding in infancy. Drs. Pless and Terry Nolan examined the role of specialized nursing care in preventing behavioural problems in children with chronic illness.

Drs. Francine Ducharme and Francisco Noya study factors that cause acute asthma and identify improved treatment methods. Drs. Geoffrey Dougherty, in Intensive Ambulatory Care, and Alicia Schiffrin, a diabetologist, conducted a randomized clinical trial of traditional hospital treatment versus ambulatory care of children with new onset diabetes—a radical concept in the early 1980s.

Dr. David McGillivray has investigated which diagnostic tests are least invasive and most crucial for children in the Emergency Department. Drs. Ciarán Duffy, Francine Ducharme and Sylviane Forget investigated how chronic disease affects a child's perception of illness and quality of life. In the 1990s, Dr. Duffy developed the first quality of life measure for application in children with rheumatoid arthritis. Known as the Juvenile Arthritis Quality of Life Questionnaire (JAQQ), it is recognized as the best functional measure for use in clinical trials.

Important community-based research has been conducted for over 25 years by Dr. Alice Chan-Yip, who has published on health promotion research in Montreal's Chinese-Canadian community; Dr. Emmett Francoeur, who has published on recurrent abdominal pain and colic in infants; and Dr. Denis Leduc, who has focused on health outcomes research.

During 2004, CDE researchers participated in clinical studies with implications for children of all ages. Dr. Dougherty examined early response services for refugee mothers after pregnancy. Dr. Ducharme participated in three randomized controlled trials evaluating asthma medications and a community-based program to improve life for children with asthma. Dr. Pless evaluated the effectiveness of helmets in protecting skiers and snowboarders from injury.

Learning disorders

Genetic disorders, severe illness, or head injury in a young child may cause neurological and psychological deficits, including developmental problems such as difficulties in adjustment, attention, behaviour, communication, learning, physical coordination, and reading.

During the 1970s and 1980s, Dr. Maggie Bruck, at the MCH Learning Centre, conducted developmental and cross-linguistic studies of speech perception and the acquisition of reading skills. Her team of researchers also studied the effects of French immersion programs on children with language disabilities.

In the 1990s, Dr. Sylvie Daigneault, Dr. Judith LeGallais, Carol Schlopflocher, and Dr. Maria Sufrategui, psychologists, evaluated neuropsychological functions in school-aged children with traumatic brain injury to detect alterations in memory and concentration.

Autism affects one in 1,000 Canadian children, but no effective treatment program exists. Research into how to treat children with autism is a major focus of the hospital's Autism Spectrum Disorders Clinic, opened in 2003 and directed by Dr. Eric Fombonne (see Chapter 5).

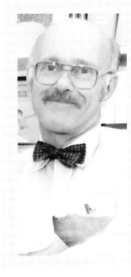

LEADER IN KIDNEY RESEARCH

Dr. Keith Drummond led kidney research as Director of the Renal Function Laboratory from 1964 until 2001. His international team determined the predictors, genetic factors, and mechanisms that contribute to kidney disease in children with insulin-dependent diabetes. These landmark studies have led to therapeutic interventions to prevent kidney damage.

Diabetes

From the 1960s to the 1990s, Drs. Eleanor Colle, Mimi Belmonte, and Alicia Schiffrin made significant contributions to studies that predicted which children would develop juvenile diabetes. In 1979, Dr. Schiffrin introduced the first intensive insulin management program in Canada for children with diabetes. Dr. Nicolas Steinmetz, former executive director, recalls that Dr. Belmonte was often criticized for advocating too much control in diabetes, "but she turned out to be right."

Dr. Constantin Polychronakos and his team of endocrinology and metabolism researchers are defining the genes that predispose children to juvenile diabetes. They have discovered an important protective gene that prevents the destruction of cells that produce insulin, the body's sugar-regulating hormone.

Cystic fibrosis

The MCH has a well-established reputation as an important centre for clinical, mechanical, and experimental research on cystic fibrosis (CF). During the 1980s, Dr. Allan Coates studied how the lungs function in children with CF and what natural or pharmacological treatments would improve their breathing.

Infectious diseases

When Dr. Melvin Marks directed the Research Institute's Infectious Diseases division in the 1970s, attention was focused on herpes simplex, meningitis, *Pseudomonas aeruginosa*, gastroenteritis, and the use of antibiotics in newborns.

Beginning in the early 1980s, Dr. Elaine Mills studied childhood infectious diseases, and as Director of Infectious Diseases, in 1991, she established the Vaccine Study Centre in Pierrefonds to evaluate the safety of vaccines in infants, toddlers, and children. By participating in over 25 clinical vaccine trials, MCH researchers have contributed significantly to the development of vaccines against once-common childhood diseases, including whooping cough (pertussis) and bacterial meningitis.

Since the 1990s, Dr. Jane McDonald has been involved in research to fight respiratory syncytial virus (RSV), a dangerous threat to children with chronic lung disease. Today, she conducts clinical trials with the participation of community-based pediatricians at the Vaccine Study Centre.

In the late 1980s, Dr. Mark Wainberg, working out of the Lady Davis Research Institute in Montreal, began to study how the human immunodeficiency virus (HIV) works to suppress the immune function in children. These studies initially focused on how HIV affected the thymus gland. His work progressed to studies assessing the effect of antiviral drugs on HIV reproduction in particular thymus cells. Today, he is an internationally renowned expert in AIDS research.

Surgical research

The interdisciplinary work of surgeons, anesthetists, intensive care specialists, and others, at the bedside or in the laboratory, has led to significant improvements in the care of children undergoing surgery.

In the 1990s, Drs. Karen Brown and Davinia Withington developed anesthetic methods for use during complicated surgery. According to Dr.

Brown, one of the great challenges of the future lies in the delivery of anesthesia during Cesarean section to infants with life-threatening but correctable birth defects. Over the years, she has also studied the quality of breathing after anesthesia, and Drs. Withington and Josée Lavoie have evaluated the safe, efficient use of tranquilizers in children after surgery.

Children with congenital heart defects that are corrected surgically have a higher risk of serious heartbeat irregularities (arrhythmias) as they age. Dr. Marie Béland has studied electrocardiograms to determine the degree of post-operative risk in children after congenital heart surgery.

Since 1977, Dr. Pierre Lachapelle has directed the Visual Physiology Laboratory in the Department of Ophthalmology. Its research aims to refine the process of diagnosis to be able to identify visual dysfunction at a much earlier stage. In particular, Dr. Lachapelle has investigated the causes and treatment of strabismus, which occurs when the eyes are misaligned and fail to fixate properly, and which, when not treated early, can cause irreversible visual damage.

A nerve injury can deprive a muscle of electrical stimulation during the lengthy period that it takes for nerve regrowth, often causing loss of muscle function. In 1995, using a small electrical implantable device to stimulate muscle in a patient after a nerve injury, Dr. Bruce Williams succeeded in keeping the muscle healthy until the nerve grew back. Since then, this technique has been adopted in 10 major university centres in Canada, the United States, and Japan for the treatment of nerve injuries and facial paralysis in children.

Thanks to the expertise of Drs. Jean-Pierre Farmer and José Luis Montes, and with the recent addition of Dr. Jeffrey Atkinson, the MCH has developed a world-class program in pediatric neurosurgery. About 65% of pediatric brain tumour cases in Quebec are referred to the MUHC, where these neurosurgeons operate on 40 to 45 children per year using sophisticated microscopic technology. Surgical treatments for cerebral palsy and epilepsy undergo continuous evaluation and revision under their direction.

Beyond the bedside

At the MCH, nursing involvement frequently goes beyond the bedside to reach into the realm of clinical research. In 1978, Dr. Celeste Johnston was appointed as the hospital's Nursing Coordinator for Research, the first such position in a Canadian hospital. A year later, the MCH Nursing Research Council was founded to screen research studies in clinical care.

Celeste Johnston's studies focused on the control of pain in children, particularly in infants. By the late 1990s, nursing-initiated research projects studied subjects such as the adjustment of children following critical illness and exposure to invasive technology (Janet Rennick, nurse, PhD; Celeste Johnston, nurse, PhD; Geoffrey Dougherty, MD; Judith Ritchie, nurse, PhD; Robert Platt, biostatistician); the value and efficacy of follow-up phone calls after ambulatory surgery (nurses Thao Lee and Elvie Parayno); and feeding problems in babies after cardiac surgery (nurses Kristina Wells and Linda Blanchard).

During the 1990s, nursing research findings presented at international conferences included work by Janet Rennick and Celeste Johnston, who studied how children in critical care adjusted to invasive technology, as well as by Franco Carnevale, nurse, PhD, and Céline Ducharme, nurse, who studied children's adverse reactions to sedation and analgesia.

THE ADOLESCENT YEARS

Adolescence is not an easy time, and MCH researchers have helped teenagers adjust to situations that go well beyond the usual problems of growing up.

In the 1970s, Drs. Robert Kinch and Peter Benjamin sought the best ways to care for pregnancy in an adolescent care centre of a children's hospital. They studied the backgrounds and emotional reactions of pregnant teens and their parents and participated in studies of the effects of recreational drugs on pregnancy.

During the 1980s, the Learning Centre sought effective treatment strategies for teenagers with learning disabilities. Dr. Renée Stevens studied the effectiveness of the Centre's after-school program in developing cognitive, academic, and social competence in learning-disabled teens.

> "Clinical research is the final common pathway through which all other research travels before it benefits children. It is the culmination of all other efforts; the pay-off for all the hard work at every other step in the chain."
>
> DR. BARRY PLESS, SCIENTIFIC DIRECTOR,
> McGILL–MCH RESEARCH INSTITUTE, 1987–1988
> *Growing together and achieving excellence into the 21st century,* October 1999

In the 1990s, Dr. Cécile Rousseau, Department of Child Psychiatry, studied how immigrant children, including children of war, integrate into their new environment, and Dr. Klaus Minde examined the attachments between children and parents in immigrant communities.

Since 1992, Dr. Brian Greenfield has been studying the effectiveness of a crisis team for suicidal youth. He has shown that the interventions of a crisis team decreased hospital admissions by 16% at a time when psychiatric emergency visits had risen by 37%.

Dr. Mark Zoccolillo investigates the effects of drug and alcohol abuse in teens and young adults, particularly the heavy use of marijuana during adolescence. He also studies how exposure to early risk factors, such as prenatal smoking and the parenting behaviours of inexperienced teenaged mothers, influences the development of antisocial behaviour.

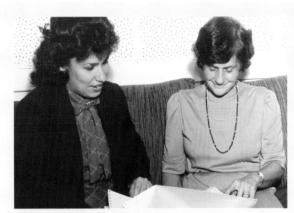

Drs. Lily Hechtman (left) and Gabrielle Weiss

ATTENTION–DEFICIT/ HYPERACTIVITY DISORDER

Research in child psychiatry at the MCH began in 1960, when two junior residents, Drs. Gabrielle Weiss and John Werry, conducted short-term trials of drug treatments for children from six to 12 years of age with attention-deficit/hyperactivity disorder (ADHD). Drs. Klaus Minde and Virginia Douglas joined the research team, measuring attention, self-esteem, and school performance in hyperactive children. ADHD research expanded when Dr. Lily Hechtman joined the department in 1972.

Together, Drs. Hechtman and Weiss conducted long-term follow-up studies of the children, who had grown into young adults of 19 to 25 years of age. These pivotal studies showed that young adults do not outgrow ADHD, and laid the groundwork for the recognition of ADHD in adolescence and adulthood.

THE FUTURE OF CHILD HEALTH RESEARCH

New knowledge earned by years of painstaking medical research is reflected in undeniable improvements to our health-care system. Newborns, children, and teenagers are better able to cope with their illnesses and now lead healthier lives because of advances made by the Montreal Children's Hospital's research community.

Dedicated physicians at the Children's Memorial Hospital sparked an interest in research within the students and fellows whom they taught. This legacy of curiosity, exploration, and hope continues today. MUHC pediatric researchers have won numerous grants, countless awards from prominent medical societies, and national and international honours and recognitions of merit.

What does the future hold for child health research at the Montreal Children's Hospital? Bringing together clinical investigators and research laboratories at the new Glen campus will help to build a synergy between researchers in all fields of childhood and adult medicine. It will create a critical mass of investigators to facilitate the exchange of knowledge and ideas; to harmonize information systems; to obtain common access to data; and to enable the accurate, comprehensive tracking of patients throughout their entire life spans. Since most researchers at the Children's are practising physicians, bringing their research facilities closer to their areas of practice will be a distinct advantage, both for them professionally and for those they serve.

By searching for the causes and cures of childhood diseases that may have consequences in the adult years, such as diabetes, obesity, and hypertension, Montreal Children's Hospital researchers help to ensure a richer and healthier future for all.

ORDER OF CANADA

The Montreal Children's Hospital has earned a worldwide reputation as one of the leading pediatric research centres in North America, and a number of MCH physicians and alumni have received the Order of Canada for groundbreaking research:

Mimi Belmonte (1999, Member)
Louise Chevalier (1987, Officer)
Caroline Clow (1982, Member)
F. Clarke Fraser (1985, Officer)
Richard Goldbloom (1987, Officer)
John Richard Hamilton (2001, Member)
Julius D. Metrakos (1986, Member)
Barry Pless (1993, Member)
Charles Scriver (1996, Companion; 1985, Officer)
Mark A. Wainberg (2001, Officer)

Other MCH alumni who have been named to the Order of Canada:
Anthony R.C. Dobell (1997, Member)
Donald Arthur Hillman (1994, Officer)
Elizabeth Sloman Hillman (1994, Officer)

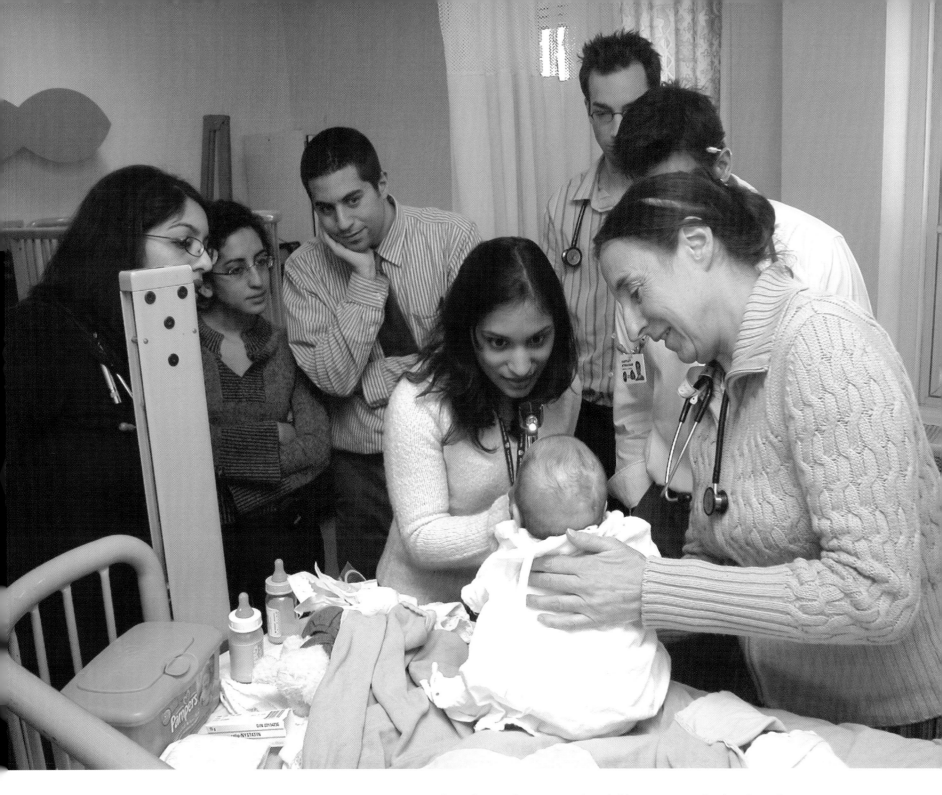

All professional groups at the Children's are involved in formal and informal teaching of students in medicine, nursing, and other health-care professions. Here, neonatologist Dr. Claudette Bardin instructs McGill medical students and residents.

"In every year since this Hospital was established, it has functioned as an educational institution, where all of us have learned from each other and from our patients and from the nursing and medical students alike."

DR. ALAN ROSS, PHYSICIAN-IN-CHIEF, 1953–1968
1955/56 Annual Report

7

Advances in Teaching and Learning

The Montreal Children's Hospital has always been a teaching institution. Just a few months after it opened, the hospital began training nurses in the special care of children, and by 1920 it had become a teaching hospital of McGill University's Medical School. Since then, the Children's has become intricately associated with a number of universities and colleges, as well as with other health-care institutions, in the training of doctors, nurses, and a wide array of other health-care professionals.

Education is a cornerstone of the MCH mission, and an integral part of the hospital's daily activities. Students can be found throughout the hospital, attending formal and informal teaching sessions and playing an active role in the care of patients. Staff members, in addition to training post-secondary, undergraduate, and graduate students, are involved in continual professional development activities to upgrade their own qualifications, knowledge, and skills. They also share their expertise with other health-care professionals throughout Quebec and beyond.

A TRAINING SCHOOL FOR NURSES

When the Children's Memorial Hospital opened in 1904, the training of nurses did not include courses in pediatrics. To provide nursing staff with the specialized knowledge and skills required to treat its young patients, the hospital launched its own training school for nurses in 1905.

The course was advertised locally and abroad, with the following notice circulated in Great Britain:

> ## AN EXCEPTIONAL OPPORTUNITY FOR GENTLEWOMEN WHO WOULD LIKE TO EMIGRATE TO CANADA
>
> Wanted by the CHILDREN'S MEMORIAL HOSPITAL, Montreal, Canada, applications from gentlewomen of good education who desire to enter a TRAINING SCHOOL FOR NURSES. Courses of training, three years. Board, lodging and a small salary allowed during term of training. Nurses, after graduation, can easily earn in Canada or the United States from eight to twelve shillings a day.
>
> For further particulars apply to The Head Nurse, Children's Memorial Hospital, 500 Guy Street, Montreal, Canada.

Successful applicants had to be healthy, strong, and well-educated, and provide a certificate of moral character. All their vaccinations and dental work had to be completed prior to the start of courses. Students were paid $7.00 per month in the first year of training, $8.00 per month in the second year, and $9.00 in the third. They were expected to pay for their own textbooks and uniforms.

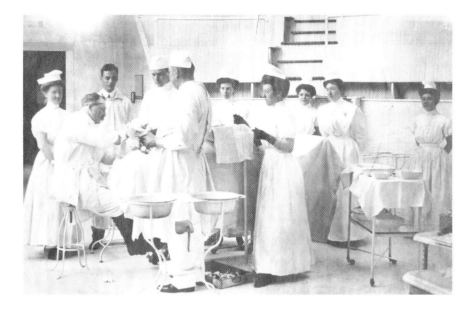

six months of their three-year program learning about adult health care. This initially took place at the Postgraduate Hospital in New York City, with the course transferred to the Montreal General Hospital in 1918. Courses in midwifery and maternity work were held at the Montreal Maternity Hospital starting in 1916.

NURSING STUDENTS AT CMH

"With regard to the education of nurses, no training is now considered complete that does not include work among children."

ANNE S. KINDER, SUPERINTENDENT OF NURSES
1925 Annual Report

The first nurses hired by the Children's Memorial Hospital were trained solely in the care of adults, as there were no pediatric nursing courses available at the time. The Children's opened its own training school for nurses in 1905. In this photo from the archives of McGill University, student nurses attend a surgical demonstration early in the 20th century.

The school's first class, consisting of five nurses, graduated in September 1907.

The life of a nursing student at the training school was not an easy one. For the hospital's 90th anniversary, Elaine Grant, then Assistant Head Nurse on 6C1, described those early days in *Au Courant*, the MCH nursing newsletter:

"Their working hours were 7 a.m. to 7 p.m. with 2 hours off during the shift, ½ day off per week, and 5 hours off on Sunday to go to church. They lived in residence, and had to be in bed by 10:30 p.m. ... One late leave per month was permitted, when they could stay out until 11:45. Lectures were given by the Head Nurse (equivalent to our Director of Nursing), her assistants, and by the medical staff at the Children's Memorial. It was not until 1924 that the first trained nursing instructor was hired."

The course of instruction, according to the 1915 Annual Report, included "lectures or demonstrations in Medicine, Surgery, Anatomy, Hygiene, Massage, Physiology, Obstetrics, Bandaging, also demonstration and practical work in the preparation of food for children and the ill."

To be registered as fully qualified by the Canadian Nurses Association, the students also had to spend

The Children's itself became an affiliate for other nursing schools starting in 1923, when several out-of-town institutions requested that their nursing students be allowed to gain pediatric experience at the

IN THE ISOLATION WARD

Connie Cloutier, a nurse at the Children's from 1961 to 1997, was trained at St. Mary's Hospital and did her pediatric affiliation at the Children's Memorial Hospital in the 1950s. She was part of the last class of student nurses to train there before the hospital moved to Tupper Street, and recalls her experience in the isolation ward:

"I can remember working night duty by myself with about 18 kids, most of whom were babies with diarrhea and vomiting. Most had those darn IVs [intravenous lines] where you had to count the drops per minute to assure that the child was receiving the correct amount of solution. It was not unusual to have a small baby on one drop per minute in order to receive 60 cc's per hour.

"Some wards were separate wooden huts set amidst the trees. At night time it was really dark, and when the wind would whistle through the ward and the night supervisor came around with a flashlight, it was pretty scary. What an experience!"

CMH. In the 1930s, the hospital decided to close its own training school and to open its doors instead to nursing students from a greater number of affiliated schools. The nursing school closed in May 1934, having trained a total of 213 nurses during its 29-year history. By the time the last class graduated, 10 affiliated schools were sending students to the Children's for pediatric experience.

The hospital also launched postgraduate courses for nurses during the Depression, when a number of private-duty nurses from other parts of Canada, unable to find employment, offered to volunteer their time to further their nursing experience. The CMH developed a three-month training program in pediatrics for them, with a certificate upon completion. The course was so popular that from the beginning applications exceeded available positions.

"The student nurse must learn and practice many of the techniques peculiar to pediatric nursing and begin to apply them skillfully and with judgment. She must learn to be comfortable with children of all age groups and to apply her knowledge of growth and development as she works with them. She must always be aware of safety hazards and accident prevention. She must meet with families and learn to support them—and all this within 12 weeks."

ROSELYN SMITH, DIRECTOR OF NURSING
1965 *Annual Report*

By the early 1950s, approximately 350 students per year came to the Children's from 20 schools of nursing in Quebec, Ontario, New Brunswick, Vermont, and Bermuda for a 12-week course in basic pediatric nursing. Students taking "Teaching and Supervision in Maternal and Child Health" at the McGill School for Graduate Nurses also came for their practical experience.

By the early 1960s, there were about 550 students a year from 13 affiliated schools, in addition to postgraduate trainees from the McGill School for

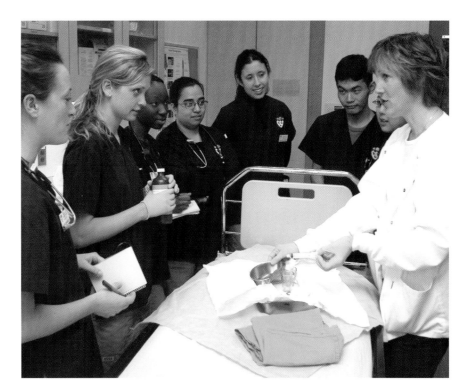

Graduate Nurses and from other provinces. (Although the number of students had increased, the number of affiliations had decreased as nursing schools found placements for their students closer to home and smaller schools closed.)

CEGEPS, UNIVERSITIES REPLACE HOSPITAL SCHOOLS

In 1970, Quebec moved away from hospital-based nursing schools to CEGEP and university programs. Since then, students wishing to become nurses in Quebec have had to complete a three-year diploma course at the CEGEP level or a baccalaureate or master's nursing program at a university. They must successfully pass a registration exam to receive a license to practise from the *Ordre des infirmières et infirmiers du Québec* (OIIQ).

These programs focus on general nursing, with pediatrics being only one area of study. CEGEP students typically spend only 10 to 12 days in a children's hospital, while the usual rotation for a uni-

Today, Quebec nurses are trained at CEGEPs and universities, and part of their practical experience takes place in a pediatric hospital. Here, second-year McGill nursing students take part in an informal teaching session on sterile vs. non-sterile techniques with MCH clinical instructor Debbie Meldrum.

PROFESSIONALISM IN NURSING

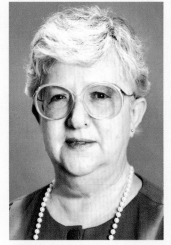

The move away from hospital-based training programs has meant an increased focus on the importance of well-trained nurses and recognition of the vital role they play in patient care. At the Children's, nurses are better educated than ever before. This is in large part due to the efforts of Evelyn Malowany, Director of Nursing from 1976 to 1997. With a teaching background, Mrs. Malowany hired university-trained nurses whenever possible, and encouraged nursing staff to upgrade their academic qualifications and take part in regular professional development activities.

versity undergraduate is approximately 24 days. At the Children's, trainees are assigned primarily to the surgical and medical units, with duties ranging from observation to total patient care with supervision. Those wishing to specialize in pediatrics receive more in-depth training once they are hired.

Each year, the MCH Nursing Department now helps train roughly 200 CEGEP students, 50 to 60 undergraduates, and 25 to 30 master's-level trainees. The hospital's primary sources of CEGEP students are the nursing programs of John Abbott, Vanier, and Dawson colleges, with baccalaureate and master's trainees largely drawn from McGill University and *l'Université de Montréal.*

During the past decade, the percentage of MCH nurses with a baccalaureate degree has been just under 50%, with the percentage steadily growing. There is also an increasing number of master's-prepared nurses, who work in specialized hospital clinics. Some—a total of 14 in 2004—are clinical nurse specialists, who have received additional training in a specialty such as pediatric neurology or rheumatology.

Today, some areas of the hospital are moving towards the nurse-practitioner model of nursing. Nurse practitioners are specially accredited master's-prepared nurses who have the authority to carry out some medical procedures and make certain medical decisions. Because the number of medical and surgical residents in the hospital has decreased dramatically in recent years, nurse practitioners fill some of the gaps. Their special training has so far taken place in the United States or other Canadian provinces, with accreditation programs in Quebec slated to start in 2005. By the end of 2004, there were seven accredited nurse practitioners working in the MCH Neonatal and Pediatric Intensive Care units.

As nurses become better educated, they increasingly raise research questions and take part in research studies. These examine, for instance, the effectiveness of various nursing practices and the results of specific treatments on children and their families. Since the early 1990s, PhD nurses at the MCH have been doing significant research in areas such as the long-term effects of hospitalization on children, particularly in the intensive care units (see Chapter 6).

PEDIATRICS BECOMES A SPECIALTY

The education of MCH physicians and surgeons has also changed a great deal over the past century.

Prior to 1930, when the American Academy of Pediatrics was founded, pediatrics did not exist as an official medical specialty. Anyone who graduated from medical school could set himself up as a pediatrician. No special certification was required, and there were no professional standards for the health care of children.

Medical school was a five-year course that could be entered directly from high school, and the curriculum included virtually no instruction on the diseases and conditions of children. At McGill, the number of hours designated for pediatric teaching in medical school was at the discretion of the Professor of Medicine and was rarely more than 20 hours during the five-year program. In his book *Small Patients*, Dr. Alton Goldbloom, who graduated from McGill University's Faculty of Medicine in 1916, described the pediatric instruction he received:

"At the bedside it consisted mainly in demonstrations on the preparation of the complicated formulas of the day, usually by an obstetrician, of a few hopeless cases of malnutrition, cases of rickets or scurvy of which there was a great abundance and a good deal of stool science."

There was no official link between the Children's and McGill University prior to 1920. With the evolution of the CMH into a truly general hospital for children, however, members of the medical profession, as well as medical students, came to observe and learn about the health care of children. In 1920, the CMH became an official teaching hospital of McGill University's Medical School, recognized as "a Canadian teaching centre for diseases of children." According to Dr. Goldbloom, it happened this way:

"Dr. Cushing [Physician-in-Chief at the Children's] decided that if the University did not want us we would invite its students to come to us on a voluntary basis. A notice was posted in the medical school offering a three weeks' course in pediatrics free to fourth-year students immediately after the conclusion of their classes. Virtually the entire class registered, and then lightning struck.

"The dean sent for Dr. Cushing; how dared he do such a thing without first consulting him? Cushing gave the dean one of his gentle, protracted, disarming smiles then told him that since we were not a teaching hospital, we could hardly come under his jurisdiction. The flustered dean blurted out 'then, this must be corrected immediately.' The course was then officially announced by the University; it was an instant success and we became a teaching hospital."

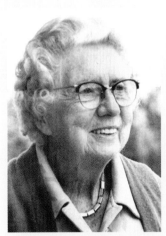

DR. JESSIE

Dr. Jessie Boyd Scriver (1895–2000) —or "Dr. Jessie," as she was affectionately called—was one of the first five women to graduate from the McGill University Medical School in 1922. Montreal's first female pediatrician, she was affiliated with the Montreal Children's and Royal Victoria hospitals from 1926 to 1967. She served as President of the Canadian Pediatric Society, and in 1979 published the book *The Montreal Children's Hospital, Years of Growth*. A dedicated physician, she made house calls far and wide, answered calls for advice at home around the clock, and always put her patients first. A brilliant student herself—she placed second in her class of 126—Dr. Scriver also became a role model for her own students.

At the hospital's 90th anniversary celebration, Dr. Elizabeth Hillman fondly recalled the day in the early 1950s when she walked with Dr. Scriver to one of the Cedar Avenue outbuildings.

"I was a first-year resident and we didn't make very much money in those days. I had a pair of shoes that the toe had come out of and I was using them for the winter weather because I didn't want to ruin my good shoes. Jessie Boyd stopped me in the middle of the snow and gave me a proper lecture that a doctor should be properly dressed at all times, while the snow fell around us and my toes got colder and colder. I have never forgotten that, nor have I forgotten all the good, sound, useful pediatrics I learned from Dr. Jessie, who was an excellent teacher and role model."

Today, roughly half of McGill's medical students are female, with the number increasing annually. Women are more likely than men to specialize in pediatrics—a fact readily observable at the Children's, where there are more women than men on the medical staff.

In 1945, with financial support from the Knights of Pythias, a medical library was inaugurated to help with post-war retraining and research. Dr. F.W. Wiglesworth, Director of the Department of Pathology, was appointed Honorary Medical Librarian, a post he held until his retirement in 1963, when Dr. John Blundell took over. Open 24 hours a day, the MCH library has been in continuous use by staff and students since its inception. Current librarian Joanne Baird has been in charge since 1983.

It was not until 1937 that a separate Department of Pediatrics was established at McGill. Dr. Cushing, still CMH Physician-in-Chief, was also appointed Professor and Chairman of the new department. This ensured that the teaching of pediatrics, which had previously taken place in six local hospitals (the Montreal General, Alexandra, Royal Victoria, Royal Victoria Maternity and Montreal Foundling and Baby hospitals, in addition to the CMH), would be largely centred at the Children's. The exceptions were training in newborn care and infectious diseases, which continued at the Royal Victoria Maternity and Alexandra hospitals, respectively.

EDUCATIONAL ROLE EXPANDS

When Dr. Cushing retired in 1938, Dr. Rolf R. Struthers took over as Professor and Chairman. Under his leadership, which lasted until 1946, the department flourished, with pediatrics becoming one of the four core subjects required of all medical students. (The three others were medicine, surgery, and obstetrics.) The hospital's role in training, too, continued to grow. In the late 1930s, the Children's

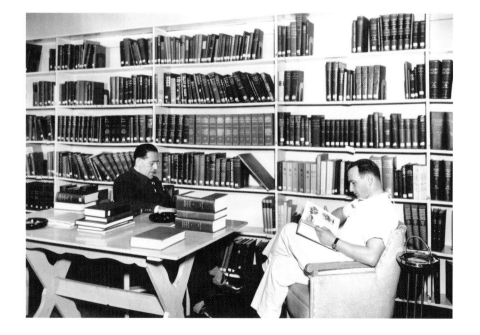

introduced postgraduate courses in pediatrics which were extremely well received by physicians in and around Montreal. During World War II, the hospital participated with McGill University in an accelerated, year-round medical course that enabled students to graduate more quickly. Then, at the end of the war, the CMH offered a three-month refresher course in pediatrics for physicians returning from the armed forces. It also established, in collaboration with McGill, a five-year diploma course in pediatrics leading to certification by various specialty boards in both Canada and the United States.

By 1946, when Dr. Alton Goldbloom became Physician-in-Chief and Chairman of Pediatrics, the number of hours devoted to pediatric teaching at McGill had climbed to nearly 200, and he was able to increase that number to more than 300. By this time, the reputation of the Children's was expanding, with applications for postgraduate training coming from as far away as China and India. Thanks to John Molson and J.W. McConnell, the first Research Fellowships were established in both medicine and surgery in 1946.

When the Children's moved to Tupper Street in 1956, it reaffirmed its commitment to education by ensuring that adequate lecture rooms, laboratories, and research facilities were available for teaching programs in medicine, surgery, nursing, and other professional and technical fields. It also restated its 1946 policy that the hospital "is constantly striving to improve the undergraduate teaching program. Closely related to this, is postgraduate training."

During the past 50 years, with the evolution of knowledge about pediatric diseases and the advent of new technologies and techniques, the training of pediatricians and pediatric surgeons has also become increasingly specialized. Postgraduates pursue specialty training in areas ranging from cardiology, neurology, immunology, and adolescent health care to emergency medicine and diseases of particular organs and systems. Typically, 50% to 75% of MCH residents today are training in subspecialties.

It was actually not until 1970 that the Children's became an approved training facility for pediatric surgery. Although as early as the 1930s there was growing recognition that pediatric surgeons required special training, only in 1970 did the American Academy of Pediatrics approve 14 pediatric surgical training programs, with the MCH one of two in Canada. Since that time, other hospitals have been added to the list, and the Royal College of Physicians and Surgeons of Canada has approved pediatric programs, including the Children's.

Since the late 1980s, the Children's has helped educate more than 300 medical and surgical trainees a year, including undergraduates, residents, and fellows.

THE LIFE OF A MEDICAL STUDENT

Dr. Alton Goldbloom remembered his first year of medical school in 1909 as a disappointment, for "instead of living subjects, there were cadavers in the foul-smelling dissecting room; instead of men and women with problems, there were mice and guinea pigs and rabbits, instead of clinics, there were tiring lecture-room benches." He did not see a living patient until he was in his third year. "In teaching the morphology and cultural characteristics of, say the streptococcus," he wrote in *Small Patients*, "no one ever thought of showing the students patients with streptococcal infections, that they might at the same time learn what the streptococcus does to the human patient."

Although didactic lectures continue to play an important role in medical education, today's medical students are exposed to patients and clinical settings much earlier and much more extensively. In their first year at McGill, undergraduates are assigned a patient to follow throughout the year, and towards the end of their second year, they are introduced to clinical medicine at one of McGill's teaching hospitals. For some students, these experiences bring them to the MCH.

In their third and fourth years, all McGill medical students, whether or not they plan to go into pedi-

DOING WHAT WAS NEEDED

Even before the CMH became a McGill teaching hospital in 1920, its staff relied on medical students to assist with laboratory work and other hospital tasks. In her book *The Montreal Children's Hospital, Years of Growth*, Dr. Jessie Boyd Scriver tells of one such case:

"The Medical Superintendent's duties were many, and to assist him a senior McGill medical student was appointed. When not attending university lectures and clinics, he did what was needed at the hospital and served as night relief for the Medical Superintendent. Dr. Arthur Henderson, who was the incumbent in his junior year 1911–12, recalled his duties, sixty years later, in a personal interview. He assisted Dr. Mackenzie Forbes with plaster casts; he was responsible for the patients at night; he did any clinical laboratory work which was ordered; he gave lectures in anatomy and physiology to the nurses. There was little or no free time, but Dr. Henderson recalls that the social atmosphere was very pleasant. Dr. Evans and he ate their meals with the Lady Superintendent, Miss Barnard, and her assistant, Miss Matthews, and occasionally after dinner they gathered around the piano in Miss Barnard's sitting room for a singsong."

atrics, are required to do an eight-week clerkship in pediatrics. Because the Children's is the only comprehensive pediatric teaching hospital in the McGill system, it is the only hospital that receives every McGill medical student—currently about 160 per year. Students spend two weeks of their pediatric clerkship in the perinatal nurseries at either the Royal Victoria or Jewish General hospital.

The clerkship at the Children's includes both formal and bedside teaching. It is also an apprenticeship, with students learning by doing. They participate fully in the life of the hospital—seeing patients, taking part in multidisciplinary meetings, tracking down laboratory results, performing examinations, and talking with families. On nursing unit teams of eight or nine people, four or five are

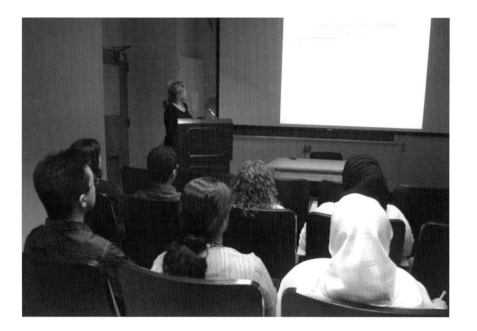

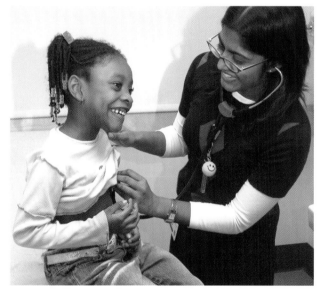

Dr. Laura Russell gives a lecture entitled "Approach to the Dysmorphic Child"—reviewing important points required to evaluate a child with multiple anomalies —to medical genetics residents, MSc genetic counselling students, and medical students and residents taking an elective in medical genetics. These lectures can also be attended by anyone on the staff, medical geneticists and genetic counsellors alike.

Christine Sabapathy, a fourth-year medical student planning a career in pediatrics, examines patient Kiara. Christine's clerkship at the Children's, like that of other students, involved practical training in a number of different departments.

"The Children's is a great place to learn about a wide range of medical conditions and see patients from many different backgrounds," she says. "There's a real drive towards teaching here; everyone puts in the extra effort to help students."

typically students. The MCH clerkship is extremely popular, and McGill usually has more students applying to pediatrics than any other medical school in Canada. When these students go on to residency training, they are much respected because of their extensive undergraduate pediatrics experience.

THE POSTGRADUATE EXPERIENCE

Prior to the 1980s, medical school graduates in Canada were required to do a one-year rotating internship, after which they could either go into private general practice or enter a specialty program. In the early 1980s, internships were eliminated across the country, and additional training was incorporated into the clerkships at the under-graduate level. Today, medical school graduates have two options: to go into general practice they must complete a two-year family medicine residency pro-gram, or they can enter a residency program in a specialty of their choice, entailing several more years of training.

Those who choose family medicine currently spend two months of their training in pediatrics. The Children's established Montreal's first family medi-cine unit specifically for the training of McGill resi-dents in 1972. By the late 1970s, similar units had been established at many of the city's adult hospitals. As the training model evolved, the MCH's family medicine unit was closed in 1981, and family medi-cine training was incorporated into the hospital's other teaching units.

Training in surgery on children is a vital part of accreditation by the Royal College of Physicians and Surgeons in all surgical specialties and sub-specialties. Graduates who elect to become pediatric surgeons face six to eight years of specialized resi-dency training after medical school. First, there is a two-year core program, including one rotation of two to three months in pediatric surgery. This is followed by three to four years of specialty training (in orthopedics or cardiac surgery, for example), of which two rotations, or between six and eight months, are spent in a pediatric setting. Those further specializing in a pediatric surgical specialty spend yet another year or two training at a children's hospital.

Graduates who go into pediatric medicine follow a core program of three years, then pursue an additional two to four years of residency training in a subspecialty (such as pediatric endocrinology or nephrology) or do advanced work in general pediatrics.

The life of a resident has changed a great deal since the 1950s and '60s. In those days, residents usually lived at the hospital and were rarely married. Their hours were extremely long, with a "one in two call schedule"—meaning that, in addition to working during the day, residents were on call every second night, so it was not uncommon for them to work 36 hours at a stretch.

Salaries were low. A chief resident in the early 1960s earned $85 per month plus uniform, room, and meals, increasing to $125 with experience. The few residents who were married and lived outside the hospital received an extra $50 per month for rent.

In 1967, residents across Quebec withdrew their services (except for emergencies), seeking higher wages from the provincial government and recognition not only as students but also as professional providers of health-care service. They achieved their main objectives, and subsequently working hours were also improved, with call schedules reduced in 1972 from every second night to one night in three. Since 1993, residents have been on call for a maximum of six nights per 28-day period, and are not permitted to work more than 24 hours at a stretch.

While their on-call schedules may be less gruelling, the overall responsibilities of today's residents are no less demanding. They are on the front lines of patient care in every area of the hospital: neonatal and pediatric intensive care units, medical and surgical nursing units, emergency room, and outpatient clinics. Many also work in community clinics and

IN RESIDENCE

Winnifred Jones worked at the Children's from 1953 to 1982, first as secretary to the executive director and later as the hospital manager. In an interview for the hospital's 90th anniversary, she described the residents' living quarters before and after the move to Tupper Street in 1956:

"Up the hill, as we called it, the women residents were tucked in tiny little rooms over the admitting office. They needed bedspreads and drapes, which I helped to get. The male residents lived in a beautiful house on Redpath. They had a groundsman and a housekeeper and a swimming pool and their own room and bathroom. But once they moved down the hill, everyone was in the residents' residence and they were all just in rooms, with one sitting room for everybody."

IN THE "PIT"

Dr. David McGillivray, Associate Director of Medical Emergency, remembers his days as a resident in the early 1970s in this excerpt from *A Fuzzy but Affectionate Look at the History of the Emergency Department* (1997):

"As a resident you were on call in the 'pit'. This was the 'affectionate' term used for the emergency by residents and staff in the 1960s and 1970s. It conjured up images of a Roman Gladiator ring where you lived or died, but in any event you came out a changed man ... At 23:00, the same time as the surgical emergency closed, the clean faced pediatric resident came on to be 'night float', by him or herself! ... I can tell you that this was baptism by fire. Not only were you alone (I mean, I have never felt so alone), you had to do all your white cell counts on bloods and CSFs [cerebrospinal fluids]. The resident could count white cells in his sleep and some did! ... The resident's best friend, as always, was the nurse who kept encouraging you, telling you what to do (what else is new) and offering you more coffee. If fun can be terrifying, this was great fun. It made a 'man' out of us. We were finally real doctors who made real decisions that made a difference."

outreach programs, where they can develop a better understanding of the social determinants of health, and there is a compulsory rotation in the under-privileged community of Hochelaga-Maisonneuve (see Chapter 11).

With medical knowledge developing at a tremendous pace, there is great pressure on residents to keep up. Fortunately, modern technology also makes information more readily available than a generation ago. With a laptop or a handheld device, or at computer terminals throughout the hospital, the resident can quickly research the side effects of a medication, access articles related to a teaching session, or get the most up-to-date information, on a newly admitted patient with a challenging medical problem—even at 3:00 a.m.

In addition to looking after patients, residents generally also carry research and teaching responsibilities, spending roughly a quarter of their time teaching medical students, trainees from other specialties, and residents more junior than themselves.

Since the 1980s, when the Quebec government established quotas for residency spots in an attempt at manpower planning, the number of provincially funded residents has decreased substantially. To

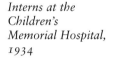

Interns at the Children's Memorial Hospital, 1934

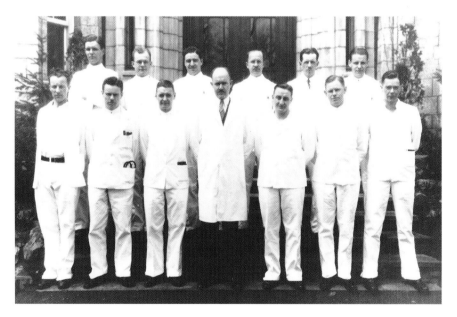

IN THE GULF
Since the early 1990s, the Children's has had a special relationship with Sultan Qaboos University in Oman, with the school sending a number of trainees to the MCH. Pediatric Program Director Dr. Saleem Razack likes to joke that "we're sending back a whole faculty this year!

"This whole group of pediatric trainees," he continues, "will occupy leadership positions there, will set up programs, and will hopefully provide us with collegial links for many years to come."

TRAINING IN ANESTHESIOLOGY
Anesthetics have been used at the Children's since its inception, but in the early days they were often administered by doctors or nurses with no anesthesia training, and in any case, very little was known about the specific requirements of young patients. This changed in 1940, when Dr. Morton Digby Leigh, the father of pediatric anesthesia in Canada, became CMH Anesthetist-in-Chief. He established a training program and published the first textbook on pediatric anesthesia in 1948. (The first three North American textbooks on pediatric anesthesia, in fact, were published by Children's staff members; Dr. C.R. Stephen produced the second in 1954, and Dr. H.T. Davenport, the third in 1967.) Dr. Leigh also instituted teaching programs in clinical anesthesia for McGill undergraduates, interns, and clinical fellows.

Today, a career in anesthesiology requires a medical degree plus five years of specialized training, including a minimum of three months in a pediatric setting. As children behave differently during anesthesia and recovery than adults, physicians specializing in pediatric anesthesiology require further training. In Canada, pediatric anesthesiologists undergo at least one additional year to gain expertise in the management of premature infants and babies and complex pediatric procedures and techniques.

make up for the shortage of residents, the hospital now takes in an increasing number of foreign trainees, many of them from the Gulf States, who are funded by their own governments or sponsoring agencies and return to their home countries at the end of training.

Today, the Department of Pediatrics trains an average of 30 residents in pediatrics per year, in addition to 24 in adult emergency medicine and 85 in family medicine. The Department of Pediatric Surgical Services receives an average of 40 residents. The Children's is also a training site for doctoral and postdoctoral fellows in many medical and surgical subspecialties, such as pediatric nephrology, rheumatology, critical care, and emergency medicine.

TRAINING OF OTHER PROFESSIONALS

In the hospital's earlier days, many of the functions now requiring specialized training were performed by volunteers or untrained personnel, or were part of the workload of doctors, nurses, or students.

In the early decades of the 20th century, for instance, most hospital administrators were doctors and nurses who ran the hospital in addition to caring for patients. In the 1930s, the creation of the American College of Hospital Administrators spurred the development of masters-level training programs across the U.S. and Canada. Trained health administrators study health-care policy and law, finance and budgeting, management processes, strategy development, environmental issues such as equipment and facilities planning, and a variety of related subjects.

"Hospitals are among the most complex environments to manage—physically, culturally, financially, and politically," says Donna Riley, MCH Director of Planning and Development, 1987–1995, and MUHC Director of Planning, 1995–2000.

"The job of an executive director, and of the senior management staff, is primarily one of advocacy and vision: ensuring services for patients and

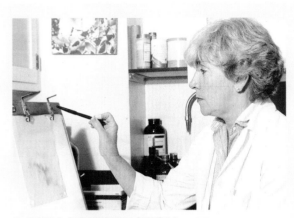

A PATH OF DISTINCTION

Not many high school drop-outs end up as part-time associate professors in a department of human genetics, but that's the path Carol Clow's career took. She quit school at age 14, got a clerical job, then married. One of her children died of leukemia, and when a second child died of SIDS, she went to see her old friend Dr. Charles Scriver, hoping he could give her some answers. He gave her something more—a job. He needed help with a research project on the incidence of phenylketonuria (PKU).

Dr. Scriver trained her to be a lab technician in the newborn screening study. Then, whenever a baby was identified as having the gene for PKU, she talked to the parents. As a mother, she understood their concerns. "I had to assure them the child would be OK," she says.

She also helped set up a food bank in Alexis Nihon Plaza near the MCH (the National Food Distribution Centre for the Treatment of Hereditary Metabolic Diseases, run by part-time university students), where parents could get the special formula and other items allowed on the strict diet that is the treatment for PKU. In 1982, she received the Order of Canada in recognition of her work on the food bank.

Over the years, she attended conferences with Dr. Scriver and presented papers on their work, and eventually McGill University made her a part-time associate professor in human genetics. But she says her greatest satisfaction came when the children she had helped grew up and invited her to their weddings.

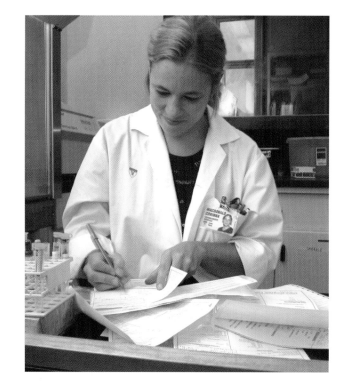

their families; removing hurdles and going after resources for staff; and influencing policy and legislation that affect people's health and well-being."

The Children's long tradition of doctors, and in recent years, nurses, at the helm, continues with the April 2005 appointment of Linda M. Christmann, MD, MBA, as Associate Executive Director for the Pediatric Mission, MUHC. Dr. Christmann's senior administrative team is made up of professionals in many fields—including doctors, nurses, and health-care administrators. In addition, the Children's supports the development of professional administrators by serving as a residency site for students from Canada's six master's programs in health administration, as well as from diploma and baccalaureate programs more locally.

The teaching role of the MCH also extends to university and CEGEP students in fields such as respiratory therapy and pharmacology; biochemistry, microbiology, and pathology; medical imaging and neurophysiology; laboratory technology; psycholo-

gy, social work, pastoral services, and child life; occupational therapy and physiotherapy; audiology and speech and language pathology; clinical nutrition; and hospital administration.

As an example, respiratory therapists do a five-week rotation at the MCH in the final year of their three-year CEGEP program. A second-year introductory phase at the hospital has recently been added, to allow the therapists-in-training a chance to get used to working with severely ill children. Their academic program has also been upgraded to include additional pediatric training and evaluation. Advances in technology have changed their training in recent years, too, reflecting the fact that respiratory therapists need to have expertise in both technology and clinical care. They may have to test children's breathing capacity and set them up on a ventilator, in addition to making sure the equipment functions properly.

There are now about 50 respiratory therapists in various MCH departments—a far cry from the mid-1950s, when Bob Baker, the hospital's first inhalation therapist, worked with just a cleaning aide and an orderly, setting up and maintaining ventilators, teaching nurses how to use them, dealing with suppliers, and all the other tasks required to keep children breathing well.

Prior to the 1940s, physicians and residents, sometimes with untrained assistants, were responsible for much of the hospital's laboratory work. Starting in the 1940s, this was increasingly delegated to technologists, freeing up residents for patient care. It was not always easy to find trained or even partly trained technologists, however, as many preferred to work for private companies offering better salaries and shorter working hours. (This is still a concern today.) Even as late as the 1970s, residents working alone in the ER at night were responsible for carrying out routine laboratory tests.

Today, MCH medical technologists have a CEGEP diploma or baccalaureate degree in medical technology or a related field. CEGEP training for biomedical laboratory technologists consists of a three-year program in all the five laboratory specialties (biochemistry, hematology, microbiology, blood bank, and histology). The nearest such program is at Dawson College, not far from the hospital's current location. In their third year of studies, students at Dawson and other CEGEPs with similar programs spend approximately 26 weeks in different hospitals, to gain practical experience and develop competencies in the field. For some students, this brings them to the MCH. Graduates who are hired by the Children's without pediatric experience receive on-the-job training.

As medical laboratory work becomes increasingly complex, laboratories are beginning to require a baccalaureate or even a master's degree. Certain areas, such as molecular genetics, now require up to a PhD.

Another example of a department launched with untrained staff is the Social Services Department, established in 1916 by a group of volunteers. Even

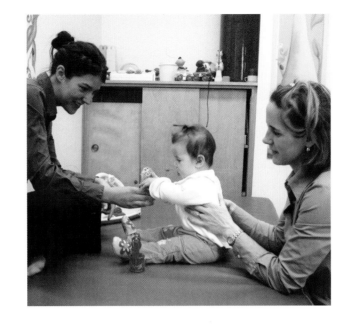

Occupational therapy trainee Nadia Gagnon-Houle (left) works with young Camille, under the supervision of MCH occupational therapist Sophie Laniel.

A PROFESSION IS BORN

Many of the specialized health-care professions that exist today were undreamed of a century ago. A clinical perfusionist, for instance, gets children onto the heart-lung bypass machine during heart surgery. This ensures that adequate oxygen is delivered to all organs, including the brain, since the heart and lungs must be stopped during the operation.

The hospital's first perfusionist in the 1950s was not a trained professional, but a 17-year-old German immigrant named Wolfgang Schroeder who was employed as an orderly. He later went on to medical school.

Today, the hospital employs three full-time, professionally trained clinical perfusionists who are a vital part of the cardiac team. Perfusionists must complete a three-year undergraduate degree with a specialization in cardiovascular perfusion, along with a fourth year of clinical training.

after McGill's School of Social Work was created in 1919, hospital financial constraints meant that volunteers remained an important part of the department for many years. These volunteers received some training from the hospital's social workers, enabling them, for example, to go into homes and help families cope with their chronically ill children (for more on Social Services, see Chapter 11).

The volunteers were eventually phased out, until today, all of the hospital's social workers have a bachelor's or master's degree in social work. Many also have specialty training in areas such as family therapy and palliative care, and play an important role in the training of social work students.

Similarly, occupational therapy at the Children's began in the 1920s with two volunteers teaching long-term patients on the rheumatic fever wards how to sew, knit, and make baskets. When the Occupational Therapy Department was established in 1936, a trained Directress was hired to develop "a scientifically-prepared occupational therapy program." Soon the department was giving lectures and demonstrations to student and postgraduate nurses, occupational therapy interns, and volunteers, dealing with equipment and procedures used to train children with cerebral palsy and other ailments in self-feeding, dressing, and simple creative occupations. By the 1950s, trainees were coming from as far away as Texas and Colorado to study occupational therapy in a pediatric setting.

Today, most MCH trainees come from McGill University, with a few from other Quebec and Ontario universities. Occasionally, the Children's provides experience for occupational therapists from France who wish to work in Quebec and need an internship to become members of the *Ordre des ergothérapeutes du Québec* (OEQ).

All MCH occupational therapists are members of the OEQ, meaning they have at least a baccalaureate degree and clinical experience. The Canadian Association of Occupational Therapists has mandated that, by 2010, the minimum educational requirement will be a master's degree.

The therapeutic use of play, today a part of the hospital's child life program, was originally part of occupational therapy. In 1936, 48 nurses and 20 volunteers took the first course in play activities that could be used during the regular nursing routine. "Eight class periods," the annual report tells us, "were devoted to a study of nursery rhymes, finger plays, songs, stories, poems, riddles, puzzles, tricks, tongue twisters, sense games, simple intellectual games, singing games, pencil and paper games and story acting." Each nurse who took part in the course was expected to keep a notebook with lists of suggested play activities, and to devote five hours a week to actual play on the wards.

Today, child life specialists use play to normalize the child's hospital experience and reduce stress levels. They also work with families. Although there is no standard training for child life professionals, they all have a bachelor's degree in a field related to child development (such as education, psychology, psychoeducation, or therapeutic recreation) and are certified by the Child Life Council.

Currently, of the 10 physiotherapists on staff at the Children's, two have master's degrees, two have PhDs and the rest are graduates of bachelor of science (BSc) programs. It is expected that within the next few years, physiotherapists, too, will require a master's degree for membership in their professional order.

MCH speech-language pathologists, audiologists, and members of the pastoral services team already require at least a master's degree, while all psychologists employed by the Children's have a PhD. Clinical nutritionists are required to have at least a bachelor's degree in human nutrition and may take graduate courses at the master's and doctoral levels.

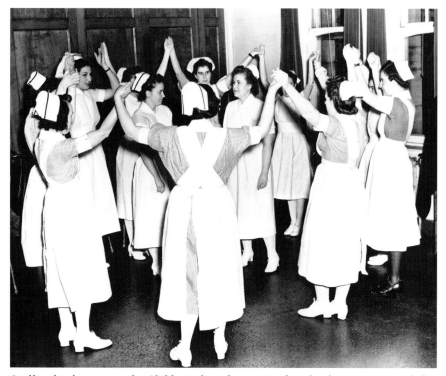

Staff and volunteers at the Children's have been trained in the therapeutic use of play since the 1930s. In "When We Go Affiliating," The Canadian Nurse, February 1940, Katherine Vaughan described the nurses' initial feelings about this training:

"Upon our arrival, our attitude towards being taught how to play 'Ring around a Rosy' and to recite nursery verses was one of suspicion and complete contempt. Now we realize that play is the great bond between the child and the adult, a common language, a medium through which the art of healing is introduced and carried on."

These and other professional groups at the Children's have seen great changes during the past 30 years, not only in the amount of training required but also in the content of the training programs themselves. Overall, they now include less didactic teaching and rote learning and more clinical involvement, with earlier exposure to patients. There are fewer large lecture hall presentations and more small group, individual, and computer-assisted learning situations. Evaluation has gone from strictly content-oriented final exams to in-training evaluation. And training is now more science-, research-, and evidence-based, as practitioners seek to evaluate the efficacy of diagnostic and remedial procedures.

CONTINUING EDUCATION

"When you finish your formal education, that's when learning really begins."

DIANE BORISOV, DIRECTOR OF NURSING

The education of MCH staff does not end with their formal training, of course; ongoing professional development is both the right and the responsibility of staff in all areas of the hospital.

The growing sophistication and complexity of patient care, along with a shortage of pediatric experience in many health-care training programs, means that graduates hired by the Children's often need additional training to fill the gaps between what they have learned at school and what is expected of them on the job. Even for experienced employees, ongoing changes in technology, medical knowledge, procedures, and philosophy mean that continuing education and professional development are an important part of the job. MCH pharmacists, for instance, keep informed about new medications produced by drug companies and their implications for children of different ages. Nurses keep up-to-date with the latest treatment techniques and procedures. Continuing education is considered so important by

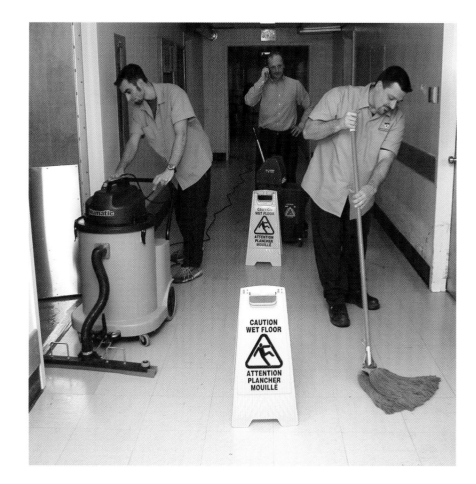

some professional orders that they are beginning to require a certain number of professional development hours per year.

Throughout the hospital's history, lectures, seminars, and informal teaching sessions have been offered to stimulate, encourage, and broaden the knowledge base of staff at all levels. Hundreds of training sessions each year, led by in-house and outside specialists, deal with everything from diagnostic and clinical procedures to communication skills, team building, youth protection, and multicultural understanding. The hospital supports professional development and encourages staff to take courses and attend conferences, or to spend time at other medical institutions to develop knowledge and skills they can bring back to the Children's.

Learning is an ongoing part of life at the Children's. Here, housekeeping section manager Leonard Johnston (centre) teaches housekeeping attendants Jean-François Cromp (left) and Dereck Moore how to clean up a flood scene safely.

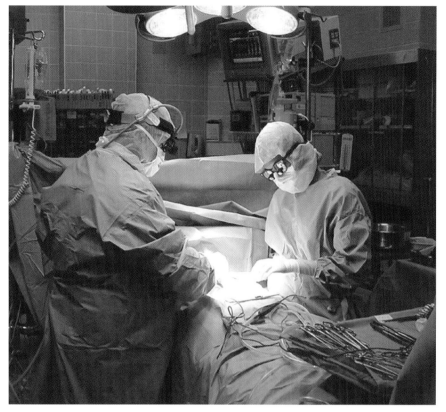

Sometimes staff training takes place "on the fly," as when a new technology or technique is used for the first time. In 2002, a multidisciplinary team from the MUHC's joint pediatric and adult cardiac transplant team performed the first mechanical heart procedure in Canada, using what is known as the Berlin heart on a two-year-old child as a bridge to heart transplantation. Although members of the team had experience in certain aspects of the procedure, most had to learn over a weekend how the mechanical heart worked, how to perform the procedure on a child and, later, what follow-up care was required. In all, roughly 100 surgeons, physicians, perfusionists, nurses, and other health-care professionals were involved in the child's care. Shown here are Drs. Christo Tchervenkov (left) and Renzo Cecere.

"We share our expertise in the treatment of disease, in the prevention of illness or injury, and in the promotion of health with other institutions and professionals in a collective effort to solve our society's health care problems."

The Montreal Children's Hospital Mission Statement

MCH staff also contribute their expertise and knowledge to professionals beyond the walls of the hospital. Since the 1920s, staff from the Children's have held formal teaching positions at universities and colleges, both locally and abroad. Community-based practitioners are invited to attend hospital lectures and demonstrations in pediatric medicine and surgery, and visitors from throughout North America and abroad have come to observe and consult with MCH specialists.

The Children's has a dynamic group of speakers (physicians, nurses, and other health-care professionals) who are strongly committed to continuing education. These professionals give lectures and presentations at local, national, and international meetings and conferences on topics as diverse as genetic counselling, pediatric advanced life support, palliative care, and developmental delays.

The development of telehealth has enabled MCH professionals to provide expertise and support to difficult-to-reach regions of the province, and to work with others to solve problems of mutual concern. With its recognized expertise in telehealth, the Children's has been mandated to help expand this program across the MUHC (see Chapters 9 and 11).

The hospital is also leading the MUHC's effort to expand the Northern and Native Child Health Program. Since 1965, the hospital has provided resident staff, nurses, and consultants to First Nations and Inuit communities in the North, combining pediatric training of local staff with service to underserved areas (see Chapter 11).

The Children's has a strong tradition in international health that goes back many decades. In the late 1960s and 1970s, for instance, hospital staff participated in a CIDA–McGill program in Kenya to train students and residents who would eventually take over the new medical school at the University of Nairobi (see Chapter 11). MCH staff also went to Ethiopia to train local physicians in community health, and other initiatives have brought MCH expertise to areas of Russia and Belarus.

A WIN-WIN SITUATION

During the past century, the training of health-care professionals at the Children's has not been without its challenges. The resources required, in terms of teaching and supervision time, space, and clerical support, have been extensive and sometimes inadequate. And adapting teaching programs in response to evolving health-care needs and advances in knowledge or techniques has required constant flexibility and creativity.

But trainees—whether medical students, residents, nursing students, or others—have always been an important part of the Children's, and it would be hard to run the hospital without them. The presence of trainees on the nursing units and in the clinics has contributed immeasurably to patient care.

The students themselves appreciate the wealth of teaching material provided by the hospital's patients and families and the expertise of the MCH staff. Members of the staff, in turn, are stimulated by the students, who ask challenging questions and spur them on to be always up-to-date.

In maintaining the high standards of its training programs and actively participating in programs that promote the exchange of expertise between health-care institutions, the Children's is ensuring that the care children receive will be the best possible—not just within, but far beyond its walls, and not just now, but for generations to come.

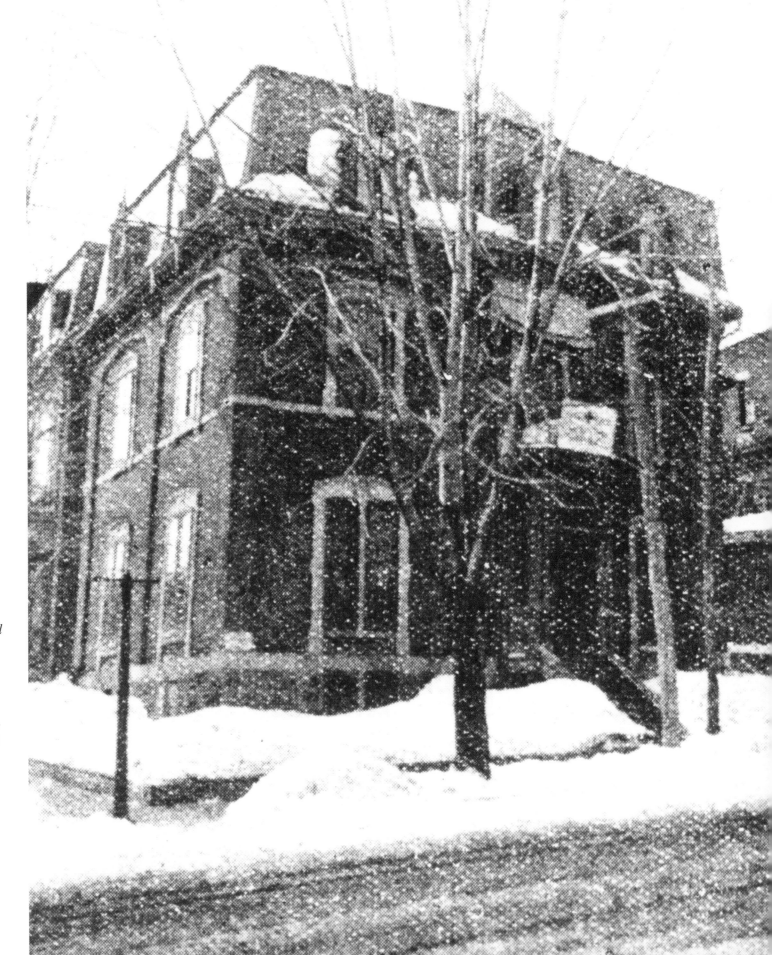

This small building on Guy Street was the original home of the Children's Memorial Hospital, from 1904 until 1909, when the hospital moved to more spacious quarters on Cedar Avenue.

"Almost from day to day the hospital has been slowly adding to its services until it has grown from a narrow and almost insignificant institution into a great Hospital—a Hospital which has far outgrown its physical facilities."

Fundraising analysis and recommendations by
the John Price Jones Corporation, 1937

8

Short on Space, Long on Devotion

From a small rented facility at 500 Guy Street, to a cluster of buildings on Cedar Avenue, to a complex of overflowing pavilions centred at Tupper Street and Atwater Avenue—the Children's has moved and expanded over the years, constantly evolving to meet the changing needs of patient care, teaching, and research.

And yet these needs have consistently had a way of keeping a few steps ahead of the available facilities.

When the Children's Memorial Hospital moved from Guy Street to its new building on Cedar Avenue in 1909, there seemed to be an abundance of space. Nevertheless, over the years other buildings were added to a burgeoning complex on the side of Mount Royal to accommodate growing needs.

In 1911, the first floor of the Arnott Memorial Cottage opened as an isolation ward. Two years later, the upper floor became the hospital's first infants' ward. The James Carruthers Out-Patient and Administrative Building was completed in 1920, the Kiwanis tuberculosis pavilion (Ward K) in 1924, and the Kinmond and Judah pavilions in 1925. This brought the hospital's bed capacity to 130. Bed capacity was further increased in 1930, with the addition of a new wing to the main building. By 1935, when the Hazel Fountaine Brown Cottage added 30 beds for children suffering from heart disease, the hospital's total bed capacity was up to 300.

The Children's Memorial Hospital also incorporated other facilities. In 1932, during the Great Depression, it amalgamated with the Montreal Foundling and Baby Hospital, which had been caring for babies since 1892, and whose occupancy had been declining. This provided 60 more beds for convalescing infants and freed up CMH beds for the care of those who were more acutely ill.

The Children's also took over, in 1940, the financially struggling Montreal Children's Hospital (also known as the Vipond Hospital after its founders) at

The Alexandra Hospital for Contagious Diseases, founded in 1903, became a chronic care institution under the Children's from 1967 until it closed in 1988.

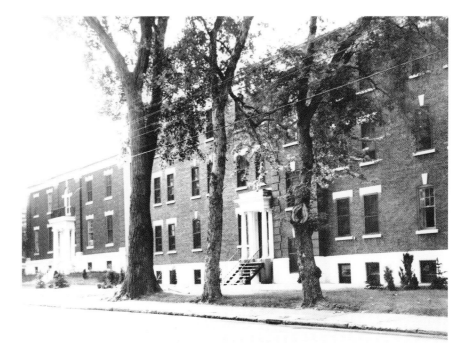

Guy and St. Antoine streets. The Vipond provided additional space for convalescents during the war and became the new, more accessible, outpatient building of the Children's in 1946.

The Alexandra Hospital for Contagious Diseases in Pointe St. Charles had been founded in 1903 to treat children suffering from such infectious diseases as diphtheria, scarlet fever, measles, and later tuberculosis. In 1967, infectious disease cases were transferred to the Children's and the Alexandra became a chronic care hospital under the MCH's management. In 1988, after the remaining 57 residents of the Alexandra were transferred to more suitable facilities in institutions and group homes, the building was sold.

Over the years, each new building was filled to capacity almost before the children and staff had moved in. With each expansion, demand for services increased dramatically. Meanwhile, as new technologies and treatment facilities were developed, these also impinged on space originally planned for patients. Non-treatment areas such as waiting rooms had to be found wherever they could, and tight situ-

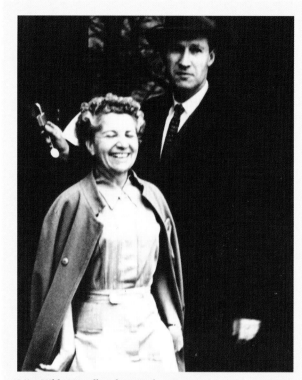

Miss Hilda Nuttall and Dr. Herbert Owen

CLOSING THE DOOR

The well-orchestrated move from Cedar Avenue to 2300 Tupper Street in December 1956 went perfectly according to plan—well, almost.

"Dr. Herbert Owen closed the door of the (old) Children's Hospital in front of the TV cameras and as he did so, the door handle—which hadn't been turned, I think, for about 20 years—came off in his hand and he tumbled backwards down the stairs.

"The next morning I went up to the hospital and looked up Carl Shivers, who was in charge of maintenance, and asked him what he did with the handle. 'Oh,' he said, 'I threw it out the back of the hospital.' I went to the back of the hospital and went through all the garbage—and shooed away about 20 cats that were out there—and found the handle. I had it mounted on a piece of oak and gave it to Dr. Owen."

Dr. Harvey Beardmore, general surgeon, *at the hospital's 90th anniversary celebration*

CATS, DOGS, AND STRIPES

The Out-Patient Department (OPD) on St. Antoine Street was crowded but efficiently run by nurses such as Orlo McInnes and her successor, Diz Wanzer, recalls Dr. Elizabeth Hillman, who was in charge of the OPD for 17 years starting in the 1950s. Dr. Hillman credits the nursing staff with creating the warm, friendly atmosphere, but it was she herself who painted the elevator doors in bright stripes and had pictures of cats and dogs put on the walls to provide a cheerful, reassuring place for children to wait. One advantage the building had at the time was an ideal location to be accessible to the public. "Sometimes too accessible," says Dr. Hillman, "as children on their way home from school would peer in at the windows at us as we sutured up their classmates."

"OFFICIAL" OPENING

The December 1956 move to the current Tupper Street site from the hospital's earlier location on Cedar Avenue was extremely successful, as chronicled in Dr. Jessie Boyd Scriver's history. However, plans for an official Royal opening were apparently disappointed. An excerpt from the minutes of the hospital's Committee of Administration meeting of May 29, 1958, reveals a typically creative MCH solution:

"Mr. Molson [John H. Molson, President] told the meeting ... that it would not be possible for Her Royal Highness, The Princess Margaret, to open the Hospital during her summer visit to Montreal ...

"Mr. Molson then said that as a matter of interest to the members, he and Dr. deBelle had visited Miss Parry [Director of Nursing] in her office, and had asked her to rise from her chair and declare the Hospital open. This had been done and the matter was now considered closed."

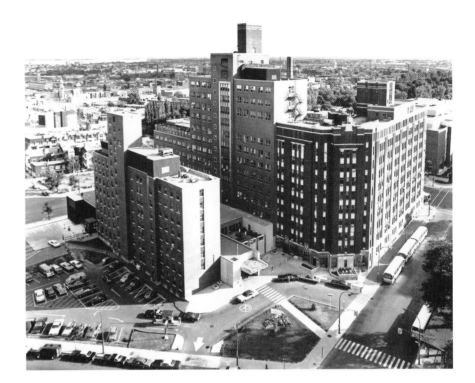

ations, such as nurses washing surgical instruments inside the operating rooms, were increasingly commonplace. In the 1940s, to make room for new departments, bed numbers were reduced and more services were provided in outpatient settings.

By the early 1950s, the hospital had grown to 12 buildings, including the main building on Cedar Avenue, a cluster of wards and labs spreading higher up the mountain behind it, and outpatient services in a separate location on St. Antoine Street.

In 1951, the Children's purchased the Western Hospital on Tupper Street from the Montreal General Hospital, added two new buildings, and in December 1956, moved to its present, more expansive location, under its new name: The Montreal Children's Hospital. At the same time, it divested itself of the other locations. The new facility offered accommodation for 385 inpatients, outpatient facilities, and residences for nurses and doctors in training. All the hospital's functions were once again under one roof—for a while.

It did not take long for the spacious new facilities to become overcrowded. Less than eight years after the move to the Tupper Street buildings, a consultants' master plan recommended expansion, particularly to meet the needs of outpatient and emergency services, research, and teaching.

By the hospital's centennial year, its main campus, bounded by Tupper and Lambert-Closse streets, Atwater Avenue, and René-Lévesque Boulevard, consisted of six interconnecting wings—A to F—totalling more than 47,115 square metres. But over the years, as activities in these buildings outgrew their quarters, the hospital has also had to find space in other nearby properties.

The Gilman Pavilion, located on Atwater Avenue just a hundred or so metres from the main hospital complex, was the home of the Red Feather Appeal until it was purchased for the hospital in 1974. It now houses Dentistry, Adolescent Medicine and Gynecology, and the Adolescent Day Treatment Centre.

This aerial photo shows the main Tupper Street complex in the late 1970s. In 1994, a third floor was added to the low B-Wing in the centre to accommodate the magnetic resonance imaging (MRI) suite. It was expanded in 1998 so the Hematology/Oncology Day Treatment Centre could move into new quarters. Also in the 1990s, bus stops were moved across the street to prevent diesel fumes from causing discomfort and health risks to patients and staff.

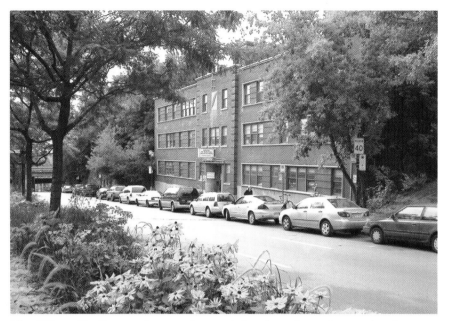

The Gilman Pavilion on Atwater Avenue is handy to the main complex, but separate enough to offer privacy to the adolescents attending clinics there. The Dentistry Department occupies the second and third floors, and also has a dental chair next to the ER for patients who cannot leave the main complex. During the 1970s, the Family Medicine Unit was located there, until it closed in 1981. From 1974 to 1997, the building also housed a school of dental hygiene.

Dr. Cynthia Goodyer's research laboratory in Place Toulon is an example of how much activity, equipment, and documentation must be crammed into small spaces. PhD student Gurvinder Kenth carries out DNA analysis while postdoctoral fellow Zak Rhani and PhD student Joy Osafo confer in the background.

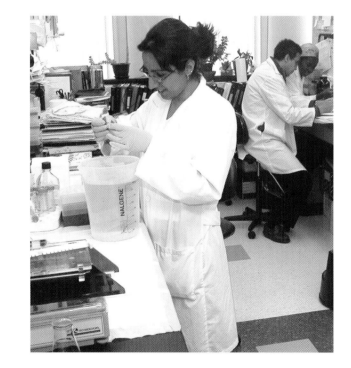

One block west of the main complex, on St. Catherine Street West, two floors and sections of two others in Place Toulon are home to the Montreal Children's Hospital Research Institute of the MUHC Research Institute, which moved there in 1979. Also on St. Catherine, about halfway between Place Toulon and the main hospital, are the premises rented since 1988 for Psychiatry and Psychology.

In 1994, some of the hospital's administrative departments, such as Finance and Accounting, moved to Les Tourelles, a renovated greystone townhouse facing the hospital parking lot from the south side of René-Lévesque Boulevard. Over the years, these departments were consolidated across the MUHC, and the MUHC payroll offices moved into Les Tourelles. In 2004, the Payroll Department was relocated to another rented property and Les Tourelles became home to Architectural Services, doctors' offices for the Emergency Department, and the administrative offices of the Institute of Human Development, Child and Youth, of CIHR (Canadian Institutes of Health Research). This trend of moving around is likely to continue while the hospital remains in its current location.

At the turn of the 21st century, despite generous response from the community for building funds over the years, the hospital continues to struggle to meet the demand for space. Closets and washrooms are converted into offices, teaching and consulting overflows into corridors, and patient rooms must now accommodate sophisticated medical equipment, storage for personal belongings, and sleeping space for family members.

NEEDS CHANGE FASTER THAN PLANS

This is not to say that the hospital is a passive victim of expanding activities. Enormous efforts have been made to foresee future needs and to cope with current limitations. Every few years, there are role studies, space studies, and proposals to renovate, build, and expand. Many of these have borne fruit. However, many more have become outdated before

Finding a Home for the Research Institute

As early as 1964, a master plan proposed new and expanded research facilities be located where either the B- or F-Wings are today. In 1966, the McGill University–Montreal Children's Hospital Research Institute was founded, with the expectation of occupying the proposed facilities in short order. However, it was not to be. The master plan underwent changes, and for the next 12 years, research had to be carried out in whatever spaces could be found. In 1979, it became obvious the Institute would need to find an off-site building if it was to have the facilities it needed, so the Board decided to rent space in a new building under construction on St. Catherine Street West. They were able to work with the architect to modify the commercial structure to suit their research needs, and they lobbied the City of Westmount to change the zoning laws to permit an animal research laboratory on the second floor.

"We didn't like the smell from the pizza place on the ground floor," recalls Dr. Harvey Guyda, director of the Research Institute at the time, "but they didn't appreciate us, either, particularly when our little white rats escaped into the lower levels. But moving into Place Toulon doubled the capacity of our research space."

In the late 1980s, the Research Institute's hopes of being repatriated to the main hospital site were set aside in the face of other construction priorities. Since then, several proposals have been explored to find facilities nearby that would provide more room for the expanding labs.

Danuta Rylski, the Institute's manager, recalls that these included the old St-Hubert Barbecue building on St. Catherine Street West, and the former Reddy Memorial Hospital facilities.

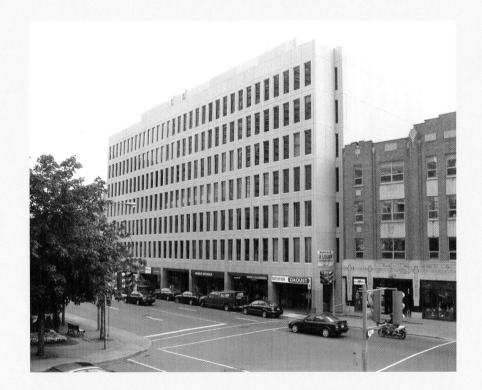

Ms. Rylski was one of the first to move into Place Toulon.

"I can still remember the day I arrived," she recalls. "I was told we were only going to be here for a short time!" Ironically, 25 years later, she has probably spent more time than anyone else working on the various plans for establishing permanent quarters.

In the end, it will be the move to the Glen campus of the MUHC that finally brings research and patient care together once again.

they could become reality because new needs and opportunities arose between planning and implementation. Meanwhile, the hospital's staff, from architects to physicians, nurses, and technical and administrative personnel, have shown enormous creativity in getting the most out of limited space, putting every nook and cranny to best use.

"Additions continued to be built—every one about 10 years too late, so by the time it was completed, we needed a new one. They should have built a new hospital!"

DR. PRESTON ROBB, NEUROLOGIST-IN-CHIEF, MONTREAL NEUROLOGICAL HOSPITAL, 1968–1976 *associated with the Children's for 40 years*

RENOVATION BOOM AND BUST

Renovation projects seem to come in waves. After the initial flurry of settling into the new buildings in 1956, there was not much major renovation until 1976–1977, when the B-Wing was built, replacing Essex Street and thus bringing the other buildings together. This construction set off a number of renovation projects in other parts of the complex, which lasted about five years.

A second wave came in the mid-1990s, following a successful capital campaign. Although this campaign had been undertaken for new construction, plans were changed in 1993, when the Children's entered into the project to create a new McGill University Health Centre. Given the proposed move to a new campus, there was no point investing in new buildings that would be used for only a few years. Donors accepted the Children's request to redirect some of the money into urgent short-term renovations and equipment that could ultimately be moved to the new location. It was expected at the time that the hospital would be in its new quarters by 2004.

Consequently, the mid-1990s saw another series of renovations and installations throughout the hos-

pital. Of course, the most high-profile changes were major equipment renewals. However, it was often the more general, mundane improvements that brought sighs of relief from staff and patients alike. Elevators ran more quickly and reliably, and air conditioning was more widely installed, now including all patient areas. While there is still too little space in many areas for the cooling equipment necessary for central air conditioning, electrical capacity was increased, allowing for more window units. The temporary boom also allowed the hospital to put into practice its vision for an environment more conducive to healing—more up-to-date design, homey furniture and curtains, brighter colours on the walls, and beautiful murals and artwork for a final touch.

FEWER BEDS IN PATIENT ROOMS

The most recent round of renovations on patient units was completed in 2004. One of the most significant, and most welcome, changes is an increased proportion of single and double rooms. Four-bed rooms were originally the norm in the old buildings, designed in the days before parents were encouraged to stay overnight and participate in their children's care. (In fact, these four-bed rooms were vestiges of the old "ward" layout of hospitals—large open rooms with lots of beds all in a row. And of course, the term "ward" has stuck, despite the evolution to nursing units with smaller rooms.)

Moreover, in the 1950s, technologies now used to monitor conditions and deliver treatment were either much simpler or did not exist, so there was little incursion of equipment into the patient's room. By the 1980s, this was no longer the case. Patient rooms were seriously overcrowded, compromising the effectiveness of personnel—not to mention privacy and comfort. While dotted lines on the floor were often the only separation between the areas assigned to each patient, including family and belongings, these lines were ineffective in blocking out sounds, sights, and more importantly, infectious agents.

Why not renovate all units, creating only private rooms capable of meeting modern technical requirements? A logical objective, but not always feasible: many of the walls in the main buildings are supporting walls, which cannot be moved. This is particularly true in the D-Wing, built in 1932. Throughout the older buildings, halls are too narrow, ceilings too low, ventilation and plumbing systems inadaptable —problems that plague older hospitals in general and contribute to the need for the MUHC and its modern, more flexible facilities.

Although it might appear that placing fewer beds in each room would deprive patients of beds, this is

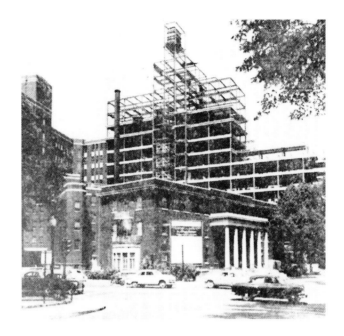

This photograph from The Gazette *in June 1955 shows the F-Wing—soon to be housing for residents—in the foreground. Behind it, the new C-Wing is taking shape.*

in fact not the case. The number of inpatient beds required has been reduced steadily since the 1970s, thanks to such innovations as new vaccines, home care, day surgery, better anesthetics, and shorter procedures. Empowering parents to provide care at home for minor illnesses and injuries, as well as chronic conditions, has also reduced bed occupation.

In 1956 there were 385 beds. By the late 1980s, the number of beds was down to about 200, and by the hospital's centennial year, it was 180. At the same time, patients who are hospitalized rather than treated as outpatients usually have more need of private rooms, either for more equipment, for family members providing care and comfort, or for isolation: they are generally sicker, and may be infectious or have low immunity to infection.

To this day, washrooms are still at a premium throughout the hospital's older complex. A number of them, along with storage closets, have been turned into much-needed office space for staff. However, even this trend had its limits. Storage space for equipment remains inadequate to this day

RENOVATIONS DEMAND EXTRA CARE

Even with the prospect of a new health centre down the road, facilities must be kept in good repair and as up-to-date as possible. This is not simple. To protect children's health, whole areas have to be completely finished with ceilings intact, and dust removed, before a patient can even be moved through them, let alone moved into them. This means renovations in a hospital go a lot more slowly than in other buildings. During renovations, whole sections between stairwells need to be blocked off with plastic sheets to keep dust and fumes from reaching patient areas. Traffic is re-directed up or down to the next floor and back again via other elevators or stairs, often for weeks at a time.

To ensure continuing hygiene in the renovated facilities, laundry and housekeeping staff are consulted to ensure the new fabric and floor coverings can be easily cleaned and maintained.

Buildings in Evolution

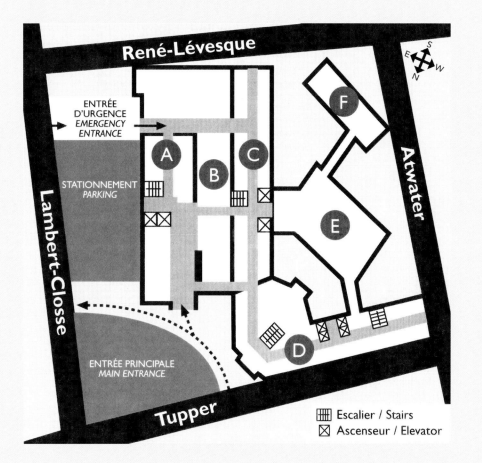

René-Lévesque

ENTRÉE
D'URGENCE
*EMERGENCY
ENTRANCE*

Atwater

STATIONNEMENT
PARKING

Lambert-Closse

A B C

F

E

ENTRÉE PRINCIPALE
MAIN ENTRANCE

D

Tupper

⊞ Escalier / Stairs
⊠ Ascenseur / Elevator

When the Children's Memorial Hospital—newly re-named The Montreal Children's Hospital—moved to 2300 Tupper Street in 1956, it occupied three existing buildings that had housed the Western Division of the Montreal General Hospital, and two that were newly constructed. The MCH's inheritance from the MGH includes the D-Wing, then called the Tupper Street Wing, which extends east along Tupper Street from Atwater Avenue; the E-Wing, formerly the service wing, connected by a narrow isthmus to the D-Wing; and the F-Wing, situated on the corner of Atwater Avenue and René-Lévesque Boulevard (at that time Dorchester Boulevard).

Of the two new structures, the taller was the 15-floor C-Wing, connected in 1956 to Wings D and E to form a rough A-shape. Once known as the Essex Wing for the street it originally bordered on, it currently houses most patient care units and operating rooms.

The other new section built for the Children's was the eight-floor Ross Residence for nurses, now the A-Wing. At the time of the move, the two new buildings, parallel to each other, were connected by an underground passageway. Completion of the B-Wing in 1977 filled in the street between A and C, and completed the current configuration of the main part of the MCH complex. A third floor was added to the B-Wing in the 1990s.

The unusual grouping of MCH buildings has been largely dictated by buildings that no longer exist. The 1876 plans for the Western Hospital, the first hospital on the site, called for an H-shaped configuration that would allow for maximum ventilation, fire safety, and organization of separate medical programs. However, over the years, plans were changed, buildings were demolished, and the site changed hands twice. The Western Hospital became part of the Montreal General Hospital in 1924 and was later sold to the Children's Memorial Hospital.

The ghosts of the old hospitals are still with us.

—as do washroom facilities and offices. During a centennial year interview, Dr. Harvey Guyda, Physician-in-Chief, was heard to note: "Office space is a disaster. There are no more toilets to de-commission."

B-WING FILLS THE GAP

The B-Wing is the newest of the MCH wings. Built in 1977, after years of anticipation, it filled in the gap—and the road—between the A-Wing and the other existing buildings. In the place where Essex Street once ran south from St. Catherine Street, children in the Emergency or clinic waiting rooms now play with toys, read books, or munch on goodies from the snack bar.

From its position at the centre of the main complex, the B-Wing feeds the hospital's patient care activities. Through its southeast entrance come families seeking relief at the ER, the single greatest source of admissions to the inpatient units. Through its north entrance come the thousands of outpatients who make up the majority of the hospital's clientele. Many inpatients also arrive through the north entrance, to go to the busy Admitting Department on the main floor. Whether arriving for a longer stay or for same-day surgery, every child who occupies a bed in the hospital comes in through Admitting.

Before the B-Wing was built, patients in strollers or wheelchairs had to be helped up a set of stairs to the old entrance in the D-Wing. This created a need for a doorman, a post ably fulfilled by Henri Desmedt. Henri stayed on for years after the new entrance was built, welcoming families, holding doors, and helping with strollers and wheelchairs.

An outdoor balcony was built just to the west of the new main entrance. It served patrons of the Tiny Tim Café, providing fresh air to families and staff alike, and—after the hospital became a smoke-free environment in the late 1980's—offering one of the last refuges to smokers. It was removed in 1994 to allow for the installation of the MRI suite. The space it occupied is now part of the café.

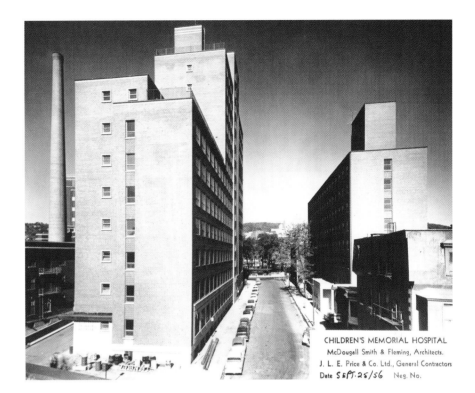

CHILDREN'S MEMORIAL HOSPITAL
McDougall Smith & Fleming, Architects.
J. L. E. Price & Co. Ltd., General Contractors
Date SEPT-25/56   Neg. No.

E-WING HAS PROVIDED RELIABLE SERVICE SINCE 1932

Formerly known as the service wing, the E-Wing is another part of the Montreal General Hospital's legacy to the Children's. It forms the short bar of an 'A' by connecting the old D-Wing and newer C-Wing. In addition to mechanical services, it houses the kitchens, the cafeteria, and a few clinical departments, such as Endocrinology, Urology, and Nephrology.

From the boiler room in the basement of the E-Wing, heat is controlled and distributed to the entire Tupper Street complex. Other mechanical operations are centralized nearby. Despite proposals over the years to relocate the mechanical services of the hospital and correct the inefficient use of space in the inner courtyard, the boiler room has been in operation continuously in its current location since 1932, when the building was constructed. There have always been higher, and less expensive, budgetary

This photo from the hospital archives shows Essex Street running north between the A-Wing (right) and the C-Wing, before the B-Wing was built, joining the two.

priorities. Nonetheless, replacement, repair, and maintenance by the hospital's dedicated personnel have kept it serving heating needs efficiently.

A- AND D-WINGS HOUSE A VARIETY OF FACILITIES

The former nurses' residence (dedicated in 1958 to the memory of Lord Atholstan, one of the hospital's major benefactors) no longer houses living quarters. Department of Nursing offices are still there, but they share the A-wing with a wide variety of other departments, serving a range of clinical, administrative, and research functions. The main floor houses the Short-Stay Unit and part of the ER. Because the floors are not the same height as in other wings, they cannot be connected to the rest of the hospital beyond the second floor. The wing is also narrow, designed for bedrooms and small common rooms, and so cannot readily be converted to in-patient units, which require more space. However, patients do visit the clinics, offices, and labs of Speech and Language Pathology, Neurology, Audiology, Medical Genetics, and Neonatal Follow-up. The Biochemical Genetics and Cytogenetics laboratories are located on the upper floors.

A QUIET PLACE

In 1957, a chapel was opened in the basement of the D-Wing. The chapel was renovated in the late 1980s to make it more accessible, removing pews to allow wheelchairs and cribs to enter easily. MCH chaplains hold mass here four times a week, with additional services held upon request. Larger services, such as memorial services, are held in the hospital's amphitheatre.

Despite proposals over the years to relocate it to a higher, brighter, more accessible location, it has not moved. Even chapels are subject to space shortages. Nonetheless, the space has managed well over the years to provide a quiet refuge for patients, families, and staff alike. It has seen a variety of ceremonies for adherents of different faiths and been a private place for reflection, prayer, and solace.

The D-Wing, while it shares the problem of inflexible configuration with the A-Wing, was built as a hospital and still contains some inpatient units. The 8th-floor Hematology and Oncology Unit does not look its age, thanks to renovations and conveniences financed by The Lamplighters, a support and fund-raising group made up of families of children with cancer. The 9th floor houses the Pediatric Intensive Care Unit, and the 10th, the operating rooms and Post-Anesthesia Care Unit. On the 7th floor, there are overnight facilities for adolescent psychiatric patients, and common spaces for younger school-aged children coming in for activities during the day. Other floors have clinical services used mainly by outpatients, such as occupational therapy services, the physiotherapy gym, respiratory therapy, and the ophthalmology clinic and offices. Much of the 4th floor is occupied by clinical laboratories. Besides clinical and diagnostic functions, the D-Wing is home to doctors' offices and conference rooms, the amphitheatre, and Medical Multimedia Services, which includes the conference rooms used for tele-health sessions.

F-WING HAS LED SEVERAL LIVES

The other building inherited from the Montreal General Hospital, the F-Wing, once housed living quarters for nurses. Dating back to 1919, it is the only remnant of the now-defunct Western Hospital, which in 1924 became the Western Division of the Montreal General Hospital. When the Children's moved in, in 1956, it became the Peter Holt House, home to interns and residents. Since the advent of salaried residencies in the 1970's, the discontinuation of internships, and the trend toward increasingly independent lifestyles, residents are no longer provided with living quarters. Only a few beds remain in the building for those on night duty.

Its life as a residence over, and not being well suited to most patient care activities because of its layout, lack of elevators, and distance from other services, the F-Wing gradually accumulated administrative activities. Central Administration, including the executive director's office, completed the shift in the 1990s, when it moved there after 40 years in the D-Wing.

Staff in the F-Wing share a special anticipation for the move to the Glen campus. The building is slowly sinking into the ground, as evidenced by the tilting windows in the executive director's office, their frames supported by wooden shims. Air conditioning is rare, and summer temperatures in many offices can reach 43°C or more—enough sometimes to close up and send people home for the day.

(More about the C- and D-wings can be found in Chapter 13.)

MONITORING THE BUILDING'S VITAL SIGNS

Whether coping with outdated facilities, enjoying new modern ones, or planning for future space, the hospital must carry on with its primary mission: to improve the health of children. Much of this mission is made possible by an invisible web of wires, pipes, and ducts that moves power, equipment, essential supplies, and information through, under, and around the buildings. These movements may go unnoticed

by patients, families, visitors, and even hospital staff, but many children's lives depend upon them.

Security is one department whose crucial work extends like a network throughout the whole hospital complex. From a hub located midway between the main and Emergency entrances, security guards keep watch over many aspects of the hospital's internal environment, with the aid of a lighted board, computer monitors, and two-way radios connected through an MUHC-wide network. (Cellular phones may not be used in the hospital because of their potential to disrupt sensitive medical equipment.)

A signal in the Security office will alert attendants to temperature changes in equipment such as cytogenetics incubators and refrigerators in the Blood Bank and research labs. Personnel can then call Housekeeping or Maintenance to correct the situation. These calls can be urgent—even a slight drop in temperature can jeopardize the results of a sensitive lab test or cause blood to be discarded.

Security officers monitor every door to the outside in every MCH building. They also manage both the room keys and the often multiple alarms for such areas as the main computer rooms or pharmacy supplies. Some keys, such as those to the pharmacy's narcotics cabinets, may not leave the building. If someone forgets and exits with one, the lock must be replaced.

PICKUP AND DELIVERY

Porters and storekeepers literally keep things moving in the hospital. Storekeepers carry a wide variety of supplies from eight different inventory centres to everywhere in the institution. Their payloads can range from everyday things like stationery and hardware to heavy-duty items like beds and equipment, or carefully prepared provisions like feeding formula and medical/surgical supplies.

Porters also transport a wide range of items. They deliver the mail, as well as reports and medical charts. They also handle more delicate duties, such as transporting specimens of blood, urine, and other

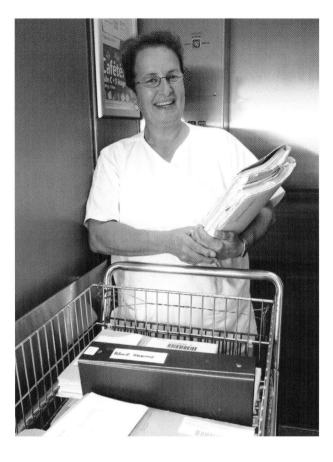

Porter Catherine (Kay) Flowers transports essential information between hospital departments.

Hematological tests were done on site at the Children's, but the technician was supervised by an MGH specialist until 1947, when Dr. Ronald Denton became director of the hospital's Hematology Department.

Test results, whether verbal or written, are easier to deliver than specimens. These days, lab results are reported back by computer, but this has only been the routine since 1992. Before then, they were usually relayed by telephone. In the very early days of the Tupper Street facilities, they might also be transported through a pneumatic chute system that ran from labs to clinics and the ER. It was phased out at the beginning of the 1970s, possibly as a result of its limited range (it never reached the wards) and possibly because of occasional accidents caused by misuse: samples themselves being sent along the system instead of paper reports, in breakable glass tubes. Not all unauthorized use of the chutes was as damaging, however. There was reportedly a small but interesting traffic in love notes!

BEHIND THE WALLS

Some essential supplies are delivered through the walls and ceilings. Oxygen is one of these. Outlets may be found in a number of locations throughout the patient care areas, including wards (now more properly called nursing units), the ER, and clinics. In the operating rooms, anesthetic gas is drawn from a column that descends from the ceiling. Altogether, four different gases are conducted through the main complex from tanks in the basement or, in the case of oxygen, from the large cylindrical tank adjacent to the parking lot.

The quality of the air, so essential in a place that houses sick children, is maintained through supply and return ducts in the walls and ceilings that ultimately connect to the cooling system located in the mechanical room in the B-Wing basement. Each patient care area has its own cooling coil for the air conditioning system.

substances to the hospital's laboratories for testing. Their timeliness, accuracy, and careful handling is important to ensure reliable results.

In the days before the Children's had its own lab facilities, transportation was even trickier. It was not until 1931 that the hospital set up its own biochemistry laboratory, which eventually came to handle work on metabolic diseases as well. Even after that, many specimens had to travel farther. Dr. Preston Robb recalled, in a centennial year interview, the summer during the 1930s when he was a medical student and had a summer replacement job as a bacteriologist. "I lived at the CMH, where I picked up the specimens in the morning and delivered them to the Pathology Building at McGill every day for six weeks."

An observant visitor will notice another system in the walls. Two lifts, much like silent butlers, are located in the walls of the C-Wing, beginning in the basement just outside the entrance to the Medical Records Department. They carry patient charts—the precious records that document every aspect of a child's relationship with the hospital. Actually a large file, sometimes containing several inches of papers, a chart includes a wide range of information such as lab and X-ray results, growth sheet, reports on procedures followed, and notes from clinic appointments and surgeries, as well as hospital discharge summaries.

The smaller lift goes only to the first floor, to the office where Medical Records keeps charts awaiting completion and re-filing, and to the second floor, where most of the outpatient clinics are located. There is a lot of lift traffic to the clinics, where charts are ordered two days before a patient's appointment so clinic staff can check for the most updated test and x-ray results. The larger lift goes all the way to the 13th-floor laboratories, with access on the floors in between for a variety of clinics, departments, labs, nursing stations, and offices.

The walls, floors, and ceilings of the MCH contain electrical wiring and plumbing, like those of any building. They also have an extensive network of computer cables, dating back to the first computer systems in the late 1970s. As new systems have come in, cables have been added. At one time, there was one cable per computer terminal; but they are much

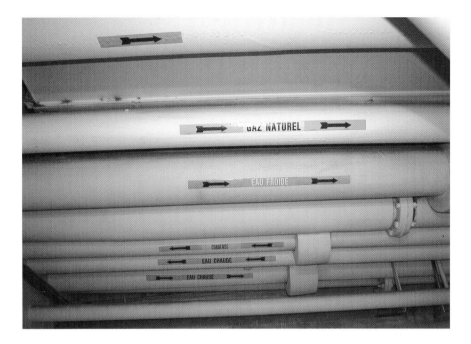

more organized now, following "main roads" in bundles through specialized tunnels and closets, and only hiving off near the equipment they serve. As with cellular phones, wireless networks don't suit the hospital environment.

The old computer cables have never been removed. Neither has another lift, no longer used, in the D-Wing walls. Years of pipes, wires, and ducts have also accumulated. And no one recalls finding or removing the old pneumatic chute system. For the health-care archeologist, there is a lot of history in those old walls.

Water and natural gas are just two of the many essential supplies that circulate through ceilings and walls of the hospital buildings. Signs and arrows here indicate the contents and direction of flow.

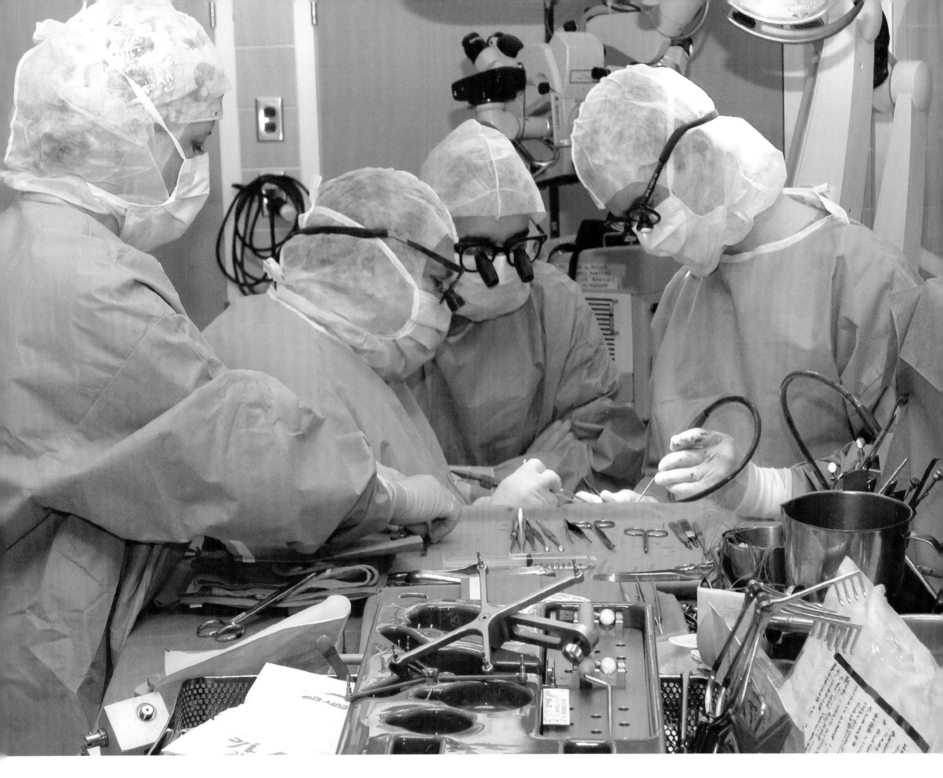

*Pediatric neurosurgeon Dr. José Luis Montes
(second from left) and the neurosurgery team have
a wide variety of instruments at their disposal.
Here they are operating on the patient's
hypothalamus, located in the centre of the brain.*

"The most useful piece of technology I've ever used? My hands!"

Dr. Preston Robb, Neurologist-in-Chief,
Montreal Neurological Hospital, 1968–1976,
associated with the Children's for 40 years

9

High-Tech Complements High-Touch

When the Children's Memorial Hospital first opened its doors, the physician's little black medical bag included just a few simple instruments: a stethoscope, an otoscope, a tongue depressor, and a thermometer. For diagnosing, he relied on his training and experience, and for treatment, on basic care, rest, and hope.

Today's hospital bedside tools include a variety of monitors, life-supporting respirators, and intravenous drips. Portable devices allow many chronically ill children to be treated at home. Sophisticated laboratory tests and million-dollar scanners are used to formulate diagnoses. Operating rooms are equipped with banks of monitors that keep track of blood pressure, blood oxygen levels, and other vital signs. And all hospital services, from the registration desk to the pharmacy, are computerized.

Patients of the MCH have benefited from a variety of technological improvements, from state-of-the-art devices such as an artificial heart imported from Germany, to new treatments for broken bones and innovative applications of video-conferencing equipment. Technological milestones achieved at the Children's include the first therapeutic heart catheterization in Canada in 1966, the first cochlear implant in a deaf child in Quebec in 1986, and the first magnetic resonance imaging (MRI) machine in a pediatric setting in Quebec in 1994.

These and other developments have had an enormous impact on patient outcomes, making it possible to treat conditions that were once inevitably fatal. But while technological advances have improved diagnosis and treatment, they have also increased the complexity of the health professions and the depth of skill required to meet ever-evolving standards of care. Professionals require many years of training to learn and apply these techniques, procedures, and technologies. Furthermore, many technologies such as life-saving devices or drugs and new genetic interventions have created ethical issues far different from those encountered just half a century ago.

THE EARLY DAYS

In his 1959 autobiography *Small Patients*, Dr. Alton Goldbloom wrote that, with few laboratory tests available, and not always accurate, the diagnostician had to rely on his training and his acumen:

"His sharp eyes would recognize a rare or familiar disease at a glance, he could pick out the one or two pink spots on a thigh or abdomen that would at once tell him that his patient had typhoid fever and, long before the Wassermann reaction, could recognize a blotchy pinkish rash as the sign of syphilis. His trained hand with 'an eye at the tip of his finger' could in a moment locate a tiny mass in the abdomen and determine its nature with uncanny accuracy. His trained ear could pick up a cavity in the lung 'the size of a hazel nut, *with the shell on*,' as Osler wrote of a colleague of his time. His nose could smell typhoid or diphtheria."

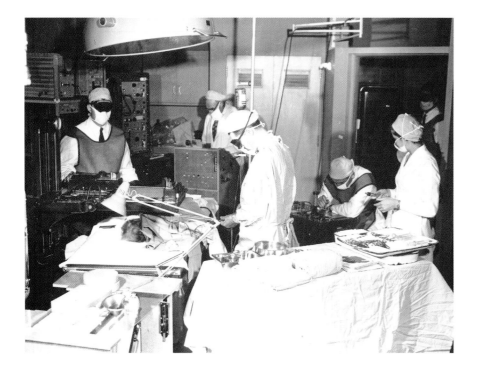

This old operating theatre in the CMH, circa 1950, appears stark compared with the well-equipped operating rooms of today.

possible to supply required fluids simply by inserting a tiny needle into the child's vein.

Blood transfusion was done directly: the blood was withdrawn from the donor and given immediately to the child. Mary Wilson, Assistant Director of Nursing Education in the 1930s, recalled, "as the blood came from the donor, it was collected in a glass container with citrate. This had to be stirred until the doctor was ready to put it into the vein of the receiver. As a probie, I was given the job on one occasion to do the stirring. I remember the feeling of nausea and faintness to this day, but I managed not to spill the blood."

"A pediatrician in those days always carried in his bag a small knife (to open the eardrum) and in ordinary households he could deftly pierce an eardrum literally in a fraction of a second, giving the suffering child instant and effective relief. The pediatrician in training had ample opportunities for piercing abscessed ears. On the wards and in the outpatient department it was an ever-recurring, daily experience. Because of the tiny size of the ear canal and the difficulties of adjusting and using the conventional head mirror with its reflected light, a simple and highly useful electric otoscope had come into use, equipped with a magnifying lens which brought the eardrum clearly into view despite the wiggling of the baby. This instrument, basically unchanged from the original models, is familiar to every mother who takes her child to a pediatrician. The ear specialists of the day, however, frowned on this new device; it made the esoteric far too simple."

Dr. Alton Goldbloom,
Physician-in-Chief, 1946–1953
Small Patients, 1959

In the 1920s, Dr. Goldbloom recalled, "Any laboratory examinations beyond the very simplest were made through the courtesy of one of the larger hospitals. An ancient X-ray machine, operated usually by the intern, was used for the comparatively infrequent pictures that were taken. Occasionally the plates (and later the films) were sent to the roentgenologist of one of the large hospitals for interpretation." In 1931, the Children's Memorial received badly needed new X-ray equipment that enabled it to carry out most procedures in use at that time.

For the most part, early hospital equipment was not only manually operated, but also cumbersome. Many devices were developed first for adults, then adapted for children; needles, catheters, X-ray machines, and anesthetic devices had to be sized and calibrated for small bodies whenever possible.

In the hospital's earliest days, fluids and medication had to be administered by repeated injections. After a New York pediatrician designed the intravenous drip in 1931, which enabled the continuous infusion of fluids, minerals, and sugars, it became

RESPIRATORY TECHNOLOGY

A terrible polio epidemic that struck Montreal in 1932 inspired desperate hospital staff members to innovation. The iron lung had been developed in the United States several years earlier to save the lives of patients with paralytic respiratory complications from polio, but there were no iron lungs available in Montreal. So Dr. Howard Mitchell, the general superintendent, and Tom Wright, the hospital carpenter, constructed a coffin-shaped respirator out of wood. It was so effective that the Nuffield Foundation in England adopted and modified the design, and shipped new models around the world for emergency use.

Children with polio also required physiotherapy, which was very difficult with these early respirators since the child's entire body was encased in a wooden box. The physiotherapist would remove the child from the respirator for a few seconds to work on an arm or a leg, but the child had to be returned to the respirator quickly in order to breathe. This difficulty prompted a very welcome technological advance in the 1950s: the Bird respirator, which enabled the child to breathe through a tracheotomy or nasal tube and freed him from the box.

The introduction of non-invasive ventilation technology in the 1980s revolutionized the field of respiratory medicine. Non-invasive ventilators are used on babies to avoid putting a tube down the infant's throat, and on chronically or acutely ill patients before trying more invasive procedures.

The BIPAP (bi-level positive air pressure) machine is a portable, non-invasive machine with a mask that can be used overnight to push air into the lungs of children suffering from a neuromuscular disorder that progressively weakens the chest. The machine can be fine-tuned to suit the child's size and the level of breathing assistance required. Although many of these children are in wheelchairs, they can now live at home thanks to this technology.

The next generation of ventilators appeared in the 1990s. These devices are made to assist breathing more gently, in order to minimize or prevent stiffness and damage to lungs from the constant pounding of the respirator, which had been serious side effects of earlier models. Computers now control the way all ventilators deliver each breath.

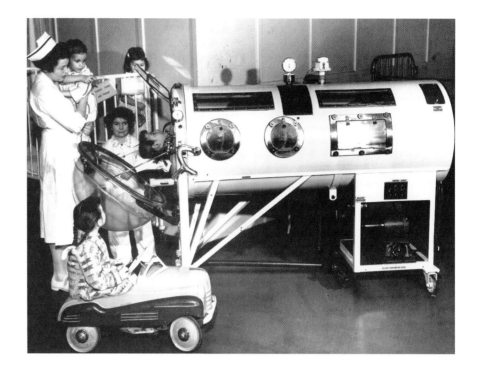

New high-frequency ventilators have proved beneficial for premature babies, whose lungs are often very stiff and can't take in normal volumes of air. High-frequency ventilators provide 500 to 600 very small volume breaths per minute, compared with 20 to 30 larger breaths a minute from normal ventilators.

Many other advances occurred in the field of respiration in the 1980s and 1990s. For example, diagnostic machines can test lung capacity and other measures of lung function, or determine whether a child has asthma.

This artificial lung machine, or iron lung, shown in a 1953 photo when the hospital was on Cedar Avenue, was used to help children paralyzed by polio and unable to breathe on their own.

ONDINE'S DISEASE

In 1986, surgeons at the Children's implanted a phrenic nerve pacemaker in Benoît, a 22-month-old baby suffering from Ondine's disease. In this genetic disease, the central nervous system fails to control breathing during sleep or when the person is concentrating on something other than breathing. The phrenic nerve, which normally tells the diaphragm to contract and relax, does not receive the stimulus from the brain to cause breathing to occur.

The pacemaker was developed in the United States in 1974, but Benoît was the first Canadian child to be treated successfully. Since then, the MCH has continued to be a leader in this field in Canada and currently has nine patients fitted with this device.

Before this approach was developed, says respiratory physician Dr. Michael Davis, the babies died the first time they fell asleep. If a newborn's sibling had died of this disease, that newborn would be checked immediately at birth, and if also affected, would be placed on a mechanical ventilator. Now the phrenic nerve pacemaker allows these children to lead normal, active lives during the day. While they sleep, a home ventilator helps them breathe so the phrenic nerve can rest.

The pacemaker consists of a receptor, a single electrode that touches each of the two phrenic nerves (one on each side of the thoracic cage). A small radio transmitter, which can be carried in the child's clothing, sends a signal to stimulate the receptor, causing the diaphragm to move. This technology is also sometimes used on individuals with neck or high spinal cord injuries.

The pacemaker has its flaws, however. When Benoît was 15, he went on a school trip to an amusement park in Toronto. His signal generator failed when it got soaked on the log splash ride, and his ventilator was at home, so to keep him breathing regularly, his schoolmates sang with him all the way home on the bus to Quebec's Eastern Townships region.

IMAGING

Imaging equipment has come a long way from the X-ray machine acquired in the early 1930s. And while X-rays can depict infected lungs and broken bones, scanners now provide images of soft tissues as well. The hospital performed the first CT scan in a pediatric setting in Quebec in 1977, and shared its scanner with Hôpital Ste-Justine for five years. Since then, CT scanners have improved considerably, using less radiation and working faster. A test that once took half an hour can now be done in less than two minutes. Ultrasound, a painless imaging technique based on sound waves, has been in use at the Children's since 1980, primarily to examine the heart, kidneys, and abdomen.

In 1994, the MCH became the first hospital in Quebec to use MRI in pediatrics. "This was a huge advance because we could look at the spine longitudinally, rather than in cross-section, and see the brain and other organs in more than one dimension," says Dr. Gus ÓGorman, Director of Radiology from 1983 to 1999.

Clinical applications of MRI technology have expanded with the development of the modality.

SOLVING A MYSTERY

In the early 1930s, improved X-ray equipment allowed CMH doctors to solve a mystery that appeared with alarming frequency in Montreal and elsewhere: children were developing lead poisoning, but the symptoms were often subtle, and similar to those of a brain tumour. One child even underwent brain surgery before the correct diagnosis was determined. Some of the children showed characteristic signs of lead poisoning, such as stippling of the red blood cells, but physicians discovered that the most reliable indicators were X-ray pictures of the ends of the bones, where lead deposits cast dense lines. Eventually, the cause of the outbreak was also discovered: lead paint on toys, and in one case, paint from a chewed pencil.

A GIANT MAGNET

The MRI, paid for by private donations, was installed in late 1994. Most of the pre-installation work involved preparing the surroundings, or "envelope," for the machine. Consideration had to be given to its extreme weight, particularly as it was on the 3rd floor; to shielding it from radio frequency; and to keeping its electromagnetic field from disrupting other equipment in nearby labs and imaging facilities. (Caution is required: anything metallic can be quite forcibly drawn to the machine's giant magnet. People going into the MRI room must remove metal objects such as watches, jewellery, and even artificial limbs!) The machine was hoisted by a huge crane and set into place from above, and had to be carefully aligned before being sealed into place.

New software has made it possible to see a wider variety of pathologies and to gather more information about them. It has also become an important tool for the surgeon. Information from the MRI—about the location of a tumour, for example—is stored in a computer, to which the surgeon's tools are also connected. As pieces of tumour are removed, the surgeon can gauge the distance to healthy tissue by checking on a display screen.

SURGERY AND ANESTHESIA

Advances in anesthesia and monitoring have gone hand in hand with new surgical techniques to make procedures better and safer. Ether, first introduced in 1846 as a highly effective anesthetic, was replaced decades ago by other agents. Some are inhaled, others given intravenously. All are safer and have fewer side effects than ether.

Fifty years ago, the anesthesiologist monitored the anesthetized child with a stethoscope to check the loudness of the heartbeat and quality of the breath-ing, a finger to check the strength of the pulse, and an eye on the child's colour. Today, sophisticated non-invasive monitors measure the blood oxygen level and the adequacy of the child's breathing and circulation.

The Stephen-Slater non-rebreathing valve, an important innovation in pediatric anesthesia, was developed at the CMH in 1948. It was initially devised by Dr. Harry M. Slater and Dr. Morton Digby Leigh, the first pediatric chief of anesthesia at the Children's. Later, Dr. Slater collaborated with Dr. C. Ronald Stephen to redesign it, and the new model became known as the Stephen-Slater valve. The significance of this device, which was adapted from valves used by underground miners, was that it could prevent a child who was breathing sponta-neously from rebreathing expired gas. Dr. Slater, who had a particular interest in anesthetizing children for dental surgery, also invented an inhaler that looked like a familiar telephone handset. It induced anesthesia smoothly and did not cause excessive anxiety.

ANESTHESIA BRINGS MAJOR ADVANCES

Since the 1970s, short-acting anesthetics have changed the way most pediatric surgery is handled. In the mid-1950s, day surgery at the Children's was restricted to children requiring dental restora-tion. Today, three-quarters of the surgical caseload is performed on an outpatient basis. This is due to the availability of short-acting intravenous or inhaled anesthetics, allowing rapid recovery from their effects.

Anesthetics are also used to sedate children when necessary in non-surgical and therapeutic procedures such as in oncology. While every effort is made to avoid or minimize sedation in children, sometimes it is essential that a child be perfectly still to obtain a reliable diagnostic result without inflicting pain. Sometimes anesthetics are also used to treat chronic pain.

NEW TOOLS OFFER GREATER PRECISION

Lasers became available about 30 years ago and the Children's was one of the earliest hospitals in Canada to use this new technique. In plastic surgery, they were used primarily in the early days to remove birthmarks known as port wine stains. Now they are used by a number of surgical specialties including ENT (for treatment of vocal cord growths), neurosurgery, and others. Over the years, lasers have improved such that they leave almost no scars.

In the early 1990s, general surgery was revolutionized with the introduction of laparoscopy, which significantly reduced the invasiveness of many procedures and also contributed to the development of

MICROSURGERY AND MINIATURIZATION

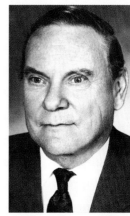

In the early 1970s, plastic surgeon Dr. Bruce Williams (now Surgeon-in-Chief) pioneered the use of microsurgery at the Children's. The first microsurgical procedures were to repair tiny arteries and veins in children who had accidentally lost fingers, or even hands. Dr. Williams made important contributions to the field with his research on the internal anatomy of nerves, ensuring that re-attached nerves would provide feeling and movement. He also pioneered the use of a pulse generator, a device implanted in muscle to keep it stimulated and healthy until the nerve grows back.

Surgical microscopes have become brighter and more powerful, says Dr. Williams, noting the latest models can magnify vessels up to 40 times. They are also much easier to manipulate, and allow several people to observe the surgery simultaneously. Microsurgery has also benefited from the development of miniature versions of tools such as scissors and clamps, and of finer suture materials.

PULSE OXIMETER

A simple device called a pulse oximeter has made it easy for the anesthetist to assess whether there is adequate oxygen in the blood during surgery. Attached to a finger or thumb, it monitors oxygen levels at all times. It is used in microsurgery to make sure the blood is circulating in re-attached vessels. In respiratory medicine, it can also be used to check whether a child suffering from severe asthma has enough oxygen in the bloodstream.

day surgery. In laparoscopy, the surgeon makes a pair of small incisions and inserts a flexible tube in each. One tube—the laparoscope—has a light on the end, the other a surgical instrument. This minimal-access surgery, used primarily on the colon, appendix, and hernias in children, is much easier on the patient and promotes faster recovery.

CARDIAC SURGERY

One of the MCH's great strengths is cardiac surgery. Miracles are made possible, not only by the hospital's team of surgeons and other professionals, but also by the technology which keeps patients alive during operations and in intensive care.

The hospital led the way in 1938 with the first operation in Canada to repair a congenital heart defect. Then, in 1946, Dr. Arnold Johnson performed the first cardiac catheterization in Canada at the CMH. In this procedure, a catheter, or tube, is inserted from an artery or vein in the leg into the heart, and a dye injected so an X-ray can identify a defect.

By 1957, after the hospital moved, the cardiac team had equipment that enabled them to induce hypothermia to cool a patient's body to 30°C, arresting the circulatory system for five minutes—just enough time for the surgeons to do their work. The acquisition of a newly invented heart-lung bypass machine, which takes over the functions of the heart and lungs, allowed open-heart surgery to be successfully established at the MCH in 1958. The use of heart-lung bypass technology eventually supplanted hypothermia in heart surgery.

Until the mid-1960s, cardiac catheterizations were used to establish diagnoses, by obtaining blood pressures in the heart or oxygen saturation levels, for example. In 1966, MCH cardiologist Dr. James Gibbons performed the first therapeutic, or interventional, heart catheterization in Canada on a patient of any age. The patient in this case was a baby with transposed great arteries of the heart. The baby appeared blue because there wasn't enough oxygen in the blood circulation to his body. Using a catheter, Dr. Gibbons enlarged a small existing hole in the heart to allow for better mixing of red and blue blood, so that the baby could survive until he was old enough for surgery. In 1966, surgery on newborns was not possible, and that meant a wait of six to 12 months. Today, cardiologists perform a similar catheterization procedure, then operate to switch the position of the arteries before the baby reaches four weeks of age.

When Dr. Christo Tchervenkov joined the hospital in the mid-1980s, he brought with him techniques learned at the Boston Children's Hospital. For the first time, newborns and infants were able to undergo reparative heart surgery directly, without waiting until they had grown, allowing them to develop more normally and reducing the disruption, stress, and cost of multiple procedures over several years.

Improved diagnostic equipment arrived on the scene in the 1970s and early 1980s, with Doppler technology for echocardiography, for example, that lets the cardiologist visualize the anatomy of the heart and watch the blood move through the heart structures. With non-invasive techniques available, the need for catheterization as a diagnostic tool decreased. However, therapeutic catheterization is increasingly being used for procedures such as closing holes or abnormal connections in children's hearts with miniature, umbrella-shaped plugs or coils. Such interventional catheterizations often save children from having to undergo heart surgery.

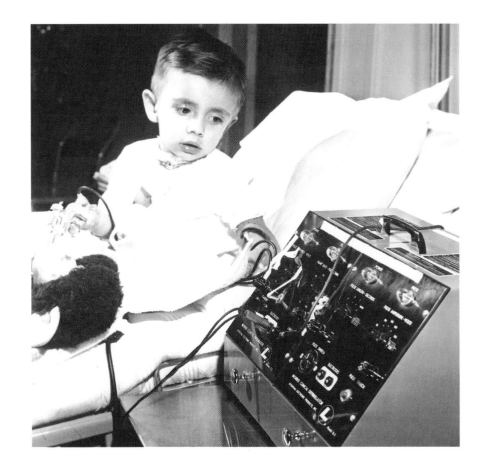

In 1994, the Children's became the first hospital in Quebec to use another diagnostic tool in young children: transesophageal echocardiography. This technique involves putting a small flexible tube with an ultrasonic device down the esophagus to visualize the heart. Pediatric surgeons find it particularly useful as a guide before and after surgery.

The combination of new life-support technology and innovative surgical procedures has saved many lives. Extracorporeal membrane oxygenation, or ECMO, a sophisticated heart-lung machine that can be used for prolonged periods, came along in the early 1990s, at about the same time as other developments in cardiac surgery. This technology, which can maintain the oxygen supply and pump blood safely for relatively long periods, was developed in

Gilles needed a pacemaker to maintain an adequate heart rate, so was inseparable from this large external pacemaker. He was three and a half years old at the time this photo was taken in 1958, several years before miniaturization allowed for internal implantation of pacemakers.

the United States for babies with life-threatening infections.

Initially, the Children's wanted an ECMO machine to help children with diaphragmatic hernias until corrective surgery could be done. In 1991, after considerable discussion between the government, the Children's, and Hôpital Ste-Justine about the value of the treatment, the Children's began a two-year trial of ECMO on the recommendation of the *Conseil d'évaluation de la technologie* that had recently been set up in Quebec. The trial program, led by Dr. Thérèse Perreault of the MCH, was successful, and the technology was subsequently adopted by both pediatric hospitals.

ECMO is now applied in different circumstances than originally envisioned. This technology makes it possible to maintain babies and children on a heart-lung bypass machine for several days after complex cardiac surgery, allowing the heart to regain strength and begin to heal from the surgical trauma. It also reduces risks in surgery to repair diaphragmatic hernias. When respiratory support is needed for newborns, however, ECMO has been largely superseded by newer medications and high-frequency ventilators.

Another recent advance in cardiology is the Berlin artificial heart. Developed in Germany, this external system provides assistance to a weakened or ailing heart and acts as a bridge until a donor heart becomes available, or until the heart recovers. MCH doctors successfully used a Berlin heart for the first time in Canada in a two-year-old child in 2002.

ORTHOPEDICS

With its roots in orthopedics, the Children's has remained at the forefront of spinal surgery throughout its history. One condition orthopedic surgeons treat relatively frequently is scoliosis, or curvature of the spine, caused by a variety of inherited or other factors. In the early 1960s, a young MCH polio patient who developed scoliosis became one of the first to have metal Harrington rods (named after the

ÉMILE AND THE BERLIN HEART

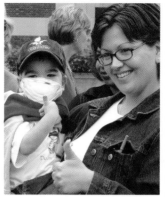

Two-year-old Émile's odyssey began in 2002 when his parents brought him to the MCH emergency room in respiratory distress after he had been treated for an ear infection. The doctors diagnosed acute viral myocarditis and put him on the waiting list for a new heart, but Émile's particular blood type made finding a match very difficult. He needed immediate help if he was to survive the expected long wait for a transplant.

For the first 17 days, Émile's heart was supported by the ECMO machine. Then his doctors obtained permission to use the Berlin heart, even though it had not yet been approved for use in Canada. As soon as it arrived from Germany, doctors attached the device to the toddler. It kept him alive for 109 days until he received a heart transplant. A team of roughly 100 people, led by cardiologist Dr. Christo Tchervenkov, cared for Émile during his long ordeal.

Above, Émile gives the "thumbs-up" sign as he leaves the hospital in the arms of his mother, Sherley Grondin.

Texas surgeon who developed them) surgically implanted to keep his spine in the corrected position.

Since then, the technology has continued to evolve. "There has been a major breakthrough in terms of implants for scoliosis," says orthopedics chief Dr. François Fassier. The hooks that were used to attach the rods internally to the spine 20 years ago have since been replaced by more reliable clamps and screws. These attachments are so strong that the child is no longer encased in a body cast for weeks, as in the past, and can stand and walk within days of surgery. Currently, about 50 children a

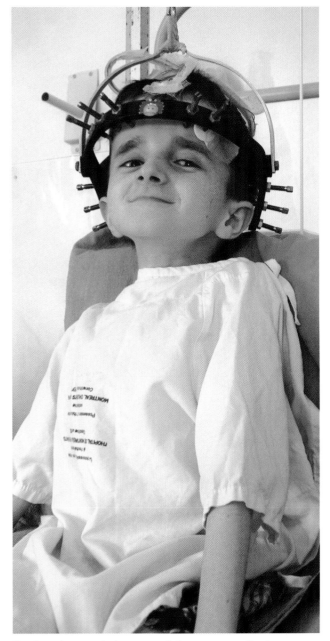

Justin, who was being treated for severe scoliosis (curvature of the spine) as a result of a genetic disorder called osteogenesis imperfecta, or brittle bone syndrome, was fitted with an apparatus he called his "crown." The device was attached to his skull by a series of screws and linked to a system of weights and pulleys, permitting tension to be exerted on his head and spinal column to correct the body as much as possible.

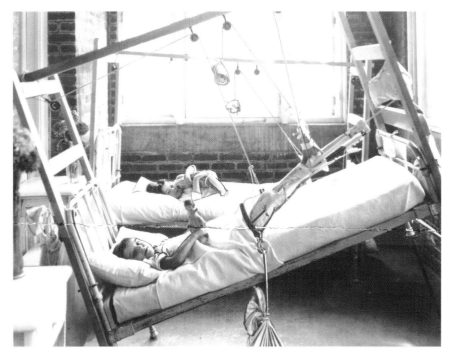

Elastic rodding is a new technique that has completely changed the treatment of fractures of the thigh bone or forearm. As recently as the early 1990s, such fractures required the child to be in traction for three weeks, then in a large cast for another three weeks. No more. A rod made of strong, but elastic, titanium is surgically inserted in the canal of the bone to hold it straight while it heals, and the child can return home within several days. The rod is later removed. This photo, from 1934, illustrates the traction endured by children with fractures before these advances.

year undergo surgery for scoliosis, while others are treated without surgery.

Several MCH orthopedists have also been involved in designing a software program called Scolisoft that they hope will lead to improved treatment options for scoliosis. The Quebec Scoliosis Network helped them set up a database of about 200 cases, including X-rays, photos, pre- and post-surgical analyses, and other clinical data. This information about how cases have been managed is made available to orthopedic surgeons to assist them in determining the best treatment for new patients.

In the 1990s, Dr. Vincent Arlet introduced thoracoscopy, an alternative technique in spinal surgery, to the MCH. In this procedure, the surgeon approaches the vertebrae from the front by making small holes between the patient's ribs. This is much less invasive than making a wide opening in the chest, and the procedure does not interfere with breathing or muscle function.

One key to the Children's excellence in orthopedics is its close collaboration with the Montreal Shriners Hospital, as the two centres provide complementary services and a multidisciplinary approach to care. For example, children with cerebral palsy undergo surgery on the spinal nerve to reduce spasticity at the MCH, and then have rehabilitation therapy at the Shriners. Dr. Fassier, head of pediatric orthopedics at both hospitals, has also performed complex bone-lengthening surgery in both settings.

NEUROLOGY AND NEUROPHYSIOLOGY

Neurology has come a long way from the day in 1935 when Dr. Herbert Jasper, of the Montreal Neurological Institute, looked at the electrical activity of the brain with an electroencephalograph (EEG machine) for the first time in North America. Early EEG machines had only four channels, says Dr. Bernard Rosenblatt, Director of the Division of Pediatric Neurology and the Department of Clinical Neurophysiology; today's models may have up to 120 channels, as well as digital readouts. Results are no longer printed on metres-long strips of paper, but appear instead on a computer which can identify unusual spikes in electrical activity or brain seizures.

The ability to monitor neurology patients has also improved. A child sometimes has to stay in the hospital for several days so doctors can see the form the seizures take and correlate EEG activity with outward behaviour. Around 1950, this involved setting up a 16 mm movie camera, an EEG machine, and a mirror, to record the patient in bed and the EEG machine readout simultaneously. Today things are much simpler. The computer synchronizes the video camera, microphone, and EEG machine, identifies possible seizures in the EEG recordings that may not be outwardly noticeable, and helps the neurologist

get through large volumes of data from several days of monitoring activity.

Different methods can be used to study brain activity. The EEG technician can place electrodes on the child's scalp or, in epilepsy surgery candidates, the neurosurgeon can open the skull and place a sheet with electrodes in a grid pattern right on the brain. This gives more accurate localization of those parts of the brain which generate the seizures. The head is closed and bandaged, and the child goes back to his room for several days of monitoring prior to surgery.

The neurologist maps the brain to identify areas responsible for essential functions, such as movement, sensation, and speech; if such an area is the source of seizures, it may not be possible to remove it. In one mapping method, somatosensory evoked potentials, the doctor stimulates a nerve (in the child's wrist, for example) and watches the grid to see which area of the brain responds, thus differentiating sensory regions of the brain from motor regions. This helps the surgeon avoid damaging regions related to movement.

In 1980, Dr. Rosenblatt founded one of the first evoked potentials labs in Canada devoted to pediatrics. This lab was equipped for evoked potentials in all sensory systems—visual, auditory, and sensory—and was the first lab in Quebec to do spinal cord monitoring of children who had Harrington rods implanted for scoliosis.

In 1992, the MCH became one the first hospitals in the world to place an electrode into a tumour in the centre of the brain. This made it possible to confirm that the tumour, growing in the child's hypothalamus, was the origin of his epileptic seizures. Although the tumour was not malignant, it was causing terrible behaviour, which disappeared when the tumour was removed.

In 1997, Dr. Rosenblatt and Dr. Ron Gottesman, Director of the PICU, collaborated with neurologists in the U.S. and Australia to identify seizures in infants, since seizures do not look the same in babies as in older children. Based on this data, Dr. Jean Gotman, at the Montreal Neurological Institute, developed the first commercially available software for detecting seizures in newborns.

PEDIATRIC NEUROSURGERY

Before the advent of new imaging techniques, neurology and neurosurgery patients were sometimes subjected to painful diagnostic tests. Until the mid-1970s, air or dye was injected into the spine or brain to create contrast between the structures inside the skull, which could then be recorded using X-rays. If the structure was not in the normal place, the neurologist inferred that something was pushing on it. These techniques were abandoned in the late 1970s when the CT scanner allowed the neurologist to see the actual lesion for the first time. Then after 1994, the hospital's MRI machine added new imaging possibilities.

The Children's got its first Cavitron ultrasonic aspirator in 1987. This machine, used to remove tumours from delicate tissues, emits high-frequency sound waves that pulverize tumours into a wet paste, then suctions them out. Neurosurgeons were the first to use this technology at the hospital. The Children's has had a succession of three Cavitrons over the years, as the technology has become more powerful and precise.

New technology in surgical drills has also made it much easier for surgeons to gain access to the interior of the skull. Today, says Director of Neurosurgery Dr. José Luis Montes, "we use high-speed drills and saws, and they have so many attachments that you can almost do designs in the bone."

The biggest risk in neurosurgery, says Dr. Montes, is that there is no margin for error: even a small mistake can cause paralysis. Here again, technology is reducing the risks. A new technique, neuronavigation, allows the surgeon to be more precise than ever, by combining information gathered through MRI prior to surgery and stored in the computer with images obtained during the operation.

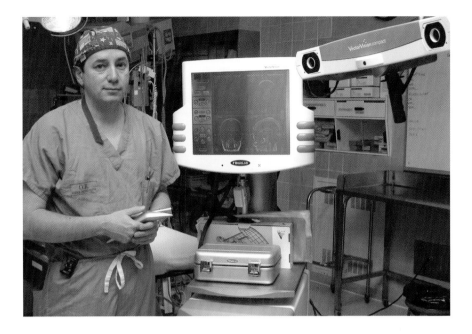

The surgeon uses a specialized wand—a mechanical arm linked to a computer—to map the brain. A sophisticated microscope, equipped with an antenna and a receiver, acts as a virtual pointer to guide the surgeon to the critical point. Neuronavigation is currently used to treat about 50 children a year at the MCH, mainly with epilepsy and brain tumours. Applications to navigate the spine are now available, as well as real-time correction updates with ultrasound.

The next development in pediatric neurosurgery will be the use of functional magnetic resonance imaging (fMRI) in the operating room. In fMRI, if the patient moves a muscle or thinks of a word, for instance, a hot spot lights up on the brain. The goal is to use this technology in the operating room to identify regions of the brain that control different functions. With the 2003 recruitment of neurosurgeon Dr. Jeffrey Atkinson, who specializes in this emerging field, the MCH is becoming a leader in applying this technology to pediatrics. The use of MRI scanning during surgery is becoming standard to assess complete mass of tumour removal or brain dysconnection in epilepsy.

Pediatric neurosurgeon Dr. Jean-Pierre Farmer demonstrates the neuronavigation equipment that helps him perform brain surgery with precision and lessens the risk of damage to healthy brain tissues.

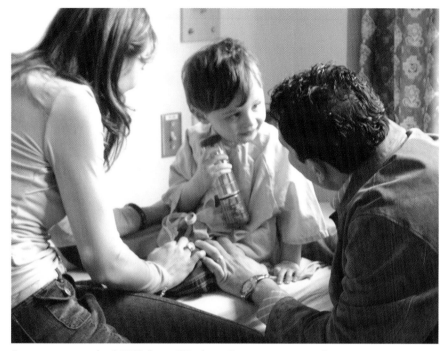

Lucas came to the MCH from Windsor, Ontario, in 2004 for surgery to remove a benign tumour in his brain. The tumour was attached to the hypothalamus, the brain's hormonal control centre, and caused an incessant stream of short-circuits that were preventing him from developing normally. He had up to 15 epileptic seizures a day.

Dr. José Luis Montes and his team carried out the highly complex and very risky operation. The tumour was melted using the Cavitron ultrasonic aspirator and the debris carefully vacuumed out. The team had to be extremely careful to avoid harming any of the healthy brain cells that surrounded the tumour.

Three weeks after surgery, Lucas was ready to go home with his parents, Dennis and Anita (above). He had stopped having seizures, and the slow restoration of his body's capacity to regulate his hormones had begun.

EXACT IMAGES

Dr. John Blundell, who retired as Director of Neurosurgery in 1990, assesses the impact computerization techniques have had on his field:

"Looking back, my sort of neurosurgery was essentially freehand. You had to have a very exact three-dimensional idea of the anatomy of the brain in the normal state and, if you were dealing with a tumour, in the distorted state. Now computerized images provide that information. It's a significant change."

PEDIATRIC INTENSIVE CARE AND EMERGENCY SERVICES

Intensive care is a relatively recent phenomenon. In the hospital's early days, intensive care basically meant intensive nursing. Today, patients and their families in the PICU are faced with an intimidating array of machines surrounding the child's bed, including a respirator, a cardiac monitor, and up to a dozen infusion pumps, each administering a different drug or nutrient. A child whose kidneys do not function properly may be on continuous renal replacement therapy (CRRT), a machine that provides slow, continuous therapy 24 hours a day. Members of the PICU team make every effort to help families, who are often a constant presence at the child's bedside, to understand and find reassurance in the technologies supporting their care.

Significant changes in recent years include improved ventilators and non-invasive monitors, as well as better drugs that maintain blood pressure, for example. These innovations support children recovering from surgery or suffering from acute illness. Meanwhile, the need for monitoring equipment has increased, because while more powerful drugs are available to control pain, they have potentially more side effects.

The hospital's high level of expertise in emergency care earned it designation as a tertiary care Pediatric and Adolescent Trauma Centre in 1993. In 2001, the crash room in the Emergency Department was renovated, and an overhead X-ray machine was installed that moves on tracks across the ceiling. The room is ready with oxygen masks, monitors to measure vital signs, IV pumps, heat lamps to warm a child in shock, and a defibrillator to restart the heart.

A recent addition to the Emergency Department is an image intensifier called a mini C-arm. When a child comes in with a broken arm, for example, this radiology machine allows the physician to check that he is setting the bones properly as he works. Until this machine was installed in 2004, the doctor had to manipulate the fracture, send the child for an

X-ray, wait for the X-ray image to arrive, and reset the bone if it wasn't done properly the first time, before putting on a cast. Now it is possible to see what is going on "in real time" and apply the cast immediately. This saves time, reduces the child's pain, and leads to more accurate care. Overall, it allows for better use of resources within the department.

The Children's has been providing innovative burn care since it opened the first pediatric burn unit in Quebec in 1971. Today, the Emergency Department treats more than 200 burn patients every year. There is no longer a separate burn unit; children with severe burns go into special beds in the PICU. The majority of burn victims are now treated on an outpatient basis, partly because the number of severe burn injuries has markedly decreased, not only in Montreal, but across Canada. Also, burn dressing products have improved. With the traditional treatment, the burn area requires daily cleaning and dressing changes. The new dressings, made of a silver-coated nylon fabric, only require changing every four or five days, thereby reducing pain and stress for the child. In addition, these dressings are less bulky so the child can move about more freely, and they allow for better air circulation, which promotes healing and results in fewer infections.

NEONATAL INTENSIVE CARE

Nurse Marguerite Bateman recalls the early treatment of premature infants in the 1940s and '50s: "We had two wooden boxes with a lid that lifted up and an electric light bulb continuously on to provide warmth. We made jackets of cotton wool and gauze to keep the heat in ... Our orders were to handle the babies as little as possible, and it was necessary to feed them by dropper ... Only the determined ones survived."

Newborn medicine saw a major advance in 1958, when Dr. Robert Usher, at the Royal Victoria Hospital, came up with a way to give intravenous fluids to tiny babies. In the late 1950s, Dr. Usher,

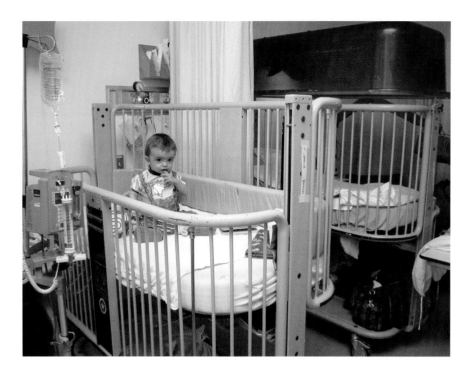

then a research fellow (and later director of neonatal intensive care at the RVH for more than 30 years, as well as a staff member at the MCH), discovered that premature babies with respiratory distress syndrome died, not simply of respiratory failure, but of a metabolic disorder when the potassium levels in their bodies rose to toxic levels. He also discovered that giving intravenous fluids was a very effective way to prevent these deaths. However, it was impossible at that time to give premature babies intravenous fluids over prolonged periods. The needles available were too large, too long, and too straight.

"In order to administer fluids to babies as small as one and a half pounds, a needle was developed, according to my design, by Mr. Hassell, the instrument shop engineer at the Royal Vic," says Dr. Usher. "It was of small calibre, short, and curved, so that it would lie flat on a baby's scalp." The "Usher needle" came into wide use everywhere, whenever a small baby required intravenous fluids. "It is very simple but it has saved a lot of babies' lives," says MCH neonatologist Dr. Louis Beaumier.

The rounded sides on these new cribs, such as the one occupied by young Gabriel, are a major improvement over the old, rectangular cribs: when lowered, they allow staff to reach babies and toddlers from more than one angle.

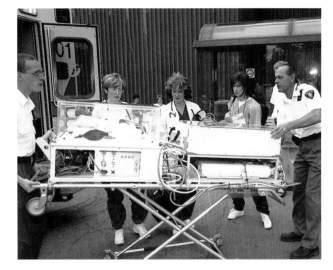

Members of the neonatal transport team use a specially designed stretcher, equipped with an incubator, a ventilator, and monitors, when they need to bring a sick baby to the Children's. Pictured (left to right): an Urgences Santé attendant; Pat Leroux, neonatal transport nurse; Claudette Lefebvre, respiratory therapist; Diane Lalonde, nurse educator, transport/outreach; and another Urgences Santé attendant.

When a call comes in asking for the Children's to pick up a sick baby from a referring hospital, a nurse and a respiratory therapist from the NICU are ready to go, equipped with one of three specially designed transport incubators. These incubators can't be ordered off the shelf. Designed in 1990 by MCH staff and ambulance service provider Urgences Santé, each unit consists of an incubator with built-in monitors, a portable ventilator, and other equipment, all sitting on a folding stretcher that can be loaded into an ambulance. This equipment allows the team members to stabilize the infant right away, rather than having to wait until they reach the Children's.

Incubator technology has also advanced in recent years. In the hospital's NICU today, incubators automatically provide sick babies with controlled heat and humidity. If the baby is cold, an overhanging radiant heater provides warmth, and if the baby has a fever, the incubator cools down. Monitors check the infant's pulse and oxygen levels, making frequent heel pricks for blood samples a thing of the past. In addition, new micro-technology methods, which allow the lab to do several tests with a very small sample, minimize blood loss.

New ventilation technologies, along with the use of surfactant (an agent that makes the lungs more elastic) and nitric oxide to improve the lung function of premature babies, have had a major impact on the survival rate of premature infants. In the late 1990s, high-frequency ventilators came into use in the NICU, although conventional ventilators are also still used.

ENDOCRINOLOGY

The most important technical advances in endocrinology have been in the treatment of diabetes, says Physician-in-Chief and endocrinologist Dr. Harvey Guyda, adding that, again, the Children's is leading the way. Since almost all of the hospital's diabetic patients require insulin, the hospital opened a new Insulin Pump Therapy Centre in April 2005, the first comprehensive resource of its kind in Quebec.

In the 1960s and '70s, controlling type 1 diabetes meant at least two insulin injections a day, but the trend was towards three or four. When Dr. Alicia Schiffrin came to the MCH in the 1980s, she took the first step towards continuous subcutaneous insulin delivery in an experiment in which some patients left a needle under the skin for several days at a time and delivered insulin through an attached catheter.

About 10 years ago, the insulin pump was introduced. This computerized device, about the size of a pager, delivers a steady infusion of fast-acting insulin. Not only does it better control fluctuations in blood sugar, it vastly improves the patient's quality of life. The child can click the device for more insulin as required at mealtimes, and adjust insulin levels when engaging in sports or otherwise physically active.

Nurse-educators at the Insulin Pump Therapy Centre teach patients and their parents how to use the pump, and respond to phone queries about technical matters. A minimum of education is necessary to use the pump, and it is not for everyone: patients who have learning problems, eating disorders, or who do not need to monitor their blood glucose frequently are among those who are not encouraged to use it. About 45 patients from all regions of Quebec, or 10% of the hospital's diabetic population, currently use this device, and it is becoming increasingly popular.

Great progress has also been made in blood glucose testing devices. At one time, testing meant sticking a needle into a fingertip several times a day. Now the needles are so fine they don't hurt, and glucometers are so sensitive they can check glucose levels in just microspots of blood. Furthermore, with an appropriate software program, they can be linked to computers at home to show a graphic analysis of blood glucose levels over a period of time.

The diagnosis and treatment of other hormone-related diseases have also benefited from developments in lab technology and biotechnology. Tests using samples from blood, saliva, or urine can detect levels of specific hormones within hours, something which 20 years ago might have taken a week. Furthermore, labs can now manufacture synthetic hormones which are identical in composition to the natural form and safer to use than hormones derived from living sources.

SPEECH, LANGUAGE, AND HEARING

By far the most significant advance in the fields of speech and hearing was the introduction of the cochlear implant, an electronic device surgically implanted behind the ear that can create the sense of sound in someone who is profoundly deaf. The first Quebec child to receive a cochlear implant did so at the Children's in 1986.

The device consists of a microphone, a speech processor that selects and arranges the sounds picked up by the microphone, a transmitter, a receiver/stimulator that converts these sounds into electrical impulses, and electrodes that send these impulses to the brain. The device is usually implanted as soon as possible after severe deafness is diagnosed.

In 1990, a team from the Children's implanted another type of hearing device, a bone-anchored hearing aid, for the first time in Canada. This device,

which can be used in children born without outer ears or ear canals, conducts vibrations through the skull.

Therapists in the Speech and Language Department help children with hearing and speech difficulties learn to speak properly. Software introduced in the early 1990s helps speech therapists evaluate speech problems. This software, used to supplement the therapist's observations, is designed to evaluate voice samples and provide objective measures of pitch, among other things.

DENTISTRY

Advances in dentistry over the last century have been dramatic. In the late 1950s, high-speed drills replaced the slower models. Other improvements include new methods of placing implants to replace natural teeth and enormous advances in cosmetic dentistry. Today, a root canal treatment can be achieved in a painless half-hour session, and discoloured teeth can be whitened within a few hours. Panoramic radiographs show the whole curve of the jaw on one film, and teeth can be aligned without braces.

Dr. Stephane Schwartz, Director of Dentistry, suggests that the biggest advance was the development of white bonding agents in the late 1960s. When she started practising, dentists had to shape the cavity and fill it with amalgam. The cavity form itself held the filling in place. But nothing would stay in place when, for example, a shallow cavity was on the vertical surface of a front tooth. "Bonding was a real breakthrough," she says.

The hospital also sees many children who have lost teeth through accidents of various types. Today, fast and efficient bonding agents, implants, and recently developed biocompatible materials to help tissue regeneration allow dentists to reuse broken pieces to fix fractured teeth, and young accident victims to keep their smiles.

The central importance of mouth function to overall health is strikingly apparent in the results of studies carried out by Dr. Schwartz to improve the eating abilities of children with cerebral palsy (CP). She and several colleagues adapted an oral appliance from a European device and tested it on 20 Canadian children with CP. Its purpose is mainly to stabilize the jaw and so improve eating skills. Resembling an orthodontic appliance, it is made to measure for each child. Until it was developed, these children had to practise jaw exercises, supervised by a clinical professional.

Children in the study, ages four to 13, simply wore the appliance every night for a year. At the end of the study, they all showed improvement in overall health because of better nutrition, and most had experienced significant growth spurts. In addition, half were able to keep their mouths closed when at rest.

There were also some unexpected improvements: the children were better able to sit and move around, demonstrating the connection between oral position and body posture. As Dr. Schwartz observes, "It goes to show what the old song says is right: 'the head bone's connected to the neck bone, the neck bone's connected to the back bone …'"

PEDIATRIC OPHTHALMOLOGY

The technology used in pediatric ophthalmology has been greatly improved in recent years. When the MCH Children's Vision Centre opened in 1997, it was equipped with some of the most up-to-date equipment available to treat a number of conditions, from cataracts to cancer.

Cataracts (clouding of the lens) may be present at birth, or appear later on, and require prompt surgical removal. The development of miniaturized instruments made this procedure easier and safer, as small incisions can heal quickly. In the mid-1970s, when an instrument was developed that was less than 1 mm across and could simultaneously cut and suction out cataracts, the MCH was one of the first hospitals in Canada to use it. Most children treated for cataracts require subsequent therapy to ensure

they develop good vision and may need to wear contact lenses or glasses.

A new panoramic digital camera in pediatric ophthalmology makes it easier to document and manage several eye conditions, including retinoblastoma, a cancer of the eye. The Retcam 120, a wide-field digital imaging system, was acquired in 2000 at the instigation of Dr. Rosanne Superstein, a specialist in retinoblastoma. These tumours affect one in 15,000 children and are usually diagnosed within the first two years of life. Detected too late, they can cause blindness and death. Since about 1995, treatments have been developed using new combinations of chemotherapy and radiation therapy which have led to significant progress against this disease.

Like other cameras used in ophthalmology, the Retcam, which resembles a small, pistol-handled flashlight, can produce sharp images of the retina. But because this camera is digital, the ophthalmologist can also view and manipulate these images on a computer monitor, store them on a CD, compare them with subsequent images to monitor progress, and e-mail them for a second opinion. However, these cameras have not entirely replaced the old methods: ophthalmologists continue to make coloured pencil drawings of the retina by looking into the eye through specialized magnifying equipment.

The Retcam system is also used when the physician suspects a baby has been shaken violently. The telltale polka-dot hemorrhages in the retina are easily seen, and the images can be saved and printed for use in court, if necessary.

Fitted with a lens adapted for tiny eyes, the Retcam is also used to monitor improvement following treatment for retinopathy of prematurity, common among babies born before their eyes are fully mature. "Effective treatment of this condition, developed about 15 or 20 years ago, was a major advance in care," says ophthalmologist Dr. John Little. In the past, babies with this disorder went blind. Now, with early diagnosis, the condition is treated with laser surgery or with cryotherapy (a freezing treatment).

The surgical technique used to correct crossed eyes remains basically unchanged, although outcomes in older children (around age six and up) and adults improved after the introduction of a suture procedure, 15 to 20 years ago, that allows the suture knot to be adjusted after the patient wakes up and opens his eyes. Some other treatments, however, haven't changed much: the best treatment for lazy eye is still patching and glasses.

CLINICAL LABORATORIES

The hospital has 10 diagnostic laboratories, each of which plays a specialized role in identifying the disorders and diseases that affect the children who visit the hospital, and in marking their progress and recovery. The Biochemistry lab measures the amounts of glucose, protein, sodium, potassium, and other substances in specific organs to help diagnose and monitor diseases. The Hematology lab looks for abnormal numbers of different types of blood cells that may indicate conditions such as anemia, diseases such as leukemia, or the presence of infection somewhere in the body. Technologists in the Microbiology lab study microorganisms such as bacteria, viruses, and fungi, not only to identify those responsible for an illness and the agents that can kill them, but also to help control the spread of infection. Several of these labs, including Biochemistry, Pathology, and Hematology, have been in existence since the hospital moved to Tupper Street, while the Genetics labs, for instance, date from the 1970s.

Central Laboratories

Today, almost every stage of laboratory testing is automated and computerized. But just 30 years ago, medical technologists in the Biochemistry lab checked blood and urine samples the old-fashioned way: using hand and eye. Violeta Kramer, Manager of the MCH Central Laboratories and the MUHC

Genetics Laboratories, remembers that when she began working at the Children's in 1971, testing blood glucose levels meant boiling the blood sample in the test tube, adding a reagent to make it change colour, and then placing it in a spectrophotometer machine to compare it with a standard colour range. The sample turned lighter or darker, depending on the amount of glucose present.

An even more laborious process was the testing of liver enzymes for abnormalities that might indicate liver disease, such as hepatitis, or a liver that is over-functioning in reaction to a child's medication. The technologist had to mix the reagents from a kit, add a drop to a sample of blood serum (the clear liquid part of the blood), and click a stop watch. Each sample in the spectrophotometer had to be checked periodically over a 15-minute period.

In the 1980s, a single machine speeded up all these tests. The multichannel analyzer could test a tray of 32 samples at a time for various indicators such as blood glucose, creatinine (a measure of kidney function), and potassium levels. It graphed the readings, but the technologist still had to write them down and phone the physician with the results.

When the Biochemistry laboratory started to use dry chemistry in the 1990s, things really evolved. Today, each reagent comes already prepared on a separate slide. As each slide goes through the machine, it receives a tiny drop of a patient's specimen. The machine gives the results in a printout, highlighting any abnormal readings. It can also forward the results automatically to the physician.

Some tests have now become point-of-care procedures, done at the child's bedside or in the diabetes clinic, for example. The technologist pricks the child's finger, puts a drop of blood on a strip, and feeds the strip into the instrument. This machine, a glycated hemoglobin analyzer, is about the size of a bread-maker and can be wheeled to the clinic on a cart. The results are available right away, with no test tubes to label and no specimens to transport. If medication needs to be adjusted, this can be done instantly, cutting down on phone calls to patients after they have gone home.

Similar changes have taken place in recent years in the Hematology lab; however, this is one field where pediatric samples cannot be handled in the same way as specimens from adults. While the automated hematology analyzer can automatically prepare and stain slides when using a blood sample from an adult or older child, a small child cannot provide the quantity of blood the machine requires, so the technologist has to prepare about 75% of the slides manually. Then a laser beam inside the machine counts the different types of blood cells in the specimen, indicating the presence of any abnormal cells. A trained technologist still has to look at samples under the microscope, however, to make sure the cells, which are sometimes hard to tell apart, are identified correctly.

Immunology is concerned with how the immune system responds to allergens and infections. Major advances in the Immunology lab have all but eliminated the uncomfortable and sometimes risky procedure of skin testing in children to identify sensitivities. In the past, allergic sensitivity was tested by scratching the skin, putting tiny amounts of allergens, such as pollen, on the scratches and waiting to see which areas became red or itchy. Now the technologist programs a machine to test various allergens directly on a patient's blood serum sample. The results are faster and more accurate than skin tests and the process much less invasive.

TINY IMPROVEMENTS

Sometimes small improvements can have big impacts on safety. Such is the case with blood testing. Today, the needles used for testing are fine-calibre so they don't hurt the child, and they retract, reducing the chances a technologist will be accidentally stuck by a needle and exposed to a blood-borne disease.

Endocrinology

Endocrinology focuses on the body's glands and the hormones they secrete, which regulate everything from growth to blood sugar levels. Laboratory testing here is also evolving in a new direction, as the radioimmunoassay (a test using a radioactive substance to create fluorescence used to measure thyroid function and other hormone levels) is becoming obsolete. Handling and discarding radioactive substances have always carried significant risk. Now, most tests are done with chemically produced fluorescence. The result is accurate testing and a safer working environment for staff.

Pathology

In the Pathology lab, technologists examine tissue samples under the microscope to make or confirm diagnoses. Samples are sliced to the desired thickness by a machine, then placed on glass slides and stained. Since the 1980s, new electronic technology has greatly improved the capabilities of microscopes, not only for viewing but also for recording. In the past, hand drawings were used to show biopsy results; now accurate and detailed photographs are available. But some things have not changed: while a child undergoes surgery to remove a tumour, someone still has to run from the 10th-floor operating rooms to the 4th-floor Pathology lab with a tissue sample to determine whether it is malignant.

Renal Function Laboratory

The Renal Function lab does routine screening of urine samples of children from the inpatient wards, clinics, and ER. Bladder infections are fairly common sources of pain and fever in children, and emergency physicians find it quick and easy to rule them out as causes of these symptoms. The technologist puts a dipstick, coated with several different chemicals, into a sample containing at least a tablespoon of urine. The reagents on the dipstick react, indicating the levels of white blood cells, red blood cells, protein, acetone, and glucose in the sample. In the past, the technologist had to assess the dipstick results visually; now a machine reads the intensity of the colours produced and reports them in a printout. The computer sends the results directly to the physician. Microscopic examination of the sediment from the urine may be done to confirm dipstick findings. If observation shows there is infection, the sample can be sent to the Microbiology lab to grow a culture of any bacteria that are present, and test for antibiotic sensitivity.

Microbiology

The Microbiology lab is divided into two sections: Bacteriology and Virology. Although the lab has been around for many years, two people were instrumental in developing and expanding its role between the mid-1970's and 2000: Simon Sorger, chief technologist in charge of Bacteriology, and Patrick Quennec, chief technologist for Virology.

"Virology went from nothing to a lab that does all virology testing for the MUHC," says Dr. Jane McDonald, Director of the Department of Microbiology.

Children tend to have a lot more viral infections than adults, and the lab has specialized equipment to deal with them. Tissue culture facilities allow cells to be grown and maintained so the technologists can see what effects different viruses have on them.

It used to take several weeks to identify the type of respiratory virus affecting a child. Over the past 20 years, however, viral diagnostic techniques have become so rapid that now technologists aim to have the answer the same day. In some cases, molecular techniques are used, especially to diagnose common viruses that are usually relatively harmless but that can seriously affect children with suppressed immune systems.

The Bacteriology section of the lab is set up to identify bacteria that commonly affect children, such as pertussis, using classic microbiology techniques. A sample from the back of the child's throat, for example, is put on a Petri dish and the bacteria are

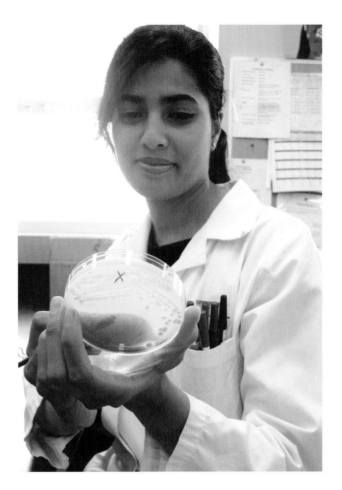

Laboratory technologist Kamal Patel examines a culture in the Microbiology lab.

allowed to grow. Although some procedures are more automated than in the past, most are done manually by skilled technologists. The lab's computerized information system disseminates results automatically.

Microbiology's role is not just diagnostic; it is also important in surveillance testing. For example, the hospital's infection control nurse looks for clusters of cases of *Clostridium difficile* (bacteria that cause diarrhea), or for *Staphylococcus aureus* that can cause wound infections, in order to control outbreaks. If cases of *Salmonella* (bacteria that cause digestive upsets) or other communicable diseases appear, the lab transmits the information to public health authorities.

Genetics

The genetics laboratories are the newest additions to the hospital's clinical diagnostic facilities. The Cytogenetics lab performs prenatal diagnosis, testing fetuses for conditions such as Down syndrome, associated with advanced maternal age; familial diseases such as Tay-Sachs; and, recently, an inherited form of deafness. The Biochemical Genetics lab examines blood or urine samples to test, for example, for essential enzymes or proteins that are missing in inherited metabolic diseases such as Tay-Sachs and thalassemia.

In the Molecular Genetics lab, in Place Toulon, technologists grow tissues, extract DNA from tissue samples, and study the chromosomes for defects. This approach helps identify not only what enzyme is missing, but what chromosomal abnormality is responsible for this condition. If a child is suspected of having an inherited disease such as cystic fibrosis, either because of the results of biochemical genetic tests, or because of symptoms, the Molecular Genetics lab always examines the chromosomes to confirm the diagnosis. When a child is found to have an inherited disease, family members—siblings, parents, grandparents, and sometimes others—are also tested to see whether they are carriers of the same genetic defect.

TRANSFUSION SERVICE

The Blood Bank, or Transfusion Service, as it has been officially known since the MCH became part of the MUHC, is the heart of the hospital, says assistant chief technologist Irene Lawlor, who has worked there since 1973. It provides blood products to children undergoing surgery, as well as children with anemia or who have suffered serious injuries, and others.

In recent years, attention to quality and safety in this service has become paramount. "We were always concerned about quality and followed the standards of the time, but now the level of standards has changed," Lawlor explains.

In the early days, blood products were kept in regular refrigerators. Now storage facilities are monitored and a central alarm goes off if the temperature deviates above or below the proper temperature. Satellite refrigerators in areas of the hospital that frequently need blood products, such as the operating room, are also monitored, and transportation times must be tracked to ensure these products are not out of cold storage for too long. If they are, they must be discarded.

All blood products are supplied by Héma-Québec, which took over this role from the Red Cross in 1998, and are screened by them for the presence of infections such as hepatitis. The Blood Bank stores these products and makes them available in the hospital. The recipient is tested for blood type, and a sensitive gel testing system is used to ensure compatibility between the donated product and the recipient.

In the 1970s, it was common for the recipient of a transfusion to receive whole blood. Today, the child gets only the products needed, whether plasma, red blood cells, or platelets, and only the minimum required volume.

Another relatively recent innovation is that, if their blood is compatible with the child's, family members are able to give blood for a child's surgery through Héma-Québec's directed donation program. To minimize risks involved in exposing babies and young children to disease via blood products from multiple donors, one donor's blood can be divided, whenever possible, into many small pedipacks, using a new sterile connecting device.

TELEHEALTH

Telehealth, a method of delivering health-care services at a distance through communications technology, originated in the early 1960s. It was adopted at the Children's in the late 1980s when MCH biomedical engineer Steve Retfalvi began working on a link between Baffin Island and the Children's to transmit electrocardiograms via modem. Other individuals worked on developing clinical applications from these technologies, including the late Quebec City pediatric cardiologist Dr. Alain Cloutier, who founded the Eastern Quebec Telehealth Network in 1992. "He got me interested," recalls MCH cardiologist Dr. Marie Béland, who has been caring for children in the North for many years. She saw the value in being able to see and discuss an echocardiogram as it was being done, rather than waiting for a tape to be shipped.

Encouraged by the work of Drs. Cloutier and Béland, and their colleagues from Sherbrooke and Hôpital Ste-Justine, the Quebec government set up a provincial telehealth program in pediatric cardiology in 1998. It installed equipment in 32 hospitals across the province, and in four referral hospitals where specialized pediatric cardiology services were available, including the MCH. Each site is equipped with cameras, microphones, and television screens so that patients and health-care professionals can see and hear each other and interact in real time. Participating hospitals were initially located in English- and French-speaking communities in Nunavik, Val d'Or, and the lower north shore of the St. Lawrence River, and the program has since expanded to involve more than 100 health-care facilities. The province pays for the infrastructure and for telecommunications charges, which may include satellite or landline links between health-care establishments.

Now Dr. Béland's pioneering work in telehealth cardiology has been expanded to other applications. MUHC telehealth services coordinator Madeleine St-Gelais, a former nurse-practitioner who worked in an isolated region of Quebec for 20 years, is helping people to apply the technology to many other purposes, including training and consultations in both pediatric and adult medicine.

Eleven rooms in the Children's have been hooked up to the provincial network to deliver telehealth services, including teaching and training sessions for professional teams working in remote or isolated areas. Operating rooms have also been cabled so

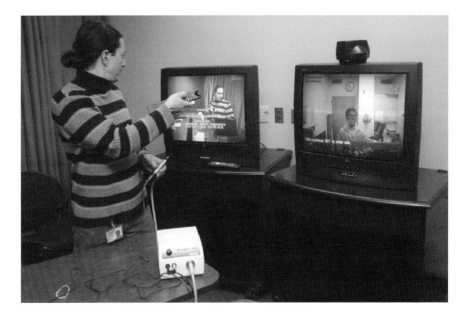

surgeons in outlying areas can learn new techniques without travelling to Montreal. A surgeon at the Children's can receive and respond to questions as a surgical intervention proceeds.

This technology is also frequently used for consultations. An MCH expert can not only discuss a distant case with the health-care team there, but can also see the patient—to evaluate a wound, for example. X-rays can be transmitted digitally. Other examples include a speech therapist who meets weekly via telehealth with a patient in Val d'Or, a social worker who coaches other social workers working with young patients with mental health problems in Nunavik or elsewhere, and a psychologist who provides weekly follow-up therapy to the families of children with feeding disorders in Quebec City. For families, teleconferencing saves time and money and reduces the disruption of routines by eliminating travel to Montreal for weekly one-hour sessions. (Read more about telehealth in Chapter 11.)

The uses of telehealth are limitless, says Johanne Desrochers, Telehealth Network Administrator. "We just have to have a bit of imagination." But telehealth is not appropriate for every situation. Some-

Laurent Soussana, MCH telehealth technician, tests the two-way video system to make sure everything is in working order.

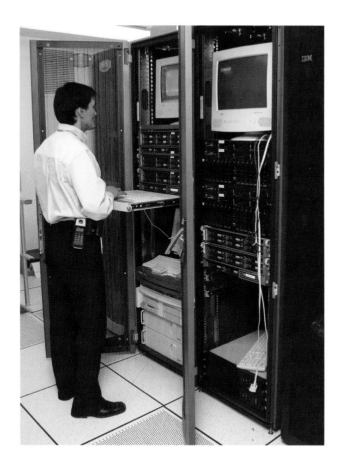

José Hernandez, site management team leader for network development and administration, in the room that he calls the "brain" of the hospital's computer network. This room houses the servers and routers.

times the quality of the image or sound is poor, and sometimes the health-care professional decides the patient should come to Montreal and be seen in person. Also, regional hospitals may not have the necessary resources in an emergency.

"The technical part is easy," Ms. Desrochers notes. "The hard part is to organize care around it to maintain the same standards of care.

"Telehealth is never a first choice. The first choice will always be human-to-human contact."

COMPUTERIZING THE HOSPITAL

The MCH first stepped into the computer age in the late 1960s when it rented time on a mainframe at the Royal Victoria Hospital for accounting applications. "You filled in forms, key-punch operators entered the data on punch cards, and the cards were

MEDICAL MULTIMEDIA SERVICES

Medical Multimedia Services coordinates telehealth communications. It was known as the Audiovisual Department when it opened in 1957. At that time, "magic lantern" visual presentations (large-format glass slides projected on the wall) were still in use. Soon, however, 35 mm colour slides replaced them. Photographers arranged presentations on twin slide projectors for teaching and conferences. Today's presentations incorporate everything from photos to animations and videos, all digitally mixed. Boxes of Letraset gather dust on the shelf, while the graphic artist does his job with the click of a mouse. In 2001, the department changed its name to Medical Multimedia Services.

sent by courier to the Vic," recalls Myer Kwavnick, former manager of Systems and Data Processing (now Information Services).

By 1978, computers had become somewhat smaller and affordable enough that it was time for the Children's to have its own mainframe. Known as a mini-computer, it was nevertheless still big enough that it had to be housed in a specially constructed room of its own. Now the operators were able to do away with punch cards and enter data directly into the computer. Because terminals were expensive and

EARLY WORD PROCESSORS

Former manager of Systems and Data Processing Myer Kwavnick remembers the days before personal computers were common, in the late 1970s and early '80s: "We had a very crude word processor on the mainframe computer. People would call on the phone and ask if a terminal was available, then come down to the computer room to type something. They would save the file in an account we gave them. We had a typewriter printer that— wow!—printed the text right-justified. There was only one font. People would take that copy, read it over, and come back to make corrections."

Technology has been applied to building maintenance and architectural services in the form of very sophisticated Autocad programs introduced around 1990. Computerizing all the architectural drawings and blueprints, and adding in the locations of all the wiring, ducts, vents, and plumbing helps staff manage essential functions of the hospital, from building security to infection control.

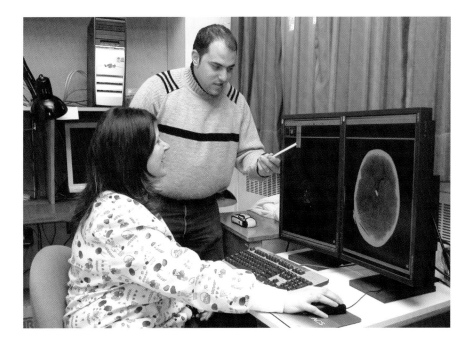

required lots of connecting wires, in the beginning there were only six in the whole building.

The MCH was one of the first hospitals in Quebec to use the computer for clinical applications. The first services to be computerized were registration, admitting, and clinic appointments, in 1978. Payroll came onstream in 1983. The following year, the OR, Radiology, and a number of labs were computerized. The Teddy Bear clinical viewer was also introduced, which allowed doctors and nurses to look up patients' basic information, lab results, and various other clinical information. Printers were installed on every ward and lab results were sent directly, instead of over the telephone, to avoid errors in communication. Security features prevented access by non-authorized personnel.

In 1985, computerization of the Pharmacy automated the calculation of dosages of medications prescribed in the ER and on the inpatient units. The ER was computerized during the same year, making it possible for the MCH to track its emergency visits.

The hospital's mainframe has been replaced twice, in 1992 and 2003, each time by a smaller and more powerful computer. Replacing the mainframe is a major event, says systems analyst Anna Badia. "We have to move over all the applications and make sure everything is running smoothly." And of course, all of this has to be done with minimal disruption to normal and vital hospital activities, meaning that it must usually be done during the night.

At first, the hospital's own programmers designed computer systems in-house to meet specific requirements. Because much of the clinical software being developed for hospitals in the 1970s and '80s was for the U.S. market, and hospitals in Quebec function in a very different context, it was generally not feasible to install ready-made programs from outside vendors. By about 1990, the technology had evolved so that off-the-shelf programs could be adapted to different environments, and the early 1990s saw the MCH acquire and implement, in quick succession, clinical applications for Medical Records, Laboratories, Radiology, and Pharmacy. As more such software became available, Information Systems staff spent less time programming and more on helping hospital departments determine their needs and shop for software, and then on adapting and maintaining it.

Despite tight budgets, the hospital was able to accomplish a great deal over a relatively short period of time, says André Rousseau, manager of Information Systems (now Information Services), Biomedical Engineering, and Telecommunications between

Domenico Loria (standing), an information specialist with Information Services, discusses the picture archiving and communication system (PACS) with PACS coordinator Manon Leclair. Introduced in 2004, the system eliminates the use of X-ray film and allows for images to be accessible to all professionals who need to see them, throughout the hospital and beyond.

1988 and 1996. For example, he recalls purchasing in 1991 an inexpensive software system for the labs from New Zealand that provided good service for more than a dozen years. Much of the hospital's software was also legitimately obtained for free by joining a group of Quebec hospitals using the same Hewlett-Packard technology and sharing their development work.

In 1996, several hospitals, including the Children's, formed a partnership with software supplier MediSolution to develop an outpatient appointment system which is now used across Canada.

In 2000, the hospital started to migrate to MUHC-wide systems. Future developments, such as the Clinical Information System, will ultimately lead to computerized patient charts. There will also be more clinical workstations so that attending staff and other members of the treatment team can enter their notes on the spot. Eventually, digital files will replace paper charts, although probably not before the move to the Glen campus.

The increased use of computer technology in clinical medicine offers significant benefits. For physicians, having laboratory reports and other test results delivered electronically means treatments can be started or adjusted more quickly. They can also use Internet access to look up information, such as the contraindications of a drug. Ultrasound, nuclear medicine, MRI, and X-ray images are readily displayed on computer monitors, where their levels of contrast and magnification can be adjusted for better interpretation. These digital images can be viewed from anywhere in the hospital, and if necessary, consulted by several doctors at once.

THE HUMAN ELEMENT

There is no disputing the fact that the trend over the last decade and a half has been to more technology, and particularly digital, in every facet of medicine. This trend will certainly continue, but nothing will ever replace an experienced doctor's intuition. Dr. Goldbloom wrote, "To be a good physician required long training and long experience, and to become truly great was given to only a few. Today, the laboratory makes the diagnosis in many cases, even for the less endowed physician. The patient, too, comes to rely on the test more than on the doctor. He will ask: 'What does the test say?,' not 'How do you interpret the results?'"

Former Executive Director Dr. Nicolas Steinmetz echoes Dr. Goldbloom's thoughts. "The big challenge," he says, "is not to allow technology to take over and drown out the human element."

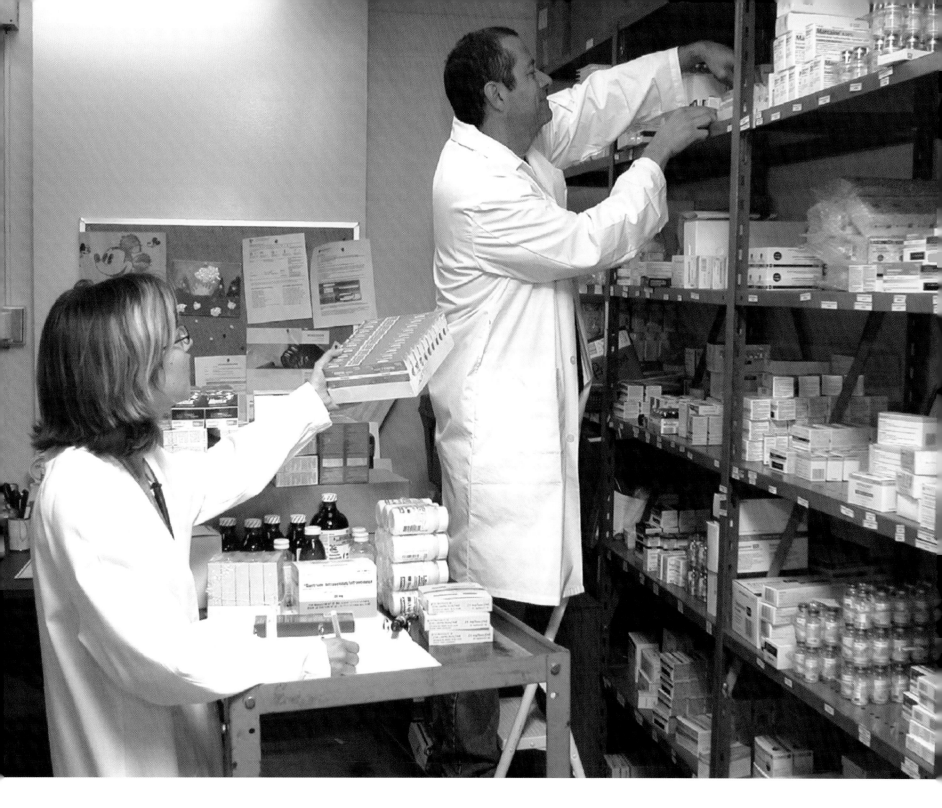

Resource allocation issues created by the rising costs of new drugs, technologies, and therapies are among the challenges facing hospitals as they enter the 21st century. One area of medicine that is evolving rapidly is the development of newer, more complex, and often more costly medications. Here, senior pharmacy assistant technicians Chantal Vermette and Serge Gauvreau stock incoming drugs in the pharmacy store room.

"At the MCH, our guiding ethical principle is the child's well-being.
We must always be asking ourselves: what is in the best interest
of each child, what *can* we do, and then, what *should* we do?"

DR. LOUIS BEAUMIER, DIRECTOR,
NEONATAL OUTREACH TEACHING PROGRAM AND TRANSPORT TEAM

10

Making Difficult Decisions Together

In the hospital's first decades, complex issues such as when to stop life support seldom came up because there were few such options. Also, because the hospital's population was relatively homogeneous, ethical issues arising from ethnic and cultural differences were uncommon.

But over time the community changed, as did medicine. As new technologies and drugs were developed that saved lives or had an impact on quality of life over the long term, increasingly complex ethical issues arose. Underlying many of these situations was the basic question: just because a treatment is available, is it in the patient's best interests to undergo it?

Two committees associated with the hospital have mandates specifically concerned with ethics. One is the Research Ethics Board (REB) of the Montreal Children's Hospital Research Institute of the MUHC Research Institute, which deals with ethics in research. The other is the Pediatric Ethics Committee (PEC), created in the mid-1980s to address issues concerning treatment of patients. At that time, there was increasing recognition of parents' rights to make decisions about their child's treatment, especially when it was a question of life support.

The hospital also has a clinical ethicist, a position created in 1984. Dr. Kathleen Glass, who has filled that post since 1997, explains that the job is multi-layered. Working with the PEC, the ethicist helps create policies that assist health-care professionals in making decisions about treatment options and procedures. The ethicist keeps up-to-date with new developments in biomedical ethics, shares this information with hospital staff, and accompanies doctors, nurses, and other clinical personnel through the more sensitive cases they encounter. She is also available to meet with patients and families. Anyone in the hospital, whether a patient, a patient's family, or a staff member, can call on the clinical ethicist for an ethics consultation. On occasion, a case may also be presented for discussion and advice by the PEC. The attending physician is always notified of any request for ethics consultation.

The PEC occasionally forms subcommittees on an ad hoc basis to investigate the need for policies and to develop them. For example, in 1992 the committee formalized guidelines for decision-making regarding the initiation, escalation, or withdrawal of treatment in complex, life-threatening situations. This policy was revised in 1995 and resuscitation guidelines were added in 1996. There are also policies on the type of consent required to take and use photos of patients, and on the use of blood products in treatment. This latter policy was developed not only in response to safety issues around blood products, but also because the hospital serves a number of families whose religion prohibits blood transfusions.

Every year, the PEC invites health-care professionals from throughout the MUHC to a one-day conference on ethical issues. Nurses, social workers, physiotherapists, doctors, administrators, students, and others hear presentations on themes such as involving the child in decision-making, dealing with religious issues, multiculturalism, and ethical issues in resource allocation.

The majority of problems arise out of difficulty in communication between health-care professionals and patients or their families. The second most common issue is waiting time to get an appointment, to have surgery, or to be seen in Emergency. All complaints are treated as confidential matters and are not documented in the patient's medical file. The people involved in the complaint are also involved in resolving it.

DIFFICULT CHOICES

The most difficult ethical issues generally surround the treatment of a critically ill child, especially when a positive outcome is not a foregone conclusion. Factors taken into consideration in treatment situations include the patient's preferences, medical condition—for example, would the proposed treatment definitely help, or could it

THE OMBUDSMAN

Whenever parents have a complaint about their child's care, they can go to the hospital ombudsman for help in formally resolving the situation. The MCH created this position in the 1980s, with the aim of helping families through the health-care system. In the mid-1990s, the provincial government decided that every hospital in the province should have an ombudsman. The official title then became Service Quality Commissioner, and in 2005 the government proposed changing it to Complaints Commissioner. "But we still refer to the ombudsman," says Elisabeth Gibbon, who has filled the position since 1992. "People feel comfortable with it, and they don't like to be labelled as complainers."

prove useless or even harmful?—and quality of life with and without treatment.

Cardiologist Marie Béland admits, "It is difficult not to intervene and to let nature take its course. A couple of times a year, there's a child who has been through a lot, been in the ICU for months. Knowing that the child will remain severely handicapped, we have to ask, when has the child suffered enough?"

Frequently the doctor decides to convene an ethics consult in this kind of situation. It might include 10 to 12 staff members, including the ethicist. They discuss the case and present alternatives to the parents, and when possible, to the child or adolescent, assessing with them the potential impacts of each decision.

In rare instances when the family and hospital staff disagree, says Franco Carnevale, the hospital's Critical Care Coordinator and Chairman of the PEC, "our goal is to do everything we can to understand where the family is coming from and find common ground, while at the same time to try to help the family understand where the hospital is coming from. We are bound by professional duties and responsibilities, but at the heart of the issue is always the best interest of the child."

CONSENT ISSUES

One of the most fundamental issues in ethics is that of obtaining consent for treatment. In Quebec, children must sign their own consent as of age 14. Many parents express surprise when their teenager has to sign a consent form prior to an operation, observes Dr. Bruce Williams, Surgeon-in-Chief.

Dr. Williams makes an effort to explain to even very young patients what will happen during surgery. "Children of four years and up, even a little younger, can understand and accept what is going to happen to them, and I always give them an opportunity to ask questions. They ask good, common-sense questions like, 'How do they put me to sleep?' or 'How long will the bandages be on?' These are important things."

CHRISTINE

The case of 11-year-old Christine posed the dilemma of whether to try to prolong a child's life. Christine underwent aggressive chemotherapy and the amputation of an arm to arrest her bone cancer, but, after 18 months, the cancer returned and spread to her lungs. Her parents insisted on additional bouts of treatment, despite the fact that her chances of full recovery were less than 20%. Christine, however, was self-conscious about her prosthetic arm and upset that she'd had to give away her cat because it posed a risk for infection. She refused further treatment. The nursing staff, who had seen her painful struggles during previous sessions of chemotherapy, were reluctant to pressure her into undergoing treatment.

Her health-care team felt Christine's ability to make decisions about her care was impaired by her high anxiety level and poor understanding of the reality of death. Nevertheless, Christine took part in discussions with her parents and doctors of various treatment options, and spoke with other patients undergoing similar experiences. Eventually she, her parents, and the health-care team agreed that discontinuing chemotherapy was a reasonable choice.

The focus of Christine's treatment then shifted from cure to care. Supported by the palliative care team, she went home, was able to enjoy a new kitten, and died peacefully.

Families are more involved than ever in making health-care decisions, he adds. "They read a lot, they know the possible complications, and they are involved in the child's care." Dr. Williams realizes that parents often remember only part of what he tells them, so he usually suggests they do some reading and research about the child's condition at home, then come back with questions.

Neonatologist Dr. Louis Beaumier emphasizes the importance of the parents' role. "We ask them to be very active and we inform them of how their child is and the potential prognosis." Most of the time, he

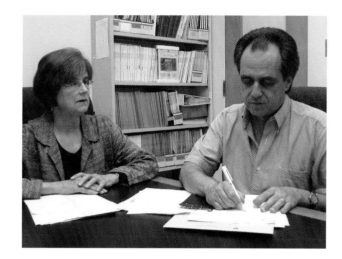

The hospital's clinical ethicist, Dr. Kathleen Glass, shown here with Dr. Franco Carnevale, Chairman of the Pediatric Ethics Committee, serves as policy advisor to the PEC and the Research Ethics Board, as well as consultant to hospital staff, patients, and their families.

says, everyone agrees to carry on with treatment. But sometimes parents have to choose whether to operate or not—if there is only a minimal chance of survival, for example, or if the child will be deeply handicapped afterwards. Then, he says, the difficult choice is up to the parents. "The quality of life differs for everyone and, as doctors, we cannot make that decision. We have to know what the parents want."

Sometimes, especially when the family belongs to a cohesive and supportive cultural group, the discussion involves more than just the family. One such case involved an aboriginal family. The parents listened to the pediatrician propose a course of treatment for their sick child, and then they returned home to ask the advice of their community's traditional healer. After he approved the procedure, the family agreed to let the treatment begin.

Hospital staff are careful to refrain from making value judgments about practices that differ from their own. In one case, Haitian-born parents insisted their child could not undergo medical treatment unless the curse that they believed was causing his illness was lifted. Working with the pastoral services and multiculturalism staff, the parents and the care team located a voodoo priest/shaman of the Haitian community who suspended the curse until it could

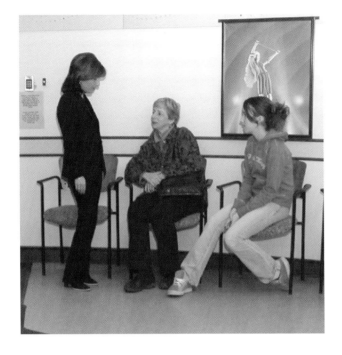

be entirely removed in Haiti. Then they were able to proceed with conventional treatment.

While there are basic guidelines, every case is different, and what is considered an ethical solution in one situation might not apply in another.

ETHICS AND MEDICAL RESEARCH

For many years prior to 1980, the Committee for Medical and Dental Evaluation of the Council of Physicians, Dentists and Pharmacists (CPDP) received and reviewed morbidity and mortality reports and research protocols. After the Children's became a founding member of the Pediatric Oncology Group in 1980, it became clear that the existing system did not give adequate attention to protocol review. In 1984 the Institutional Review Board (IRB) split off from that evaluation committee to concentrate on protocols, says Dr. Patricia Forbes, who chaired the IRB from 1984 to 1989. Initially, the IRB only reviewed protocols funded in the United States and followed strict guidelines set out by the American government, with particular emphasis on

informed consent. Gradually the IRB expanded its mandate and became responsible for all protocol reviews. The process eventually split into two components, scientific and ethical. The body that dealt with ethics was the Research Ethics Board (REB), composed of scientists, clinicians, an ethicist, a lawyer, and members of the public.

Every experimental procedure and research project involving children has to be approved by the REB before it can be carried out. First, the protocol is examined by three scientific reviewers who are experts in the field. If necessary, it is returned to the researcher for response and rewriting. Then it goes to the REB, which must be satisfied that the scientific review was well done. In their deliberations, the members follow guidelines outlined in the *Tri-Council Policy Statement: Ethical Conduct for Research Involving Humans*, issued by Canada's three research funding agencies, the Canadian Institutes of Health Research (CIHR), the Natural Sciences and Engineering Research Council (NSERC), and the Social Sciences and Humanities Research Council (SSHRC). The main principles underlying these guidelines are the minimization of risk and a well-balanced risk–benefit equation.

In reviewing each case, Board members first look at whether a study has both scientific value and validity: has it been designed in such a way that it will contribute to science in general and benefit children? They also try to determine whether the investigator has fully explained to the child and the family what the study's objectives are, what procedures are involved, and the potential risks and benefits. "It is parents who authorize participation, but both by law and according to ethics policy, children are supposed to have a say," says Dr. Glass. Since a child might agree to participate just to please the doctor or other authority figure, it is important that both the child and the family understand that participation in a research project is entirely optional, and that if the child or parent says no, their decision won't affect the care the child receives.

The REB also considers the protection of patient confidentiality. They look, for example, at how personal data is stored, and whether the research respects the hospital's policy on disclosure and consent. The issue of consent is particularly important in genetics research, when tissue samples may be taken and stored for future studies, or in cancer research, when tumour samples may also be stored for future use. If a sample can be identified as coming from a specific individual, that patient cannot give open-ended consent, but must at least specify that it is to be used for cancer research or health-care research.

Another ethical issue related to research involves patients on clinical trials that provide new drugs under study for free. The question is, when the trial ends, who is going to pay for the medication if ongoing treatment is needed, and will the institution continue the treatment if it is clearly working but the family can't afford it?

ETHICS AND GENETICS

Geneticists at the MCH have been working for more than 30 years to understand and interpret the mechanisms of genetic diseases, and to screen and counsel families at risk for those conditions, says Dr. Charles Scriver, Alva Professor Emeritus of Human Genetics at McGill University, and former director of the MCH's DeBelle Laboratory for Biochemical Genetics.

Dr. Scriver spearheaded a community medicine project in 1971 called the Quebec Network of Genetic Medicine. This project offered parents the option to take part in two screening programs, one for newborns, and one to identify carriers of certain mutations. Its aim was "to try to prevent disease, rather than wait for it to happen," he explains.

The newborn screening program is targeted primarily at phenylketonuria (PKU) and thyroid diseases, but also covers about 25 other conditions. Every mother is informed about the program and may refuse to participate, but otherwise the screening is part of standard health care for newborns.

The discovery that PKU-related mental retardation could be prevented through diet changed the medical community's approach to genetic diseases, Dr. Scriver notes. "It was the first genetic disease to respond to treatment. This changed the whole thinking of the medical world about genetic diseases. Before that, people felt that the die is cast, and there is nothing you can do about it. Now, newborns are screened for this disease around the world."

Parents and fetuses are also tested to see if they have genes that can cause Tay-Sachs disease and a severe form of anemia called thalassemia, both fatal conditions for which there is no cure.

As well as testing, the program offers counselling when a test result is positive. "Within the health-care system, people have access to reproductive counselling, prenatal diagnosis, and pregnancy termination if they so want," Dr. Scriver explains. While he admits that some people had concerns about this program when it was introduced, the people of Quebec accepted it, and he feels it was and remains ethically sound.

"It was an option for life," he says, noting that since the program has been in place, people who carry the genes for these diseases have married and gone on to have children, while the incidence of these two diseases has been reduced by 95%.

FUNDING DILEMMAS

Until the introduction of provincial Medicare, the hospital was faced daily with situations in which parents couldn't pay for their child's treatment. They were never turned away; hospital policy was to care for all children seeking treatment. Meanwhile, the community did what it could to support the institution.

Money, or the lack thereof, is still an important issue, and has been ever since the provincial government started tightening the health-care budget in the mid-1980s. Dr. Nicolas Steinmetz, Executive Director of the Children's from 1987 to 1995 and 2003 to 2004, recalls how the hospital struggled as costs rose steeply for pharmaceuticals and for acquiring, maintaining, and regularly upgrading biomedical equipment, while shrinking budgets made it difficult even to maintain existing staff and programs. Since the 1980s, because government funding for hospitals is for operating expenses only and does not include resources for capital expenditure, some of the funds raised by the MCH Foundation have been earmarked to pay for equipment. Even so, these technologies generally entail long-term operating costs that must somehow be covered within the hospital's annual budget (foundations cannot supplement operating budgets), so choices still need to be made.

During Dr. Steinmetz's tenure, the senior management team's approach to these difficult decisions was to have everyone responsible for providing a service at the hospital participate in allocating the budget. "Everyone made their needs, from their point of view, known. In the process, we included representatives from the parents. It was a large, unwieldy committee, but everyone was there. We heard everybody, we made a list of priorities, and then we made exceptions."

High priority services included emergency rooms, operating rooms, and intensive care units. It was hard to match these up against palliative care, a family resource centre, or pastoral care, but, says

ONGOING SERVICES

"Arguments have been made as to the ethics of saving lives in the Neonatal Intensive Care Unit if you do not provide the ongoing, long-term services these children need in areas such as speech therapy, psychology, or occupational therapy," says Kathryn Aitken, former Associate Director of Professional Services. "These decisions must be made in collaboration with other parts of the health-care system such as CLSCs and rehabilitation centres; the fact that the government forced all concerned to clarify their missions helped, but it was a painful process."

ETHICS AND BUDGETS

Resource allocation has to be a consensus-building process, and ethics is part of that process, says Dr. Nicolas Steinmetz. In the late 1980s, the hospital organized a one-day conference on the ethics of budget allocation, the first time such an event had been held in Montreal. Representatives of Quebec's Ministry of Health were among those who packed the amphitheatre.

Dr. Steinmetz, "regardless of where it falls on the priority list, an institution that claims to do all the things it does and be what the Children's wants to be has to have pastoral care. It's going to be funded, and we won't cut it to the point where it becomes ineffective. So you have to make those decisions if you want it to be an institution that does all the human things that people need, and not just medical interventions."

THE PRICE TAG OF PROGRESS

Kathryn Aitken was at the table when many of these debates took place. She was a senior director of the MCH for many years, first as Director of Hospital Services, then as Associate Director of Professional Services until 1997, in charge of labs, pharmacy, social services, medical imaging, rehabilitation services, child life, and other services. She recalls that professional and medical services were changing dramatically at the time, both in response to budgetary pressures, and as new scientific knowledge became available.

Some services, such as Occupational Therapy and Child Life, were able to reorganize and find ways of doing more with less. Others grew, despite the financial constraints. For example, it was becoming clear that nutrition plays a key role in children's health care, and the hospital had to increase its resources in Clinical Nutrition Services. Respiratory Therapy also expanded as new and better respirators became available, although these machines were very expensive. Even the trend to provide health care by multi-disciplinary teams brought additional costs, as someone had to coordinate the team members.

Other services, including Psychology and Speech Therapy, were stretched to the limit. Waiting lists for Speech Therapy were years long, and there were concerns that young children might miss out on fully effective therapy, since speech development peaks during a certain period of the child's first years. Many of these services were not available elsewhere in the community.

Pharmacy was another area that put tremendous budgetary pressures on the hospital, which raised a number of ethical questions. As new, complex, and potentially dangerous drugs became available, they required careful supervision. The hospital had to improve its drug distribution system and increase the involvement of pharmacists in clinical care.

Another ethical issue arose with the trend to treat more patients on an outpatient basis. While the government paid for inpatients' drugs, once children became outpatients, their families had to cover the costs of prescriptions, but many of these new medications were very expensive. This raised the dilemma: should patients be admitted to hospital to ensure access to needed medications that were beyond their ability to pay? The government did provide a budget to help chronically ill, long-term patients pay for their medications, but it became inadequate as more and more new medications became available.

Other challenges in allocating sparse resources include reducing the number of routine tests that are done, and eliminating outdated methods, especially when new technologies come along that can replace old ones, says Dr. Steinmetz. It is also important to make sure a new drug or machine is truly an improvement.

ASSESSING TECHNOLOGY

In 1988, Dr. Maurice McGregor helped the Quebec government set up the *Conseil d'évaluation de la technologie,* to carry out rigorous analyses of the costs and benefits of new technologies. Today, Dr. McGregor chairs the Technology Assessment Unit of the MUHC, a body that analyzes the usefulness of new equipment and its value in relation to its cost. There are ethical and legal issues associated with buying any item, he notes: "Anything new you buy means taking money out of something else."

COST–BENEFIT VS. VALUES

By virtue of its mission, a university hospital needs to be innovative and provide cutting-edge therapy. But what happens, for example, when a therapy is very expensive and only benefits a few children, when the money could pay for the salary of a badly needed social worker who could help hundreds of patients? Making this kind of decision on a strictly cost–benefit basis does not take into account other issues, such as the long-term viability of the institution. To attract dynamic researchers and additional or continued funding, for instance, the hospital needs to be prepared to invest in innovation and discovery. On the other hand, it can't always adopt a new technology or program just because an individual doctor or researcher wants it. The decision has to be made in terms of scientific evidence, and in light of the institution's core values.

Dr. Steinmetz recalls what happened when the hospital debated acquiring ECMO heart-lung bypass technology for infants. It invited ECMO experts from the United States, representatives from the provincial government, and a number of health-care professionals to a conference to learn about this new technology, its costs, and data on patient outcomes. The government then agreed to fund a two-year demonstration project and eventually provided an operating grant. "This is how you fund new technology: you base your decision on solid scientific evidence and a transparent process, you evaluate it, and you demonstrate that it will work."

In other situations, values are an important part of the equation. This was the case when the hospital decided to fund a program to save the lives of children with Ondine's Disease, a fatal respiratory illness. The treatment is expensive, the condition is relatively uncommon, and the Children's has the only such program in Canada. "This program arose out of a set of values, and an approach to the allocation of funds," says Dr. Steinmetz.

At the heart of that set of values is a focus on the sick child and the family. To ensure everyone shares those values takes time and a willingness to listen, to be open, and to participate. The goal is for everyone at the hospital to come to a consensus and to focus on what is best for the children.

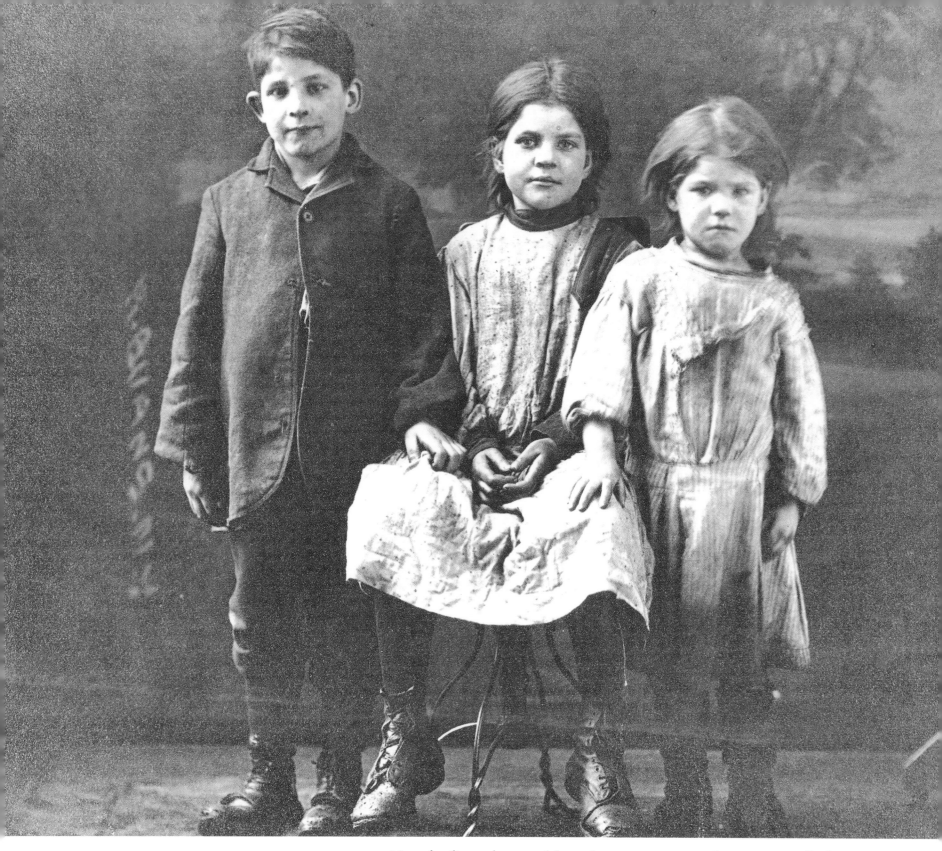

Many families at the turn of the 20th century were not only too poor to afford medical care, but lacked the knowledge of hygiene and preventive measures that would keep them from getting sick in the first place. These children, photographed in 1910, just after the Children's Memorial Hospital had moved to its Cedar Avenue location, lived in the working-class neighbourhood of Goose Village (located between the Victoria Bridge and what is now the Bonaventure Autoroute), which was razed in the 1960s.

"No doctor is ever told to go out into the community.
They just do it!"

DR. ANNE-MARIE MACLELLAN, DIRECTOR,
CHILD, YOUTH AND FAMILY HEALTH NETWORK
in a centennial year interview

11

From Pointe St. Charles to Nairobi: Connecting Children with Care

To improve the health and welfare of children, not only must highly specialized services be in place, but children and their families must also have access to them, and not be hampered by lack of knowledge, effective transportation, or financial means.

Equally important, families themselves need to know how to give their children a healthy environment in which to live, and to understand and trust the services available to them when a healthy environment is not enough.

When the Children's was new, there were many families within a short distance of the hospital who were unfamiliar with safe ways of handling food during hot weather. As a result, many babies sent home from the Children's after recovering from diarrhea or food poisoning were very soon back in hospital with the same condition. In the middle of the century, there were families in outlying areas who feared and distrusted the big-city teaching hospitals; as a result, they deprived their children of needed care. And as recently as the 1960s, the Children's was still admitting children with polio that could have been prevented had their parents had the required knowledge, confidence, and easy access to the available vaccine.

In the early 21st century, when families can get information on their children's condition from magazines, newspapers, and the Internet, keeping current on how to care for children still has its chal-

lenges. Every day's news brings new and sometimes confusing information on nutrition, exercise, and disease prevention.

Many of the hospital's most notable efforts over the past century have been geared to taking health care and knowledge out into the community—partly to ensure access, and partly because being in the community makes health care professionals better able to do their job.

One reason doctors used to make house calls was to see children who could not be transported for care; but another, equally important, was to see how people lived. Their advice could then be specific and workable given the family's living conditions. For example, a doctor could discover that the reason a young boy was frequently hospitalized with breathing problems was that he was sleeping in a damp basement, having been displaced by a sick grandparent living with the family.

House calls gradually declined over the years, largely because medicine came to require more technology than a doctor could carry in a little black bag. The advent of Medicare stopped them almost completely. However, programs that take health care close to where children live have remained a priority of the Montreal Children's Hospital and the people who work there.

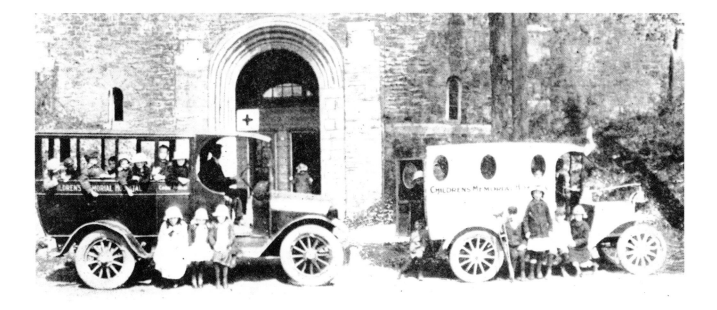

Over the decades, the Montreal Children's Hospital has initiated a wide range of community services. Some of these developed a life of their own and continued to serve the population even after the connection with the hospital was discontinued. One of the earliest of these was the School for Crippled Children.

From the first year of the Children's Memorial Hospital on Guy Street, schooling was incorporated into the daily routine of its young patients. The children's teacher at the time, Miss Sarah Tyndale, became concerned about the education of children in the community at large who could not attend school because of physical disabilities. With her suggestion as a catalyst, and considerable support from organizations and benefactors in the community, the School for Crippled Children was opened in 1916 on land belonging to the hospital. (The winning tender was for $32,500!)

In the beginning, the hospital also provided transportation and meals, and tended to the medical problems of the pupils. As the school grew rapidly—enrolment went from 7 to 97 in the first year—it gradually took over its own affairs until, in 1918, it became a separate organization. Like so many of the Children's community contributions, the school is still thriving. In 1960, it merged with the Mackay Institution for Protestant Deaf-Mutes to become the Mackay Centre for Deaf and Crippled Children—now the Mackay Rehabilitation Centre.

OFFERING CARE CLOSER TO HOME

Although by 1961 the costs of hospitalization were paid by the government, doctors' fees were not covered until 1970 with the introduction of Medicare. As a result, there were still people in the 1960s who could not afford to take their children to see a doctor. The Children's had long offered outpatient services to all children, regardless of ability to pay, but financial availability is of little help if the services are not also close to home.

The 1960s were a time of student idealism coupled with activism, and medical students were leaders. McGill medical students and residents, such as Charles Larson, Daniel Frank, Elizabeth Robinson, François Lehman, Stephen Corber, and others, set up clinics in disadvantaged areas of the city. With the active support of Dr. Elizabeth Hillman, who was in charge of outpatient services, they started to provide outpatient care for children and their families. A community clinic was established in Pointe St. Charles and was soon followed by another in Little Burgundy. In addition, on-site clinical services were offered on the Native reserve of Kahnawake, then known as Caughnawaga.

MEDICARE COMES TO QUEBEC

The intervening years have somewhat dimmed the controversy aroused by the introduction of Medicare, but at the time, it was an issue that divided the MCH community, as it did communities throughout Quebec and the rest of Canada.

It was October 1970, a time of both union and political agitation in Quebec now known as the "October Crisis." Both British Trade Commissioner James Cross and Quebec cabinet minister Pierre Laporte had been kidnapped by the FLQ (*Front de libération du Québec*). The medical specialists' association of the province (*Fédération des médecins spécialistes du Québec*, or FMSQ) was protesting Medicare's introduction in Quebec. Doctors of a different opinion, including Nicolas Steinmetz and Hugh Scott (later Executive Director of the MUHC) planned to protest against the protest. The FMSQ meeting was organized outside the province for safety reasons, recalls Dr. Steinmetz, but even so, the doctors were hassled in their cars by union activists on their way to Ottawa.

"The meeting started late," he continues. "Just as we were all wondering what the long hold-up was, the president of the FMSQ came into the meeting room and announced that Pierre Laporte had been murdered. The doctors decided not to cause the government further problems by continuing their protests. We all went home, and Medicare was introduced in Quebec."

The contributions of the MCH's medical students have been lasting ones. The Pointe St. Charles clinic, a precursor of the CLSCs (*centres locaux de services communautaires*) instituted by the Quebec government in 1971, resisted becoming a CLSC in name and staunchly maintained its independence for four decades. In June 2004, it was administratively merged with other local health services into the CSSS (*Centre de santé et des services sociaux*) for the Verdun area, in a province-wide project to coordinate local health services. It is still serving its community. The work of the Little Burgundy clinic was folded into the St. Henri CLSC, also now part of the Verdun CSSS. The clinical services in Kahnawake have grown into a full-fledged family medicine clinic and hospital.

Dr. Hillman's encouragement for pediatricians to become involved in the social milieus of their patients did not stop at community clinics. She arranged for students and residents to work with Dr. Robert Pincott in his private practice in Cowansville and the local hospital, with Drs. Donald Clogg and

A PRESCRIPTION HULLABALOO

For a brief time during the early 1970s, the Little Burgundy clinic was the scene of blocks-long line-ups as people waited for prescriptions, not for medicine, but for money!

The Montreal Diet Dispensary (MDD) had published a budget-based threshold to show what level of family income was needed to provide adequately for children. Not long after, the City of Montreal passed a by-law authorizing a $10-per-month food supplement for families whose income fell below the poverty line.

Dr. Nicolas Steinmetz, then a young resident at the clinic, met with local representatives and worked out a system whereby he would sign prescriptions for the supplement, for people who could prove that their income was inadequate to feed their children according to the MDD guidelines. The plan created a hullabaloo, as City Hall was flooded with prescription-toting parents and the medical establishment wondered whether writing prescriptions for money constituted practising medicine. Newspapers published photographs of the line-ups, making the prescriptions a *cause célèbre*.

Dr. Steinmetz's explanation that he was following scientifically established guidelines eventually satisfied the medical milieu, but did nothing to make things easier for the municipal administration of the time. After a few weeks, the city decided it could not afford to continue the dietary income supplement program. A victim of its own success, the program was discontinued.

Camp Carowanis

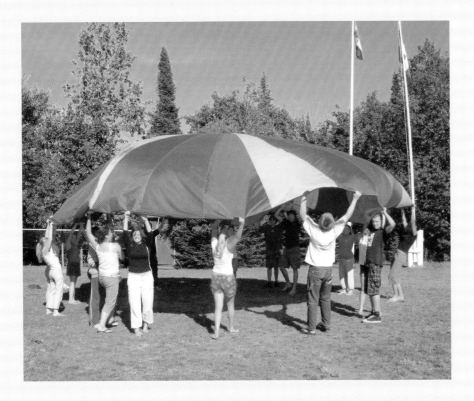

Camp Carowanis is an excellent example of the collaboration between the Montreal Children's Hospital and the community.

Located on Lake Didi in Ste-Agathe-des-Monts, the camp provides diabetic children with a fun holiday experience under the watchful eyes of doctors, nurses, medical residents, and dietitians. In addition to the usual recreational activities, children learn about testing blood-sugar levels, insulin injections (including the recently available pump therapy), symptoms and treatment of hypoglycemia, and the nutritional value of various foods.

It was in 1957 that Dr. Mimi Belmonte interested some colleagues in setting up the camp. Within a year, they had organized the first 10-day session for 20 children on rented property. It soon became obvious that the camp needed its own location, and in 1962, with the help of local service clubs, Dr. Belmonte and her colleagues were able to purchase the summer site of an orphanage that was closing down.

Service clubs and individual supporters are still depended upon to keep the camp running. At the same time, MCH and Hôpital Ste-Justine staff members provide medical expertise, and young doctors get training in a real-life, non-hospital setting. And the kids have role models to follow, because about half the counsellors are diabetics themselves, as are a number of staff.

"Diabetes is a chronic disease and a demanding one," notes Dr. Belmonte, a pediatric endocrinologist. "Children have to submit to difficult treatment, and parents are concerned about them getting into trouble, especially rebellious adolescents. Sending them to camp is not only fun for the kids, it gives parents a break, knowing their children are in a safe environment."

Camp Carowanis has grown to 180 acres and accommodates 240 children every year in two- to six-week sessions. Children from throughout Quebec go to the camp, a majority of them French-speaking. Sometimes, children from other provinces attend for the opportunity to learn French.

Dr. Belmonte, who spent 25 years as the camp's medical director, was named to the Order of Canada in 1999 for her achievements. Dr. Harvey Guyda, Physician-in-Chief at the MCH, replaced Dr. Belmonte in 2001 as President of the Board of The Diabetic Children's Foundation.

Fred Wiener in their Montreal offices. Residents also visited homes for orphans and children with disabilities. Primarily an educational experience for the young doctors, to observe how institutionalization affected children's development, these programs also provided access to medical consultations for children whose families were not in a position to pay for care.

Occasionally, perfectly normal children were placed in institutions for the mentally retarded for the simple reason that they were undiagnosed or unwanted. Birth control was limited in the mid-1960s, and the social stigma of unwanted pregnancy was so strong that even adoption was avoided: giving a child up meant admitting to having given birth.

One such child at a home in the Eastern Townships tugged at Dr. Steinmetz's heart, and he took him to the Children's, where the little boy thrived and was eventually adopted by a member of the hospital staff. The fact that this kind of unofficial transfer of care was both necessary and possible shows the enormous extent to which child welfare policies have improved in the past 40 years.

Another Hillman initiative that combined training with service to the community was the MCH's Family Medicine Unit, started in 1972. At that time, McGill University needed a place to train students in its new Family Medicine Program. Dr. Jack Charters, Executive Director, made space available in the A-Wing and placed Dr. Steinmetz in charge. Through word of mouth alone, the service soon had more patients than it could handle. It expanded into a floor and a half of the nearby Gilman Pavilion, where it offered a full range of family medical services. At its peak, it was staffed by four nurses and three staff doctors, as well as family medicine residents, a social worker, and a psychologist, with other specialists available for consultation.

By 1981, the unit had served its purpose. Family Medicine units had been set up at the Montreal General, Queen Elizabeth, Jewish General, and St.

Mary's hospitals, and it made sense to look after children with their families at the adult centres. The MCH unit was closed and the staff was spread among the other units.

By the time the Children's turned 100, many of the community needs it had served in the early and mid-20th century were being met by other institutions and government programs. But these needs have been replaced by others, many of them described in this chapter, and the Children's is always developing new ways to reach out a helping hand.

The other important aspect of community health programs that the Children's has not abandoned is the learning opportunities they offer health-care trainees. Second-year pediatric residents at the MCH currently have an obligatory four-week rotation in social pediatrics at Dr. Gilles Julien's *Clinique d'assistance aux enfants en difficulté* in Hochelaga-Maisonneuve, one of Montreal's poorest neighbourhoods.

COMMUNITY-BASED PEDIATRICIANS

The MCH's close relationship with the community is typified by the role of pediatricians who are based in private offices. These community physicians not only refer their patients to the Children's for more specialized care, but also participate in caring for children within the hospital setting. They provide patient care and teaching in the MCH Emergency Department, outpatient clinics, inpatient wards and in the perinatal units of the Royal Victoria and Jewish General hospitals. In the wider community, they also contribute at both the Lakeshore General and Herzl Pediatric Consultation Clinics, as well as the Mackay Rehabilitation Centre, Hôpital Marie-Enfant, and the Shriner's Hospital.

Their special relationship with the Children's is unique in Quebec and stronger than anywhere else in Canada. Over the years, some have participated in running special programs within the hospital. Dr. Emmett Francoeur was Director of the MCH General Pediatric Clinic (now the Pediatric Con-

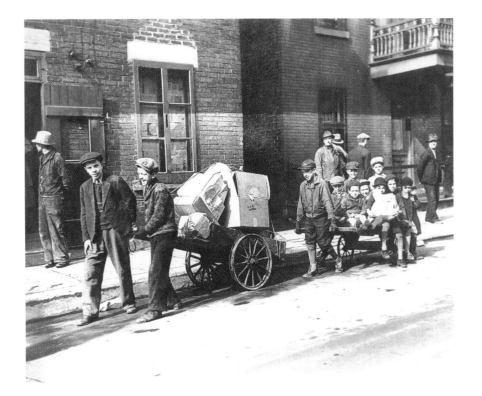

In 1930, when this photo was taken, most families did not own cars. The poorer ones often relied on non-motorized vehicles and their own foot-power for transportation. By then, the Children's Social Services Department had been operating for 14 years. At first entirely volunteer-run and funded, it offered a range of services, including car transportation to and from the hospital.

Twenty-five years ago, Drs. Denis Leduc and Richard Haber were instrumental in the formation of the Association of Community-based Pediatricians, now the Council of Community-based Pediatricians, which includes most of the MCH-affiliated community practitioners. Its aim was, and remains, to strengthen the liaison between their group and the MCH by encouraging their participation in hospital activities, and at the same time to sensitize the hospital to child health-care issues in the community. The Council has representation on the hospital's Council of Physicians, Dentists and Pharmacists (CPDP) and the MCH Physician-in-Chief attends the community group's annual meetings. The Council's 50 to 60 members see roughly 150,000 children each year, so for many families they are the first-line ambassadors for the hospital.

The Council offers its members monthly continuing medical education seminars on a wide range of topics, from autism to skin conditions. Dr. Leduc, current President of the Canadian Pediatric Society (2005–2007), observes, "The seminars not only keep us up-to-date on new developments in our field, they also allow us a forum to discuss office practice issues we have in common."

SOCIAL SERVICES: A LONG HISTORY

Of all the hospital's departments, Social Services has the longest, most wide-ranging history of promoting children's health and welfare. Established in 1916 in response to concern about home hygiene conditions for infants, it quickly took on a much wider range of responsibilities. One of the first social services departments in a Canadian hospital, it dealt with the ravages of poverty, neglect, and abuse, as well as the impact of serious illness on children's lives. It went on to send kindergarten workers into the homes of convalescent long-term patients, provide crafts sessions to inpatients, arrange for children's convalescent care at adult facilities, and offer learning opportunities to medical, nursing, and social work trainees in both clinics and homes.

sultation Centre) during the 1980s before he went into private practice part-time, still maintaining his association with the Centre and working in the ER. In September 2004, he began splitting his time evenly between his private practice and the position of Director of the Child Development Program at the MCH. A past president of the Canadian Pediatric Society (CPS), Dr. Francoeur is also a consultant to the MCH's Developmental and Behavioural Pediatric Services.

"A community pediatrician can provide a valuable link for families when their children are sick," explains Dr. Francoeur. "We can be helpful to hospital specialists, too. If a family is going through a really difficult situation, we can provide background that may bring balance to decision-making. And when specialists have to explain something complicated, they can call in the doctor the children have known all their lives, to provide support and continuity."

During the 1920s, reports Dr. Jessie Boyd Scriver in her history of the Children's, "Clinicians relied more and more on the assistance of the Social Services Department for home evaluation and follow-up surveillance of patients." Perhaps the most amazing thing about the service was that it was entirely volunteer-run. The Organizing Committee that had created the department raised funds to support their work, and even provided material help such as braces, crutches, glasses, and food. By 1926, the financial needs were so great that the hospital took over departmental operations, but the volunteer committee continued to participate.

As health and social services within the wider community developed, the hospital's Social Services Department adapted its support, always serving as the vital connection between families and the services they need to deal with, both in the hospital and in the community. It was not long before it became more professional in its outlook, becoming affiliated with McGill University's School of Social Work. During the Second World War, the department attracted its first professional social worker as director, Christina James. Mrs. James was followed in 1962 by Agnes Johnston. It was during Mrs. Johnston's mandate, in 1967, that the department became one of the first social work departments in Canada, and the first in Quebec, to offer 24-hour emergency coverage to patients and their families.

Covering most of the medical, surgical, and psychiatric services of the hospital, especially the Emergency Department, they make sure families of children with serious injury or illness get the psychological assistance they need. They intervene in cases of suspected child abuse and help people deal with an array of resources. This often involves working closely with youth protection services, police, schools, and courts, as well as community agencies and government programs.

CHANGES IN SOCIETY BRING NEW NEEDS

As the hospital moves into its second century, the needs for the department's services remain as acute as ever, and are affected by social changes. Child protection is still a growing issue. Computers have brought a wide range of new challenges, from child pornography to outsourcing of jobs overseas, which can lead to unemployment and its many consequences for families here. There are more single-parent families, increasing stress on children and parents. Extended families are no longer as cohesive. Technology and medication have become a long-term part of some children's lives—children who would have died a generation earlier, but for whom quality of life, rather than mere survival, now becomes an issue. Shorter hospitalization and home care may be better from a medical point of view, but it transfers care responsibility earlier to parents, who often work outside the home. Also in recent years, there has been increasing demand for support to new refugees or immigrants with seriously ill children.

Even as demands increase, there is competition for resources, notes Margaret Ann Smith, who

A FRIENDLY PLACE TO STAY

The things social workers do sometimes require special initiatives. In 1986, the family of two children with cancer needed a nearby place to stay, so they could be near the hospital. Margaret Ann Smith's sister, Pat Laffoley, was a manager at a nearby apartment hotel. It was low season and she offered to put them up at a preferential rate. That one-time arrangement worked out so well that it grew into a permanent one over the years, and came to include patients from the Shriners' Hospital as well. There are now eight rooms at La Tour Belvedere available to MCH families. Social workers find funding for families who cannot pay; the hotel staff are friendly and supportive; and families appreciate the opportunity to mix with other visitors to Montreal, away from reminders of their worrisome situation.

directed the department from 1977 to 2003. An ageing population places higher demands on support services for older people, reducing the available resources for children. Finding support in the community to meet families' needs remains a time-consuming challenge. "Practising social work," concludes Ms. Smith, "is like trying to empty the ocean with a spoon. But, when successful, it is one of the most gratifying tasks, particularly working with the devoted and compassionate staff of the Children's."

REACHING OUT TO THE
VERY YOUNGEST PATIENTS

The hospital's Neonatal Outreach Teaching Program is a perfect example of services built on sensitive response to community health care needs.

The program grew out of requests from staff in the 40 or so birthing centres that send newborn babies to the Children's via the MCH Neonatal Transport Team. (Its specialized equipment is described in Chapter 9.) Established in 1990 by Dr. John Hortop and nurse Diane Lalonde, the team is made up of specially trained nurses and respiratory therapists working under the direction of neonatologists. Their charge was to move sick newborns safely and quickly to the Children's for specialized care. But along the way, team members found themselves responding to more and more requests for specialized advice and training. Staff at the referring hospital would ask questions about stabilizing their tiny patients, or about caring for them once they returned from the NICU.

Ms. Lalonde soon became convinced that the need for advice and training called for a dedicated program. Training staff at other hospitals to continue the care begun at the Children's would allow the babies to go back to their own regions sooner and recover closer to their families. Thus, in 2002, the Neonatal Outreach Teaching Program was born. Under the direction of Ms. Lalonde and Dr. Louis Beaumier, the program now offers consultation, on-site teaching, case review, and conferences for doctors, nurses, and respiratory therapists of the referring centres. Course topics range from basic sciences to specific skills such as neonatal resuscitation. New training sessions are developed in response to needs expressed. But the program's advantages go much further than teaching: it enhances local expertise and inter-hospital collaboration, and increases referrals to the MCH.

As Ms. Lalonde said when the program was launched, "These institutions have been our partners in developing our new program. It's their questions that inspired it."

EARLY TRANSPORT SERVICES

Although the dedicated Neonatal Transport Team and their Outreach Teaching Program are products of the end of the 20th century, the Children's was responding to transport needs as early as the 1930s, as Dr. Jessie Boyd Scriver describes in *The Montreal Children's Hospital, Years of Growth:*

"The hospital was not equipped in the thirties with the sophisticated facilities available now for the care and treatment of premature infants, yet there was provision for the transport of such infants to the hospital should the occasion arise. A doctor and nurse would ride in the hospital ambulance with the baby who was placed in a basket constructed like an incubator."

In the 1960s, the hospital would send its ambulance to towns throughout Quebec, and as far afield as the New England states, to transport not only newborns but very sick children of all ages to the MCH for care. Government regulation forced discontinuation of transport from the New England states in the late 1970s.

"More than ever, we must be actively responsive to the needs that exist in the community and do our part in coordinating and planning for medical care ... This is the direction in which this hospital, I believe, will make a significant contribution in the years ahead."

DR. ALAN ROSS, PHYSICIAN-IN-CHIEF, 1953–1968
1967 Annual Report,

Dr. Ross's words, written nearly 40 years ago, show that the hospital had not strayed from the path it set out for itself at its founding—meeting the needs of the community. His emphasis on coordinating and planning is an indication of the increasing complexity of the health care system in the second half of the century. Canadian health care had not been created and planned as a "system" in the true sense, but was a product of the responses by different entities at different times to a range of needs. Keeping on top of its haphazard growth has never been easy, and the Children's has had to work continually to ensure that children's needs did not fall between the cracks.

A new initiative that would certainly have pleased Dr. Ross was put in place during the hospital's centennial year. The Child, Youth and Family Health Network, inaugurated in April 2004, coordinated and formalized the links among health-care providers that the Children's had been building and maintaining over the years. In preparation for setting up the network, Dr. Anne-Marie MacLellan, the network's director, reports that the hospital carried out an inventory of its support and partnership activities throughout the province with hospitals, CLSCs, schools, daycare centres, and other organizations. The list proved to be 17 pages long!

"We are really in a building process," said Dr. MacLellan a few weeks after the inauguration, "but the network has been in existence for 40 years, since Hanna Strawczynski started home care for hemo-

NEW PARTNERS— LAKESHORE AND HERZL

Under the auspices of the Child, Youth and Family Health Network, the Children's has formed a partnership with the Lakeshore General Hospital, where an Asthma Clinic and a Child and Adolescent Consultation Services Clinic opened during the MCH's centennial year. Nurses and pediatricians from both hospitals work together to provide care to West Island children closer to their home.

A partnership with the Jewish General Hospital's Herzl Family Practice Centre supports the MCH's focus on continuity of care and on treating a child within the context of the whole family. Children without family doctors may be referred to the Herzl Centre if their medical problems are not too serious or complex. The Centre will not only treat the child and arrange for follow-up by a pediatrician from the Children's, it will also assign a family doctor who will see the whole family—the same doctor for every visit, unlike other community clinics.

philiacs. We're just putting a name on something and then expanding it in whatever way we see fit—it's called flexibility."

The network's Web site, created over the summer of 2004, provides a succinct description of what it does: "The Child, Youth and Family Health Network promotes and develops a wide range of specialized pediatric services and outreach activities for healthcare providers and their communities ... [It] facilitates access to many of the programs and services available through the Montreal Children's Hospital including Northern and Native Child Health, Telehealth, Neonatal Outreach and Traumatology."

The "wide range" of services referred to can include supplying a protocol for diabetic crises to an emergency physician in a small-town hospital; interpreting an ultrasound scan being done hundreds of kilometres away in real time; developing teaching programs designed to keep health-care practitioners in outlying areas up-to-date; and sending MCH residents to community hospitals to share their expertise with the staff.

The network serves well over 100 communities in every corner of the province and has links to other pediatric networks across the country.

Dr. MacLellan is charged with tying together the pieces of the network by meeting with health-care professionals throughout Quebec, promoting the services the MCH offers, and advocating for the development of new services after listening to what professionals in the community need. "What is most important," she emphasizes, "is that it's not *our* network. The network is everybody here in the hospital doing their outreach programs. If they are doing anything new or unusual, they'll tell us or tell Public Relations so we can market it."

Nurse Johanne Desrochers is the administrative head of the network, and has seen rapid growth in its scope since she was hired to develop outreach activities in 2000. She prepares agreements with other institutions and provides an administrative framework for the many and varied outreach activities.

"Much of my work involves formalizing the information, gathering it together and putting it in a place that is easy to find," she explains. "For instance, we've published a patient referral guide that we've sent to all the communities across the province. It's now in its third edition, is in high demand, and is well appreciated by members of the professional community, who keep calling us for copies."

In addition to community outreach and network development, Ms. Desrochers' responsibilities include the Northern and Native Child Health Program (see below) and the large and rapidly growing Telehealth Service.

> "We are innovators here. The Children's has a culture that supports innovation, and that is a big strength."
>
> JOHANNE DESROCHERS, ADMINISTRATIVE HEAD, CHILD, YOUTH AND FAMILY HEALTH NETWORK

TELEHEALTH

Telehealth services involve the use of communications technology (video camera, microphone, TV screen or computer monitor, and telephony)—all in real-time interaction—to deliver health care. The applications are many and growing.

A pediatric cardiologist at the Children's can watch ultrasound images being taken by a technician hundreds of kilometres away and provide diagnosis or consultation immediately. A speech therapist can help a child learn to speak via a monitor, despite being in a different city. An audiologist can send a digitally recorded ear exam via the Internet to a specialist for an opinion. Or a doctor in an outlying region can send a digital image of a child's skin condition and get feedback from a dermatologist in Montreal.

Ms. Desrochers explains that the use of video means health professionals can also read facial expressions and body language, making telehealth services effective for psychological and psychiatric evaluations.

"They somehow feel a connection. Patients have felt a strong bond with their therapist even though they have only met by videoconference. In some smaller towns they thought it was better than regular office appointments because of the confidentiality. People who see you go into an unidentified room in a hospital don't know what is said or who you are meeting with."

The connection people feel through video applies to any kind of interaction. Cardiologist Dr. Marie Béland tells the story of meeting an Inuit family in person for the first time. She had diagnosed the child at the Children's through an echocardiogram transmitted from northern Quebec. As she started to introduce herself, the patient's mother smiled broadly and said, "Oh, yes, I know you from television!"

Telehealth consultation is not only much more convenient for patients and caregivers, it saves a lot of money. Says Dr. MacLellan, "When we train a local person to work the ultrasound probe and send the image to our radiologist down here, we can save $10,000 per patient by eliminating a plane trip. And we can organize three families in a row to use the ultrasound facilities."

Telehealth can also be used in community education. For instance, videoconferences on drugs, alcohol, and suicide have been set up for interested teens in isolated English-speaking communities. Camerashy at first, the adolescents quickly warmed to the presenters at the other end of the line and asked a lot of questions.

"Physicians are not currently paid for telehealth consultations," adds Ms. Desrochers, "but they do it because it benefits the children. We have a good team of professionals who are going way beyond the call of duty."

REACHING INTO MORE DISTANT COMMUNITIES

In the mid-1960s, Dr. Jack Charters, an MCH pediatrician and later its executive director, was travelling in the Canadian North as president of the Canadian Pediatric Society. He noticed the dismal state of health of some of the children living in the Arctic and launched an initiative to convince the federal government to fund health-care projects through Canadian medical schools. As a result, several university hospitals, including the Children's, were approached to provide specialized health care to the country's northern regions. The idea was to support health-care personnel working in the North by giving consultations in medical specialties so that fewer patients would have to be flown south for treatment.

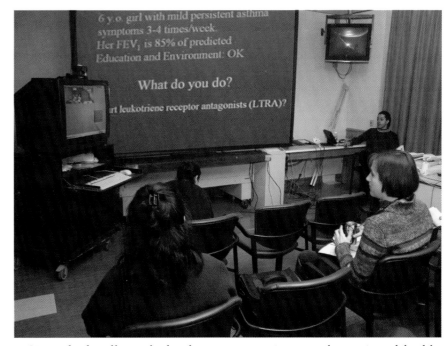

MCH medical staff attend a lunch-time presentation on asthma using telehealth technology, with the technical assistance of Laurent Soussana (far right). The interactive sessions allow them to participate in real time, with doctors in other regions of the province as far-flung as Amos, Ungava Bay, Blanc Sablon, and St. Hyacinthe.

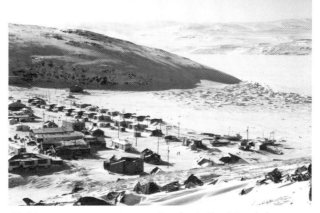

Children in communities in Quebec's Far North have received regular visits from doctors, nurses, and social workers from the Children's for 40 years. More and more can be treated without leaving their home communities, thanks to the hospital's specialized long-distance services and training for local professionals.

Dr. Gary Pekeles, Director of the Northern and Native Child Health Program, remembers the anxiety that often used to accompany flights south prior to the involvement of the Children's. "In those early days, the most frequent reason for sending people out of the community for treatment was tuberculosis. It was considered the kiss of death. People would have to spend a long time in a sanatorium, and even those who eventually recovered lost touch with their families over time. As a result, to be sent away for any kind of medical care caused morbid fear. So, understandably, offering a broad array of services right in the community reduced not only the time and cost associated with travel, but also the emotional and spiritual upheaval."

The first area the Children's became involved with was the Baffin area of what is now known as Nunavut. By its centennial year, the MCH was serving the Inuit and Cree of northern Quebec, as well as the Mohawk communities of Kahnawake and Kanesatake in the South.

Through the Northern and Native Child Health Program, health-care specialists visit children in each community. Back at the hospital in Montreal, they stay in touch, making sure Northern children have the best possible experience if they are sent to Montreal for treatment, and updating the care team in the child's community.

FIRST NATIVE PEDIATRICIAN

A particularly valuable addition to the Northern and Native Child Health Program has been Dr. Kent Saylor, who joined the Children's medical staff in 1999 after specialized training in the U.S. and Montreal and a residency at the MCH. Originally from the Mohawk community of Kahnawake, and the first pediatrician in Canada of First Nations ancestry, Dr. Saylor is not only an ideal person for outreach services, but also serves as a role model for young people in Native communities.

Visiting each community also allows them to offer training for clinical personnel there, improve services through new technologies, and work closely with public health professionals to find solutions to public health problems.

Over the years, the types of services offered by the Children's have grown and become more specialized. Pediatricians have been joined in the program by other medical and surgical specialists and subspecialists, nurses, social workers, audiologists, occupational therapists, physiotherapists, electrocardiogram technicians, and biomedical engineers, as well as other allied health professionals.

Dr. Pekeles' colleague, Dr. Johanne Morel, has been with the program for 20 years. While doctors in Northern regions may change regularly, she has been through good and bad times with families who have known her for 15 years or more. Her presence adds valuable continuity to the care their children receive.

Each year, between 3,000 and 4,000 children from Northern and Native communities consult MCH staff. Approximately 1,000 children actually come to the Children's, including 300 who are admitted because they require special care.

On the social level, the Northern community reflects its southern, urban counterpart, in that its needs are constantly evolving. As in the south, social issues are taking on greater prominence. Changing realities mean that social workers and other caregivers carry out more preventive work, through programs aimed at injury prevention (including drowning), smoking cessation, safe use and storage of firearms, substance abuse, and fire prevention in houses that use more volatile cooking methods.

Over the years, the Children's has added services to help Northern patients and families feel more at home. A special waiting room is decorated with familiar photos and art, and meals of caribou and bannock bread can be ordered from home. Interpreters are available, of course, as they are for speakers of many other languages, but their role is

SPECIAL CHALLENGES—AND JOYS— FOR SOCIAL WORKERS IN THE NORTH

Social workers in the North need a special understanding of life and conditions in far-flung Native communities.

Lee Negru, who started going north in the late 1970s, says her main interest was in establishing services that would enable children to come to the hospital with their mothers or grandmothers rather than government-appointed caretakers. Kind as these caretakers might be, children travelling with their own family members are happier and get well faster.

Mrs. Negru recalls the Anik satellite as having made a huge difference in the lives of children who had to come south for treatment. Launched in 1972, the satellite "added the human touch," she says. "The Arctic nursing station had a telephone hook-up and we could arrange for children to talk to their mothers back home. Sometimes, they were so glad to hear a familiar voice, there were no words, just sobs."

In addition to telephone links, there was radio service to the Far North beginning in January 1973. Lee Negru remembers Elisapee Davidee, the Innu broadcaster for the CBC who would interview people visiting Montreal and send reports back to their home communities so their neighbours could know how they were getting on.

even more important in the case of visitors from the North who need to navigate the streets of Montreal when they have never seen a traffic light!

Margaret Butler, who is assigned to Northern and Native Child Health Services from the MCH Social Services Department, notes that a typical quality of the MCH is "that willingness to go beyond the necessities." She remembers a First Nations family from an outlying community, who in the late 1980s faced the death of a child in the hospital. "The Children's made the Ross Lounge and its kitchen available throughout the weekend to between 40 and 50 members of the family. There, they held a

Native feast to help them cope with the impending loss."

Ms. Butler, through the program, was instrumental in the creation of Tassiutitiit, an association of cross-cultural families in Montreal that offers support to non-Native families fostering or adopting First Nations children.

REACHING ACROSS THE SEA

Through its Child, Youth and Family Health Network and its antecedents, the Children's has reached out over hundreds of kilometres to take services and knowledge to children in remote areas. However, that reach has not been limited to the borders of Quebec, the rest of Canada, or even North America.

Between 1965 and 1968, Dr. Isobel Wright established a successful pediatric service at Christian Medical College in Ludhiana, India. Shortly thereafter, Dr. Thérèse Rousseau joined a group from Hôpital Ste-Justine to help organize a pediatric service in Tunisia.

The same spirit of helping the international community has led individual MCH physicians like Richard Hamilton, Charles Larson, and Michael Kramer to carry out research, teaching, and care in places as far-flung as Bangladesh, Russia, and Belarus.

Kenya

In July 1968, Drs. Alan Finley, Colin Forbes, and Jack Charters arrived at Kenyatta National Hospital in Nairobi, Kenya (the hospital affiliated with the University of Nairobi) to set up the university's department of pediatrics. Their work was part of a 10-year project of the Canadian International Development Agency (CIDA) to establish a pediatric department, clinical training units, and postgraduate training at the medical school. Dr. Alan Ross joined them in December that year, to become Founding Professor of Pediatrics. Before long, Drs. Donald Clogg, Elizabeth and Donald Hillman, Nicolas

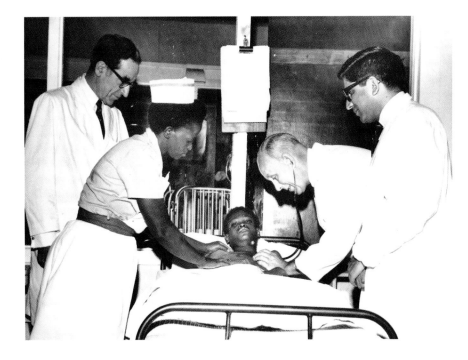

TRAVELLING WITH A FULL HOUSE

Sometimes foreign postings involve quick decisions. While their family was still young, Drs. Elizabeth and Donald Hillman were asked to replace colleagues at Kenyatta National Hospital on two weeks' notice. Arriving home the next day, Elizabeth Hillman was met at the front door by her teenaged daughter's boyfriend. "My Mum wants you to call her," was all he said. Dr. Hillman's surprise increased when she reached the boy's mother, who said, "Thank you so much for inviting my son to go to Kenya with you!" Young Miss Hillman had apparently issued the invitation. After some discussion, her parents acquiesced. Within a few days, the couple packed up and moved their own five children plus one to the other side of the world—demonstrating yet again that adaptable MCH spirit!

Steinmetz, George Collins, and Robert Hutcheon also participated.

The staff involved in the project did not embark on a unilateral knowledge transfer. Instead, they focused on an information exchange between Kenyans and Canadians. The doctors understood that to offer a curriculum suited to the Kenyans, they needed to understand the local health problems, as well as norms and values held by Kenyan doctors, and to accept Kenyan leadership. The Kenyans were taught the same curriculum as in Western medical schools, with emphasis placed on local problems: malnutrition, overpopulation, measles, and local common diseases.

Another Montreal Children's Hospital philosophy came through—the importance of understanding the community for which hospitals provide care. The MCH pediatricians took the students and residents to all the provincial hospitals, despite the difficult transportation systems, to emphasize the value of going out into the communities to see and understand local concerns. This practice allowed students to learn about the physical and socio-economic factors of diseases and enabled them to find ways of helping people prevent them.

The program was very successful, and was "Kenyanized" within 10 years. Kenyan graduates now direct pediatric services throughout the country. The new medical school created has since become the major medical training centre in East Africa. And after 35 years, Dr. Colin Forbes still practises as a pediatrician in Kenya.

Ethiopia

Another international program in which the Children's participated was the creation of a master's program in Community Health in Ethiopia, beginning in 1987. Three doctors from the Children's—Jack Charters, Charles Larson, and Nicolas Steinmetz, who acted as an external examiner—went to assist in determining the program's content. It focused on basic epidemiological principles, public health diagnosis, clean water, dealing with human waste, nutrition, organizing immunization programs, and other community health programs. A strong emphasis on nutrition for pregnant women and working in remote locations were also important parts of their education.

FAMILY EDUCATION

In addition to educating professionals, another effective way of improving the care of sick and injured children is to take the knowledge closer still to the children—to their families. Educating families is also one of the Children's oldest practices.

Sometimes this takes the form of face-to-face advice. Social workers visited homes to give advice on household hygiene during the First World War. Physicians and nurses in the outpatient department in the 1950s and '60s encouraged women to nurse their babies when the practice was in decline. At the turn of this 21st century, emergency and community physicians encourage childhood vaccinations, at a time when there is much misinformation deterring parents.

Very often, the Children's has formalized advice to parents and made it available on a wider scale. This has become particularly important as education levels continue to rise, many more sources of information are available, and people take greater responsibility for their own and their family's health.

Public lectures are offered in English and French several times a year on topics of broad interest. If there is interest in an outlying community, these lectures can be teleconferenced through the Child, Youth and Family Health Network. The Public Relations Office distributes thousands of calendars each year to all the Greater Montreal area school boards, with health tips ranging from how much toothpaste to use, to how to poison-proof a home.

Leaflets on common childhood conditions such as fever, diarrhea, or mild head injuries are distributed through CLSCs and doctors' offices, and via the hospital's Web site. The leaflets are also handed out at the *Salon Maternité, Paternité, Enfants* / Parents and Kids Fair, an annual event held in Montreal and

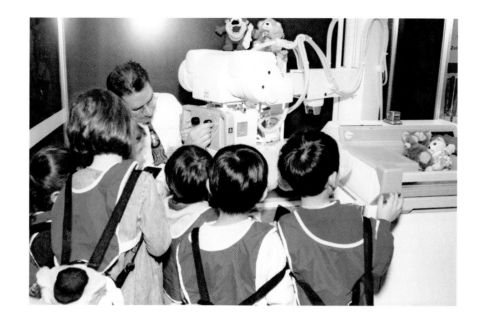

attended by more than 46,000 parents. The Salon gives families the opportunity to speak with MCH staff members, acquire health information through interactive games and displays, and even pass teddy bears through an X-ray machine!

PREVENTING SIDS

During the 1990s, the MCH organized a series of press conferences, information sessions, and workshops, and distributed documents (leaflets, booklets, and posters) to physicians, health-care practitioners, and clinics throughout the province and across Canada concerning the importance of sleeping position and other safety measures for babies. Dr. Aurore Côté took the lead in encouraging parents to put babies to sleep on their backs, to help avoid the frightening phenomenon known as SIDS (sudden infant death syndrome). Called *"Dodo sur le dos … pour la vie"* or "Back to sleep … for life," and carried out in conjunction with the hospital's Jeremy Rill Centre for SIDS, the information campaign had an important impact on public behaviour as well as on public health policy, and is estimated to have significantly reduced the number of SIDS cases.

Children crowd around a Children's staff member as he demonstrates the X-ray machine during the 1997 Montreal Parents and Kids Fair.

PREVENTING THE SINGLE GREATEST CAUSE OF DEATH

Debbie Friedman, Trauma Program Head, speaks to journalists at a 2004 news conference promoting summer sports safety. At left is neurosurgeon Dr. José Luis Montes. After noting a high number of injuries early in the season, the Trauma Program decided to focus its seasonal message to the public on safety and protective equipment, as demonstrated by (left to right) Lawrence, Jason, and Jordan.

Better public knowledge (combined with advocacy, see below) has contributed over the years to preventing such injuries as poisonings, burns, and strangulations from window-blind cords. But there are always new ways to get hurt.

Debbie Friedman, Head of the Pediatric and Adolescent Trauma Program, notes, "New trends, like snowboards, trampolines, or scooters, bring their own injuries. There is a flurry of injuries when they are first introduced because they are not always age-appropriate, children and parents are not always aware of the risks, and often they aren't supervised closely enough. Education and public awareness programs are set up and sometimes even lobbying for changes is needed. But as soon as changes are made, another trend comes along."

The interdisciplinary team running the Trauma Program participates in over 50 injury prevention and public awareness activities a year, including presentations at schools and conferences, car seat clinics, and safety displays at public events.

ADVOCATING AND LOBBYING

Public education has proved its effectiveness through the decades as the staff treating children at the MCH frequently moved beyond their clinical roles to helping prevent the types of conditions they were treating.

Sometimes, though, even public awareness is not enough. Outside organizations must play a role. To remind these organizations of their responsibilities, staff of the Children's have not hesitated to advocate for the health and well-being of children.

Dr. John McCrae was pathologist to the Children's Memorial Hospital from its opening in 1904 until he went overseas in 1914 as a medical officer. During this time, as a member of the medical board of the Montreal Foundling and Baby Hospital (which a generation later came under the umbrella of the Children's), Dr. McCrae was active in lobbying for a cleaner milk supply in Montreal. As Dr. Jessie Boyd Scriver writes, "This was the time when the shocking infant mortality rate was attributed in part to high bacterial counts in the available milk supply." Dr. McCrae is perhaps better known as author of the poem, "In Flanders' Fields." He died serving in France in 1918.

Dr. McCrae was not the only one to reach out to prominent community members for support in offering services to children. However, in the Children's first half-century, two world wars, an economic depression, and frequent outbreaks of such diseases as polio and typhoid fever meant that most of these efforts were focused on cure or rehabilitation rather than on prevention.

It was only well after the Second World War, when growing prosperity coincided with the development of vaccines to prevent diseases, and of antibiotics to treat those that could not yet be prevented, that teachers and care providers at the Children's were able to turn their focus once again on public education and advocacy. Other contributing factors included an increasingly well-read population and new developments in mass media, which enhanced

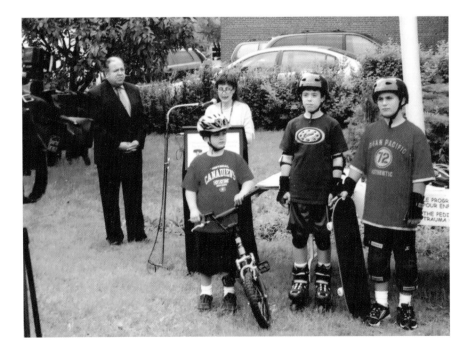

the potential of public education campaigns. At the same time, growing government involvement in health care called for closer communication with politicians and bureaucrats responsible for health-care funding and accessibility.

As a result, hospital staff sometimes found themselves going beyond providing information and advice, to lobbying for system-wide changes.

Since the 1970s, doctors from the Children's have had considerable success lobbying for simple measures that save children's lives. For instance, Dr. Norman Eade of the Poison Control Centre was instrumental in persuading pharmacists to use child-proof bottles for prescription medications.

In the same decade, Dr. Charles Scriver, Scientific Director of the McGill University–Montreal Children's Hospital Research Institute, spearheaded the addition of vitamin D to milk, with the support of Arnold Steinberg, Chairman of the Institute. Their efforts resulted in the nearly complete elimination in Montreal of rickets from vitamin D deficiency.

Dr. Barry Pless played a key role in lobbying for legislation on children's car restraints. His research on traffic injuries led to the modification of Quebec's Highway Safety Code.

Lobbying government requires support from a large network. To cast the net wider in seeking information on children's injuries, Dr. Pless and colleagues from the Canadian Institute of Child Health set up the Children's Hospital Injury Reporting and Prevention Program (CHIRPP) in 1990. The information gathered through CHIRPP has led to regulation of bicycle helmet use, the banning of baby walkers, and legislation requiring strict guidelines for playgrounds.

MCH staff have also been key movers in a network of advocates for better child protection in Quebec. In the mid-1960s, Drs. Elizabeth Hillman and Herbert Owen, who had studied numerous cases of child abuse in the Emergency Department, set up the Battered Baby Committee at the MCH, along with Margaret Ann Smith, a newly arrived

The Gazette, July 24, 1971

Montreal dairies may soon add vitamin D to whole milk

By DUSTY VINEBERG

Steinberg's Limited confirmed yesterday that it has requested Elmhurst D a i r y, its major milk supplier, to put vitamin D into whole milk.

was the best milk for babies and children.

The dairies, on the other hand, claimed they added vitamin D to skim and two per cent for two reasons.

Firstly, sales of two per cent increasing rapidly

min D is not added. The reason? "Some people will object to added vitamin D, as they do to fluoride. Crazy? Yes, but if you work with the public, you know . . ."

sorb the calcium needed for proper bone and teeth formation, especially up to the age of 18, and also especially needed by the elderly to prevent some of the b o n e s chan of old age.

said Canadian food laws are "very sensible." Whereas in the United States vitamin D had been added to many foods, including cereals, in Canada, the laws have kept

The Gazette, June 14, 1977

New law to let Quebec seize beaten children

Parents who beat their children could have them taken away without a prior court order under Quebec laws to be introduced in the National Assembly week

thorized social service centres. Each of them "will have the responsibility to intervene in all cases where the health, security or normal development of the

social worker who was to become one of the moving forces in child advocacy in Quebec. Its descendant, the Child Protection Committee, is still functioning at the hospital.

"Nothing was done about abuse at the time," remembers Ms. Smith. "No law in the province obligated reporting until 1975, and that was only after years of increasing pressure from a determined lobby of women headed by Alice Parizeau, a criminologist at *l'Université de Montréal*." A provincial committee was created, and two of its first members were Ms. Smith and Dr. Steinmetz, who were instrumental in educating social workers, physicians, teachers, police, and others about the new legislation. They travelled around the province teaching them what the issues were, how to recognize abuse, and what to do, by actually reviewing cases with them. When the extent of the problem became clear, the committee persuaded the government that child protection legislation was required. It finally came in 1979, and marked its 25th anniversary as the Children's was celebrating its 100th.

In 2001, Margaret Ann Smith launched a new initiative very much in keeping with the MCH tradition of bringing different sectors of the community together to meet children's needs. The Coalition of Education, Health, Social Work and Community Services aims to ensure that "no child falls between the cracks." Ms. Smith and pediatric social worker Rhona Bezonsky were the first MCH representatives and were later joined by Dr. Klaus Minde of Psychiatry. Although she retired in 2002, Ms. Smith still chairs the coalition. Its members include schools, hospitals, social services, and professional associations who work together to make sure children and their families are never deprived of the help they need because of bureaucracy, outdated policies and practices, or gaps in the system. They share information and professional development, and collaborate to find new solutions to social problems.

The Montreal Children's Hospital was founded by people like Drs. Forbes and Cushing, advocating for better health care for the children of the community, along with supportive community leaders such as Sir Melbourne Tait, Lord Atholstan, Messrs George Smithers and Robert Reford, and many others. In the century since then, living conditions have changed enormously. Health care has made spectacular advances. And the social, economic, and political system in which children live and seek care has attained a complexity that might have astonished the hospital's founders. But there has never been a time when people from the Children's were not reaching out into—and working with—the community to make sure that children have access to the help they need.

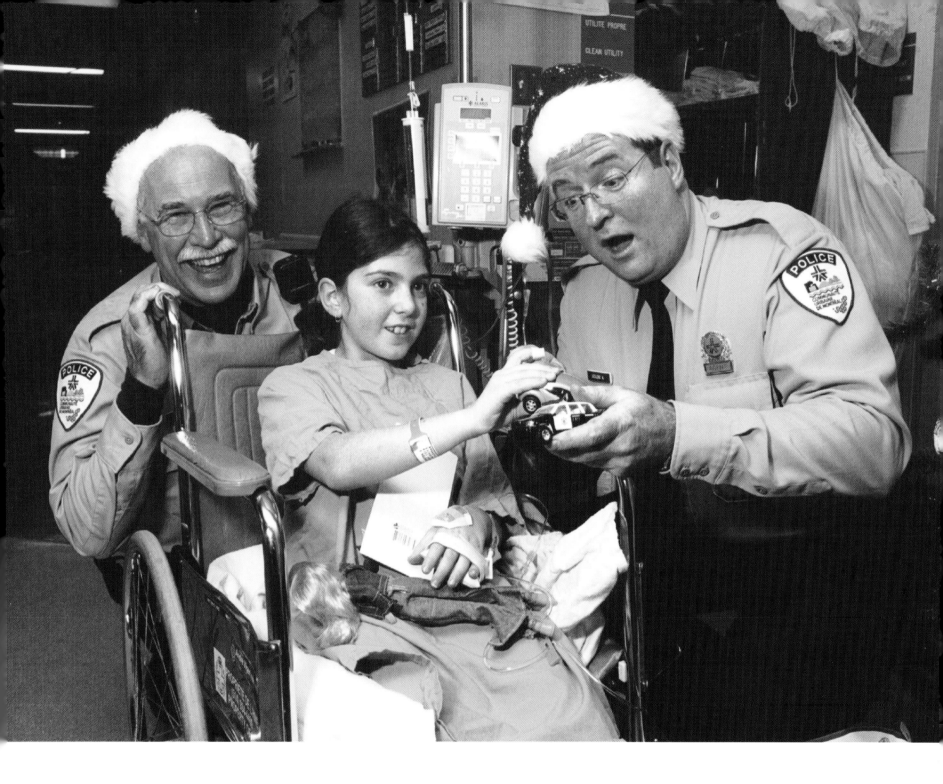

For more than 25 years, the police officers in the MCH's district have been organizing Christmas visits to its eager young patients, taking along gifts, clowns, and big smiles. In this 2004 photo, John Parker (left) and his colleague André Leclerc share a special moment with Felicia Cavuoti.

"I have had the unique privilege of spending time with patients at the Montreal Children's Hospital ... Each time, I am struck by their courage, their will to live and their spirit. Each time, I go home and hug my own healthy children. Each time, I want to do more to help the hospital's expert and caring professionals to prevent, treat, and hopefully cure illnesses. I am not alone. Individuals, private foundations, corporations and community groups have continued to show tremendous support of all hospital programs."

CLAUDIO F. BUSSANDRI, FORMER CHAIRMAN OF THE BOARD,
THE MONTREAL CHILDREN'S HOSPITAL FOUNDATION

12

A Century of Community Support

The Montreal Children's Hospital inspires fierce loyalty in the hearts of those whose children have been treated here—and in the hearts of many others who, even if they have no direct personal connection to the hospital, respect and admire the work done here over the past century. In fact, it would take a volume much larger than this one to list all those who have so generously given their time, money, and energy to the Children's through the years.

That respect and loyalty are reflected in many ways. People of all ages and from all walks of life devote their time and energy to raising funds for the hospital. Children find creative ways to raise money to help other kids get better, with dress-down or funny hair days, Halloween collection boxes, and lemonade stands. Community groups hold spaghetti dinners and benefit concerts. Corporate movers and shakers organize golf tournaments and send their employees pedalling through the streets of downtown Montreal on a bicycle built for 30. Celebrities like actors Macha Grenon, Donald Sutherland, and Rémy Girard gladly sign on to serve as official spokespersons for the hospital. Gala events organized by volunteer committees and sponsored by corporate leaders raise hundreds of thousands of dollars. Some families plan for the future by creating named or anonymous Living Endowment Funds to benefit the hospital, while other donors give quietly on their own.

What they all have in common is a fervent belief in a very good cause—making life better for sick children and their families.

HOSPITAL FUNDING AND FUNDRAISING IN QUEBEC

Historically, fundraising developed quite differently in the francophone and anglophone communities of Montreal. Most francophone hospitals

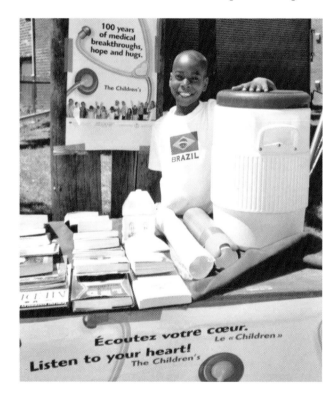

Touched by a classmate's illness, eight-year-old Stefon Julien decided to do something to help patients at the Children's. With the support of his mother, Sandra Beckles, and the principal of Cedarcrest School, Beverly Townsend, Stefon set up a lemonade stand to raise funds for the hospital.

were set up by religious institutions, usually convents, as charitable organizations supported by the church and fees for services from those who were able to pay. English-speaking Quebecers, on the other hand, had a long-standing tradition of community philanthropy. Corporations were set up to own and operate the hospitals, which were supported by fees for service. Income was supplemented by foundations that mounted regular fundraising campaigns. Although the government had taken over the funding and management of hospitals by the 1970s, anglophone hospitals continued to rely on their corporations and foundations for support. Then, as now, keeping up with new developments in hospital care required more than government grants could supply. For the same reason, francophone hospitals began setting up their own foundations and now run sophisticated and successful fundraising campaigns.

Hospitals in Quebec receive a "global budget" from the provincial government, based on various factors. Unlike most hospital systems elsewhere, Quebec's system does not fund hospitals on the basis of patients served or services provided. (The idea behind this is that payment per service might encourage overuse.) Global budgets are used primarily for the hospitals' operating expenses. Equipment, teaching, and research activities have different sources of funding—with varying degrees of adequacy.

Another difference in provincial budgeting is that hospitals in Quebec cannot depreciate their assets over time. As a result, funds are always short when it comes time to cover regular and necessary upgrades of facilities and equipment. Each year, every hospital submits to the government a list of construction or renovation projects and a list of equipment needs. Given the many needs within the province's health-care system and the limited resources to fund them, most items remain on these "wish lists" indefinitely.

Enter the Montreal Children's Hospital Foundation, without which many sorely needed projects would never get off the ground.

RISING COSTS, MORE COMPLEX NEEDS

Costs and needs have grown exponentially over the century. In 1904, the average cost per patient day was 28 cents; in the mid-1950s, it stood at $13.73. By 2004, costs had spiralled to $1,177.95 per patient day. New forms of diagnosis and treatment require new, expensive equipment, extra space, and additional training. Children are now hospitalized for more complex illnesses, requiring more supervision and costlier medications. Costs for labour and materials have also risen dramatically.

GIVING ON A STRONG FOUNDATION

The Montreal Children's Hospital Foundation was set up in 1973 to "support excellence in pediatric care ... by contributing to the advancement of teaching and research activities and by funding state-of-the-art medical and surgical equipment"—or, as the Foundation's Web site puts it, "making the Children's world a better place, one gift at a time." Donations from generous individuals, organizations, and corporations cover the purchase of specialized medical and surgical equipment, as well as the cost of some teaching and research activities.

For example, the magnetic resonance imaging (MRI) facility at the Children's, installed in 1994, was entirely paid for by private donors.

In 2004/05, the Foundation's total revenue was $15 million. About half of that amount went to purchasing equipment and services for the hospital, and the rest to research equipment and services, and to MCH special projects, such as construction and renovation. In its 32 years, the Foundation has raised an impressive total of $204 million.

JUST FOR KIDS—GIVING FROM THE HEART

In 1987, a group of enthusiastic and dedicated parents decided to band together to raise funds to purchase new, high-priority equipment for the Children's. Since then, Just for Kids (JFK) has surpassed its fundraising targets every year, raising a grand total of $4.75 million to date. The proceeds have helped to meet critical needs and acquire vital equipment for many departments and clinics in the hospital, including the dialysis unit, the dental clinic, the operating rooms, and the cardiology service.

A recent project was the refurbishment of the Pediatric Sleep Laboratory, a key facility for the diagnosis and treatment of patients with sleep-related respiratory problems. The project, proposed to JFK by the Equipment Priority Committee at the MCH, involved replacing outdated equipment that is no longer manufactured. JFK members raise money through a wide range of fundraising events, from casino nights to golf tournaments. In July 2004, 40 softball enthusiasts broke the Guinness Book world record for the longest continuous game of softball and raised $60,000 for the hospital.

LAMPLIGHTERS BRING A RAY OF HOPE

Between 1975 and 2004, the Lamplighters, a volunteer group of families and friends of children with malignant diseases, raised $1.3 million to purchase specialized medical equipment and support children being treated for various forms of cancer at the Children's. During their successful 18-year run, their efforts not only provided comfort and support to families dealing with childhood cancer, they also made possible family-friendly renovations of the Hematology and Oncology unit on 8D. One of the Lamplighters' projects was to equip children with coin collection boxes on Halloween, a popular fundraiser that is being continued by the MCH Foundation.

The Hematology/Oncology Day Treatment Centre, opened in 1998, provides a healing environment in which 7,600 young cancer patients receive

A Bicycle Built for 30

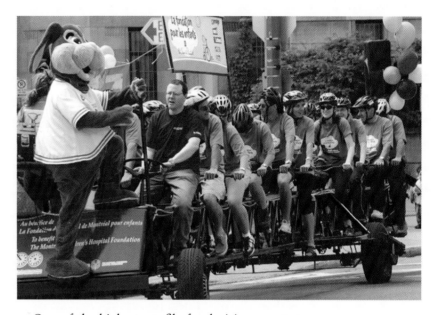

One of the highest-profile fundraising events to benefit the Children's, Pedal for Kids was started in 1992 by Michael Conway and Sylvie Lalumière-Conway in memory of their daughter Meagan. The event is now organized by an energetic committee of volunteers chaired by Paul Normandin.

Over a five-day period each spring, the big bike circulates through the streets of downtown Montreal seven times a day, escorted by the Montreal police department's motorcycle squad. Participating companies also organize other fundraising activities, such as bake sales and barbecues, to boost the total.

To date, Pedal for Kids has raised a grand total of $5,215,000, which has been used for everything from equipment, such as incubators for the NICU, to environmental improvements, such as refurbishing the recovery room where patients are reunited with their families after surgery. As of 2005, part of the funds raised thanks to Pedal for Kids will be invested in building the new Montreal Children's Hospital on the Glen site.

their chemotherapy, transfusion, hydration, and pain management treatments every year. The centre was funded by the MCH Foundation with the participation of the Lamplighters, *Opération Enfant Soleil*, the Sian Bradwell Fund, the Bruno Gattola Fund, and the Taylor James Fund.

"We have a lot of happy endings ... and some sad ones as well. It always amazes me that even parents who have lost a child still want to do so much. They find the strength to turn their grief into dedicating themselves to helping other children and parents who are battling illness."

LOUISE DERY-GOLDBERG, PRESIDENT, THE MONTREAL CHILDREN'S HOSPITAL FOUNDATION

VOLUNTEERS MAKE ALL THE DIFFERENCE

Volunteers are the lifeblood of the hospital. They're the baby cuddlers and clowns, the knitters and card players, the people who accompany sick children to other parts of the hospital for treatments

Elizabeth Sakoyannis has the best job in the world— volunteer baby cuddler at the Children's.

when their own parents can't be with them, the interpreters who help children and parents understand what's going on. In 2000/01 alone, hospital volunteers contributed 40,179 hours of their time.

The rigorous volunteer selection process includes detailed application forms, interviews, and reference-checking. Those who are accepted are given training sessions and ongoing monitoring and support. The composition of the volunteer force is changing. In the past, most hospital volunteers, especially Auxiliary members, were the wives of doctors or of other professionals, who were able to commit many hours to the hospital. Today, with a high proportion of women in the paid workforce, volunteers may be students, seniors, those who have taken early retirement, or others who make time in their busy schedules for volunteering because they "just want to help the kids."

ABOVE AND BEYOND

Some of the most dedicated volunteers are rarely seen by patients or visitors to the hospital, yet they make an incalculable contribution to the institution year after year. They are the members of strategic committees, boards, and councils. Over the years, hundreds of dedicated individuals have served the Children's, whether on the original Committee of Organization, the Corporation, the Board of Governors, the Board of the Foundation, capital campaign committees, or numerous other bodies.

As the hospital's base of support has broadened, so has the range of expertise that these volunteers bring to the table. In the early 20th century, they were a relatively small group of generous benefactors. While these are still very much involved and needed, early 21st-century board and committee members also include professionals in health care and community services, specialists in fundraising, and representatives of patients and families, as well as lawyers, accountants, and business people.

In a speech at the hospital's annual public information meeting in 1991, Board Chairman Eric

Maldoff accurately predicted, "... we will have an increasing need for people like you and me—volunteers prepared to devote time to getting to know our [health-care] institutions and their services. People who can use their knowledge to contribute to the development of policies at all levels."

Mr. Maldoff himself has been an outstanding example of the volunteer he described. Dr. Nicolas Steinmetz, who was Executive Director for much of Mr. Maldoff's tenure, says of his involvement: "He took the trouble to truly understand the complexities and the politics of how the health-care system works at the local, regional, provincial, and federal levels. He did not interfere internally but concentrated his efforts on the larger, important, strategic issues. He internalized the values embodied in the Children's and therefore was decidedly effective in helping to guide it through the long and sometimes difficult MUHC merger debates. And to do all this he has given an astonishing amount of time."

Important elements of his contribution can be seen in the current governance structure of the MUHC and the role of the Children's within it. The work of the MCH Board, disbanded on the merger, has been to a large extent taken up by the Council for Services to Children and Adolescents (CSCA), the body that represents the pediatric mission within the MUHC. The CSCA continues to advocate for the rights of children at all levels of the health-care system.

It also continues the tradition of bringing a wide variety of experience to supporting the care of children. Graham Bagnall has chaired the CSCA since 2003. The group contributes to the Children's objectives internally, he notes, by bringing in an outside viewpoint, by acting as a sounding board for staff, and by providing support, not just in assessing proposed projects, but in implementing them as well.

In addition to members of the community, the CSCA includes representatives of professional staff, families, other partners in the MUHC, and McGill University. This makes for a wide diversity of experience and opinion.

"The meetings are always very spirited, and the discussion open and constructive," reports Mr. Bagnall. "It's a joy to chair a group like this." Is there something special about the Children's that brings out enthusiasm? "Maybe a combination of the institution's mission and the people who are so passionate about it."

"TRIPLE-THREAT PEOPLE"

The Auxiliary of the Montreal Children's Hospital, originally called the Women's Auxiliary, has been an integral part of hospital life for nearly 70 years. In 1938, six young women organized a Christmas party for the 350 children in the old Montreal Children's (Vipond) Hospital on St. Antoine Street. The party was a sensational success, and the hospital asked the now growing team to form an official Women's Auxiliary and raise money to buy a refrigerator unit for the hospital. In 1940, the old Montreal Children's joined the Children's Memorial and the Auxiliary continued its enthusiastic efforts for the merged institutions, organizing rummage sales, Victory Bond campaigns, and fashion shows.

John H. Molson, President of the Children's Memorial Hospital, commended the Auxiliary in January 1950 for members' "energy, efficiency and enthusiasm." Phoebe Seely, a founding member of the Auxiliary, told the *Montreal Star* in 1958 that "Hospital volunteers are triple-threat people [engaged in] service to the Hospital, fundraising and good will ambassadorship between the Hospital and the public."

Over the years, the Auxiliary has provided the hospital with everything from station wagons and an X-ray machine to ceiling lights for the operating room and an oxygen tent. Today, the Auxiliary raises about $250,000 every year. About 10% of the funds raised go to research and the rest to the purchase of medical equipment.

The Junior Associate Group (JAGS) was born in the early 1960s, swelling the ranks of the Auxiliary

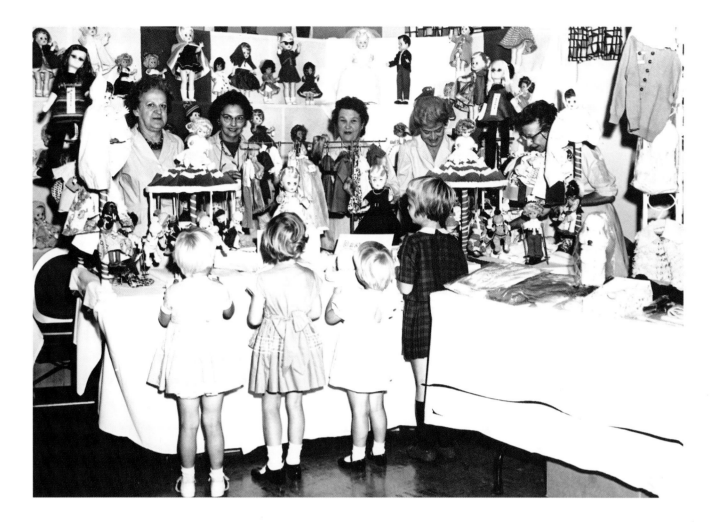

Young customers look over the merchandise at one of the Auxiliary's bazaars in the late 1950s. Sales have been an important source of income for the Auxiliary since its inception. Its first permanent point of sale came in 1945, when it started co-managing the Nearly New Shop downtown with the Montreal Maternity Hospital Auxiliary. That shop was unfortunately destroyed by fire in 1979, but locations within the hospital walls have survived and thrived. The Tiny Tim Gift Shop, now called the Boutique and located on the second floor of the B-wing, and the nearby café (evolved from a small canteen in the St. Antoine Street location) are reliable sources of funding for equipment, research, and patient needs. And the annual bazaars still attract young and old.

and helping with the snack bar, Red Cross blood donor clinics, the annual bazaar, and many other activities. JAGS formed a sewing group in its early days that made baby nighties and shrouds, jackets, and "modesty pants" to cover casts and braces. An arts group decorated the wards, made felt hand-puppets for patients, and fashioned hundreds of crepe-paper hats for patients' birthday parties.

In 1965, the Auxiliary decided to think big. In *A 60-Year History of the Auxiliary of the Montreal Children's Hospital (1939–1999)*, Joan Hofman, Auxiliary President from 1975 to 1977, recalled the staging of the first Mardi Gras Fiesta at the Windsor Hotel. "We volunteers worked for months

THE TINY TIM FUND

An undated flyer in the files of the Montreal Children's Hospital (probably from the 1960s) describes the *raison d'être* of the Tiny Tim Fund set up by the Auxiliary in 1951:

"[It] provides patient comforts and necessities not covered by government or other sources of revenue. By giving to this Fund, donors contribute to the health and happiness of children in sickness and need.

"Tiny Tim means new eye-glasses for a little girl with poor sight whose father is unemployed. He supplies a brace for a crippled boy from a low-income family, a partial denture for a child injured in an auto accident, transportation to and from our clinics for those in poor financial circumstances. Because of the Tiny Tim Fund, we are able to brighten dreary waiting areas and provide comfort and relaxation during anxious hours."

Over the years, the funds required to help families in need have increased exponentially. The Department of Social Services now manages the Fund at the hospital, and donors to the fund currently contribute close to $300,000 annually.

and months, hammering, sewing, thinking, thinking, thinking!" That event in 1965 raised $11,369 for the MCH—a huge amount at that time. After several unfortunately timed snowstorms in the following years, the date was changed and the event, renamed Spring Fling, was held annually in April or May until 1978.

Marcie Scheim, Past President of the Auxiliary and one of the centennial coordinators, calls that period the heyday of the volunteer. One of the contributors to that heyday was Marylee Kelley, President from 1973 to 1975. Mrs. Kelley, also a very active Board and committee member, continued to make lasting contributions to the hospital and to health-care services throughout Quebec, until she passed away during the hospital's centennial year.

TURNING TRAGEDY INTO HOPE FOR OTHERS: THE PENNY COLE FUND

Families never really recover from the loss of a child, but some are able to turn their heartbreak into hope for others by setting up a memorial fund through the Children's Foundation. One such benefactor was Jack Cole, a philanthropist from the age of 18, when he helped raise money to build the 600-room YMCA on Drummond Street. He and his wife Elsie had a daughter, Penny, who was diagnosed with leukemia at the age of 12. Penny spent eight years as a patient at the Children's, even working as a volunteer in her dying days.

After Penny died on her 20th birthday in 1967, her father dedicated himself to the hospital. He established the Penny Cole Laboratory at the MCH and endowed a chair in hematology and oncology for the hospital through McGill University. He is credited with the creation of the Montreal Children's

THE SIAN BRADWELL FUND

"I used to lie on the bed with her and show her beautiful coloured pictures of tiger cubs playing and, for effect, demonstrate how tigers growl. At the age of five months, she started growling at birds, squirrels, kittens, and other small animals which used to come into our garden. It was funny to hear the sound come from such a tiny girl ... Less than a week before she died ... she was still trying to growl at stuffed toy animals."

Sharon Bradwell, mother of Sian, who died of cancer in March 1986, at the age of 17 months

On October 3, 1990, the day Sian would have turned six, her parents established the Sian Bradwell Fund, through the Foundation, to help children with cancer at the Montreal Children's Hospital. To date, the fund has raised over $600,000, covering such special items as printing a handbook for parents of children with cancer and purchasing specialized medical equipment, as well as special mattresses to ease the pain of children in the terminal stages of cancer.

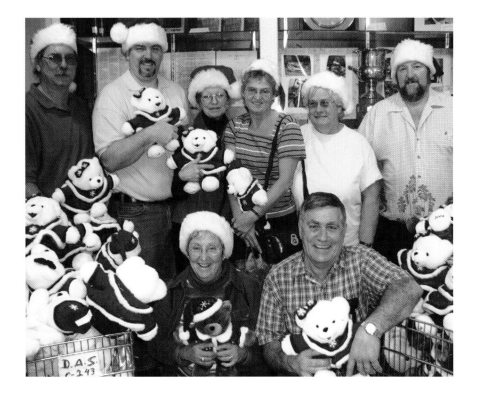

the liver that leads to severe hypoglycemia and other complications.

Dominique spent the next seven years, both at home and in school, on the very strict treatment program that kept her alive. Every three hours, around the clock, her parents fed her a glucose-based "cocktail." Although she was surrounded with care and love, Dominique's life was plagued with difficulties. On the eve of her eighth birthday, an acute pancreatitis took her life. During her final moments, she showed tremendous courage. Although she was suffering, she begged her favourite aunt and babysitter, Jeanne, "Don't tell my mom how much it hurts."

"Today, we understand the disease better," explains Dr. Robert Barnes, endocrinologist at the MCH. "Even though we still don't have a cure for it, we know that starch, a totally natural product that contains glucose, makes it possible for us to regulate blood sugar. Starch is digested over a period of several hours and thus frees up sugars on a continual basis." The treatment consists of ingesting starch several times a day and following a restrictive diet reviewed regularly on an outpatient basis. The arrival of new feeding techniques, such as gastrostomy buttons and home sugar-monitoring equipment, has made it possible to control the disease more precisely. "To find a cure, we have to wait until research discovers a way to restore the deficient enzyme," says Dr. Barnes.

Since 1993, Ross Côté Jr. (far right) and friends have organized a series of fundraising events to benefit the Montreal Children's Hospital. Every year, part of the proceeds is used to purchase teddy bears, which are distributed to patients in December. The rest goes towards the purchase of medical equipment. To date, the Township Toddlers have raised over $50,000 for the MCH.

Hospital Foundation and served as its Honorary Chairman until his death in November 2004. "He held the Children's Hospital close to his heart," Louise Dery-Goldberg recalled. "Every year, even through the time he was ill, we continued to receive his tremendous support. Even in his late 80s, he was still an absolute charmer."

FUNDING RESEARCH FOR THE LOVE OF A CHILD

In 1973, Lorraine and Marc Belcourt created an endowment fund in memory of their daughter Dominique, who died at the age of eight after a lengthy illness.

At barely five months old, Dominique was admitted to the Children's for urgent care. After a month of hospitalization, which included biopsies of her spleen and liver for possible tumours, it was determined that she had glycogen storage disease type 1, a genetic disease related to an enzyme deficiency in

GIFTS-IN-KIND

Donations take many forms. The 1927 Annual Report noted that, "We are indebted to the Sewing Committee of the Junior League of Montreal for practically monthly donations of knitted sweaters, scarves, baby jackets, and bootees; to the Needlework Guild of Canada from which we received in November last, a very large supply of babies' and children's clothes, underwear, etc.; to the Junior Red Cross Society for a wonderful parcel of mufflers, sweaters, bibs, wash-cloths, and scrap-books sent at Christmastime …"

The Belcourts had a definite goal in creating an endowment fund: to help other children suffering from liver disease by funding research. To date, the Dominique Belcourt Fund has grown to over $80,000. With this, the Belcourts have been able to establish an MCH Pediatric Medical Grand Rounds annual lectureship in Dominique's memory, at which researchers from around the world share the latest advances in liver diseases.

THE HEART OF LIFE FUND

Robbie and Gary Silverman learned during a 19-week prenatal ultrasound that one of their twins had a major congenital cardiac malformation. At birth, Benjamin was blue. Because of the malformation, he was getting only 70% of the oxygen he needed. He spent the first 15 days of his life being evaluated, monitored, and tested in the NICU.

At five weeks of age, Benjamin underwent his first surgery, to allow his tiny pulmonary arteries to grow larger—a temporary solution until he grew stronger. A few months later, a cardiac catheterization procedure confirmed that Benjamin was ready for the complete repair of his heart malformation, and on February 19, 2002, the five-month-old underwent his second open-heart surgery.

When Benjamin's heart failed during surgery, the cardiology and cardiac surgery team worked tirelessly to keep him alive. "They never gave up hope.

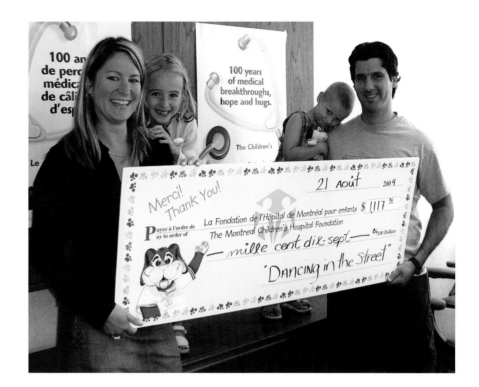

ART FROM THE HEART

Visitors to the hospital frequently remark on the cheerful artwork adorning the walls. The murals are the handiwork of volunteers, some professional and some amateur artists. The art on the main floor, near the emergency room, is by girls from Trafalgar School who were rewarded with juice and cookies, while the painting on 3D, in Respiratory Medicine, was done by Grade 3 boys from Selwyn House. Teresa Di Bartolo of Architectural Services supplied a colour palette and the students painted within it to match the décor.

That's my message to parents who discover that their child is sick: always have hope," says Mrs. Silverman.

The Silvermans have no doubt their son is alive and well today because of the perseverance and expertise of the MCH team. "In another hospital, or with a different team of specialists, or even a decade ago, Benjamin would surely not have made it," says his grateful father.

The Heart of Life Fund was created in 1997 by parents of children who, like Benjamin, had undergone a cardiovascular intervention at the MCH at a very young age. The fund's purpose is twofold: it serves as the basis for a support group for parents of children with heart malformations, and its members raise funds to help pediatric cardiac specialists acquire the best state-of-the-art equipment.

In August 2004, Tracy Mimeau-Worthington and Yannick Dion, the parents of young patient Émilie Dion, decided to turn their traditional "Dancing in the Streets" party into a fundraiser for the Children's. Two streets were closed to traffic and local families were invited to enjoy all sorts of activities. The final tally for the hospital: $1,117.

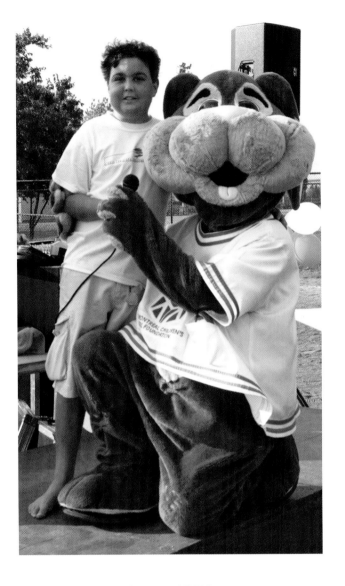

Caramel, the hospital mascot "born" in 2001, is a big, furry puppy designed to embody the warm and caring qualities that make MCH staff so special. A great favourite with children, he represents the hospital at hundreds of events. Here, he poses with Christophe Robichaud at a fundraising event for the Christophe Robichaud Fund, organized by the boy and his family in 2004 to raise funds for the MCH Hematology/Oncology Department.

TELETHONS RAISE MILLIONS

Annual telethons organized by the Foundation for Research into Children's Diseases and *Opération Enfant Soleil* have raised millions over the years to fund research and purchase medical equipment for the hospital.

Opération Enfant Soleil was founded in 1988 by *le Centre hospitalier de l'Université Laval*, in Quebec City. Its first telethon was so successful that the two other major pediatric centres in Quebec, the

Montreal Children's and Ste-Justine hospitals, joined in the following year. A few years later, the organizers decided to give 15% of the proceeds to children's health services outside the major centres of Quebec, and the rest to the three larger centres. Since its first year, *Opération Enfant Soleil* has distributed more than $70 million throughout the province. But the community has been generous in more than money. Four thousand volunteers support the work of telethon and hospital staff, and organizations everywhere in the province get involved in the fundraising. The 18th edition raised more than $13 million to support children's hospitals in Quebec.

The 24-hour Telethon for Research into Children's Diseases has been broadcast annually since 1977. It is one of several community events organized by the Foundation of the same name. Others include *le Gala des étoiles*, the Standard Life Marathon and *le Bal des Enfants du Monde*. A prime example of support by an involved community, the Foundation for Research into Children's Diseases was started by the Inter-Service Clubs Council, whose members currently include B'nai Brith, Civitan, Kinsmen, Kiwanis, Knights of Pythias, Lions, Optimists, Richelieu, Rotary, and Zonta. Service club members and corporations sponsor and participate in its events, which since 1977 have raised more than $44 million—more than $5 million in 2004 alone—for four pediatric research centres in Quebec, including the Children's.

CARING FOR KIDS RADIOTHON

The second annual Caring for Kids Radiothon, held in March 2005, raised $1,724,661 for the hospital, far surpassing the previous year's total of $1.2 million. Broadcast live from the Children's by CJAD 800, CHOM 97.7 FM, and MIX 96, the radiothon featured stirring testimonials from sick children, parents, former patients, and health-care professionals.

More than 450 volunteers manned the phones. Many of the 9,000 callers joined the Children's

Circle of Hugs, pledging 50 cents a day, or $15 a month, to help sick children feel better. Equipment funded through the radiothon includes an anesthesia machine, 50 syringe pumps, two portable ventilators, 10 pulse oximeters, two operating tables, and three portable neonatal ventilators.

CREATING A HEALING ENVIRONMENT

Not so long ago, the physical environment of the hospital was very plain, with white or pale green paint everywhere. That was considered appropriate at the time, as well as cheaper to maintain. Over the past 15 years, all that has changed, largely thanks to the Task Force on Pediatric Design chaired by MUHC Board member Mary Anne Ferguson, currently Vice-Chairman of the Council for Services to Children and Adolescents, and long-time member of its predecessor, the MCH Board of Directors. The task force includes designers, a community representative who is a parent, and a cross-section of hospital staff.

From the beginning, the hard-working task force looked into every aspect of the hospital's internal space and sought creative ideas from both inside and out. They worked tirelessly to advocate improvements, some of which were quite radical in their use of colour and design. Much of the implementation was possible only because of volunteer support, some of it financial, but most of it hands-on, on-site work. Task force members were consistently consulted on the environmental design, as they still are. They worked carefully with the hospital's health care professionals, who pointed out, for instance, that it would not be a good idea to paint a ward for respiratory cases blue, because it would be harder to see if a patient's skin turned blue!

The work of the task force has become increasingly important with the growing understanding that the environment affects healing and patients' responses to medication and treatment. Mary Anne Ferguson recalls that her "most thrilling moment" at the Children's was when she heard from PACU nurses two weeks after windows had been installed: "Nurses noted that patients required less medication, proving that a healing environment is not simply frilly window dressing, but real. It saves costs, and brings better interaction between caregiver and patient, quicker healing time, and increased patient satisfaction." These improved results are still being seen in 2005.

One of the committee's most visible achievements is the Children's Corner just outside the main entrance. With a sculpture given by an anonymous donor (pictured on the cover of this book), a large mural from the Montreal Area Decorative Painters, and a comfortable granite bench, it provides a quiet and restful place for children and their families to take a break outdoors.

"We are hard-wired as human beings to respond to nature," explains Ms. Ferguson, "and we need its restorative aspects to help us heal during that time when we are at our most fragile."

The community's involvement in creating a healing and restorative environment, not only for patients and their families, but also for staff, has become a lasting legacy for the Children's that will continue even as the hospital moves to its new home at the Glen site.

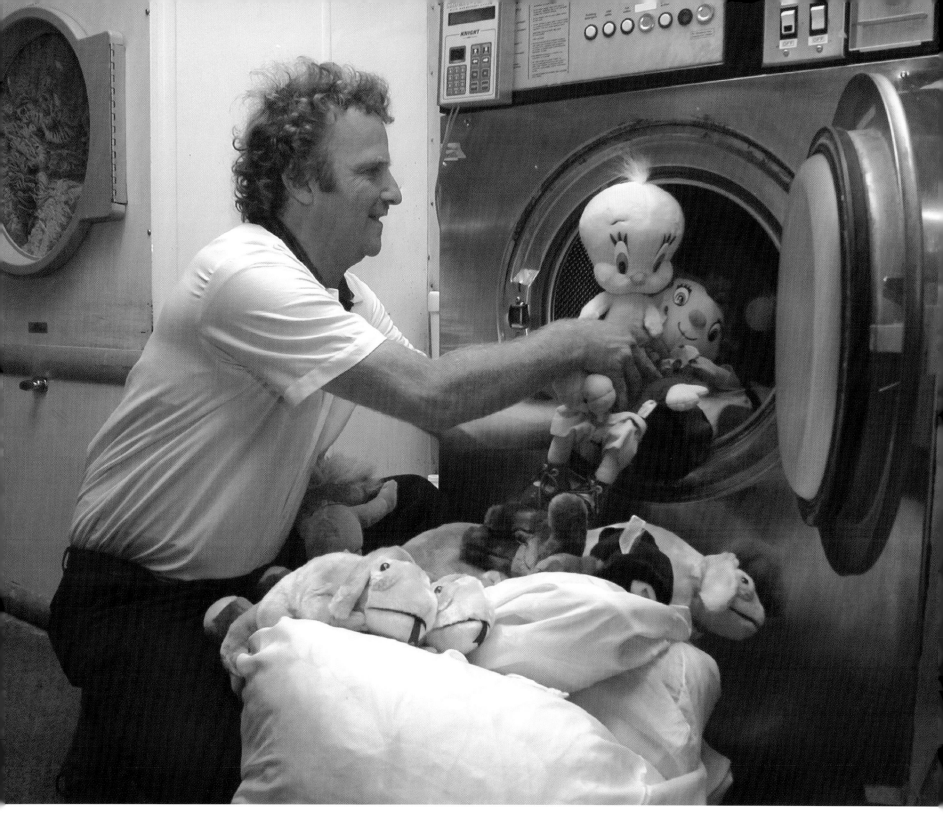

The MCH laundry sometimes handles items not found in most laundries, including plastic toys, and even stuffed animals. In this photo, laundry worker Normand Dumas loads a group of cuddly creatures into the washer. Sometimes these soft toys are forgotten in beds by their small owners and collected with the sheets, but they are not tossed away. If left unclaimed, they are given to charity.

"Hospitals have come a long way since the 1950s — it's an entirely different world!"

DR. JACK CHARTERS, EXECUTIVE DIRECTOR, 1970–1987
in a centennial year interview

13

A Day in the Life of the Children's

4:00 A.M.

In one of the busiest children's emergency departments in the country, things are slow. Only a few patients are being examined by nursing and medical staff. The wee, small hours are the only time when people working there can get a sense of control and catch their breath before the onslaught of the coming day.

More than 65,000 patients a year pass through the Emergency doors at the southeast corner of the main hospital complex. That is fewer than the 90,000 or so who came annually during the 1970s and '80s, thanks to improving child health in general, better injury-prevention awareness, increased access to health-care services in the community, and, to some extent, the reduction in infectious diseases. However, traffic still remains high at most times of the day. Most of the children admitted to the hospital arrive through the ER.

Accommodating these large numbers has required adaptation over the years.

Unlike the other departments at the time of the 1956 move, the ER, along with other outpatient services, had already left its overcrowded quarters in the Carruthers Building at the Cedar Avenue location. Some 10 years earlier, it had moved to the hospital's other site on St. Antoine Street—the Montreal Children's (formerly Vipond) Hospital site. In 1956, it was integrated into the new quarters at the south end of the C-Wing, near what is now the

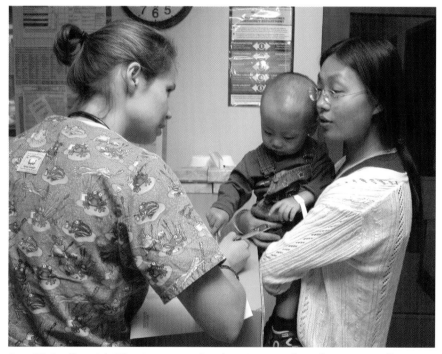

Luo Hui talks with ER triage nurse Lindsay Bryson about her son Apollo Xiu, who fell out of bed and is being checked for possible injuries.

When they arrive in the Emergency Room, children see a triage nurse, who ensures that the most urgent cases are seen right away. During peak periods—9:00 a.m. to noon, and later around 2:00 p.m. and 7:00 p.m.— others may wait a while.

"Emergency Room" is a bit of a misnomer. The ER is actually a suite of rooms, including waiting areas, triage areas, X-ray and other emergency test facilities, and treatment rooms. Extensive renovations in 1994 brought a number of badly needed changes to the ER, including new triage and examination rooms. They also added an ensuite washroom, to the relief of parents who had had to coax urine samples out of uncooperative small children in the overcrowded public facilities down the hall.

SHORT-STAY UNIT REDUCES EMERGENCY ADMISSIONS

The ER staff these days try to treat children without the disruption of admitting them. The Short-Stay Unit just down the hall was created in 1996 to accommodate children who need to be monitored or stabilized for less than 24 hours. The unit's creation erased the last vestige of the A-Wing's former life as the nurses' residence. The large room had been the Ross Lounge, originally a gathering area for nurses in what was known as the Ross Residence when it opened in 1956. Even after 1970, when nursing education was moved to CEGEPs and the residence was no longer needed, the Ross Lounge served as the locale for nursing seminars, as well as for hospital meetings and events of all sorts.

electrical intake. Then, when the B-Wing was completed in 1977, the ER was relocated to its present site and given an entrance near the parking lot that allows more room for ambulances and police cars, as well as easier access for harried parents.

6:00 A.M.

By 6:00 a.m., children and their families start to trickle in to the ER in larger numbers.

Activity picks up in other areas of the hospital, too. Uniforms and bed and patient linens are being delivered to the ER, operating rooms, wards, and clinics by laundry staff, who start deliveries early to avoid tying up elevators. (Buildings without utility elevators require some compromises.)

Surgical instruments are being taken to operating rooms in covered carts from another service in the basement not far from the laundry—the Central Supply Room, or CSR. There, the used medical and surgical instruments from the OR, the nursing units, and the clinics are taken apart, washed, and sterilized in a tunnel-washer reminiscent of a carwash. Discharged dry, they are then arranged in surgical instrument sets, prepared for particular types of

procedures belonging to the different specialties (such as orthopedics, plastic surgery, or neurology) according to hundreds of "recipes" kept in the department. Single instruments are delivered in carts with specially tagged sections.

In the near future, each instrument will be marked by a laser and scanned by an under-table camera in CSR—rather like a grocery-store checkout. There won't be a single scalpel that can't be put exactly in its right place. And that's no mean accomplishment. While the number of procedures carried out at the Children's is fewer than at most adult hospitals, the number of instruments is greater. This is partly because the Children's covers the full range of

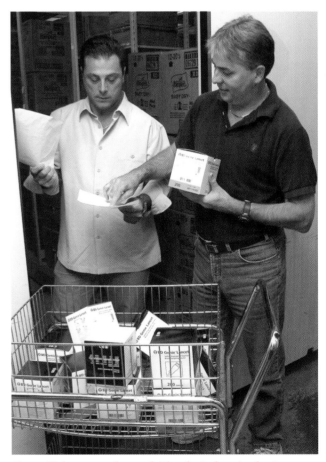

Costa Kalantzopoulos and Claude Aubry, in the Stores Department, check on supplies to be delivered.

specialties, like neurology and heart surgery, while adult hospitals specialize more, and partly because each instrument must be stocked in many more sizes to accommodate babies, children, and teens.

7:00 A.M.

The next shift of laundry workers arrives to start washing, drying, and folding laundry orders for the next day. Altogether, they serve between 35 and 40 different areas each day, including Housekeeping— they wash the mops!

The Emergency waiting room begins to fill up. Tired night staff go home and a larger contingent comes in for the day.

Surgical operations get underway in the OR on the 10th floor. "OR," like "ER," is shorthand for a suite of rooms. (It has been more than 60 years since the Children's had only a single operating room.) The suite consists of 10 operating rooms (two with a viewing gallery), offices, supply rooms, and a waiting area for children and their families near the D-Wing elevators. From the waiting room, a corridor extends past the OR doors to another entrance at the C-Wing elevators. Only OR patients and staff dressed in scrubs can enter this corridor, to keep the operating areas sterile. The C-Wing entrance is used by arriving staff and for deliveries of supplies.

There are other OR facilities on the main floor in the Owen Day Surgery Centre. Used exclusively for day surgery when it opened in 1976, the smaller OR area now handles the minor inpatient procedures, leaving the complex ones for the 10th floor. During summer months, and depending on patient volume, all surgeries are usually carried out on the 10th floor.

Seven o'clock is the time most clinical and support staff are starting work. This in turn places increasing demand on other services. One of the most peculiar flurries of activity affects the security staff, whose many responsibilities include unlocking doors. Their peak time of the day occurs between 7:00 and 8:30 a.m., as people arrive for work having forgotten their office keys!

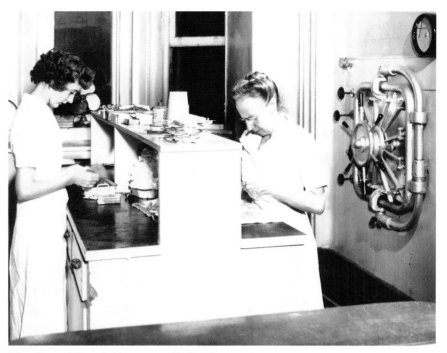

The Central Supply Room, on Cedar Avenue, in 1939

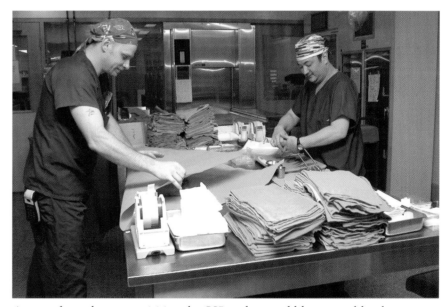

A nurse from the 1920s visiting the CSR today would be amazed by the elaborate facilities. While there were times on Cedar Avenue when surgical instruments had to be washed by hand in the OR, owing to lack of space, the modern CSR has more space and equipment than several early 20th-century operating rooms. In this 2004 photo, James Payne and José Aracena prepare surgical supply kits.

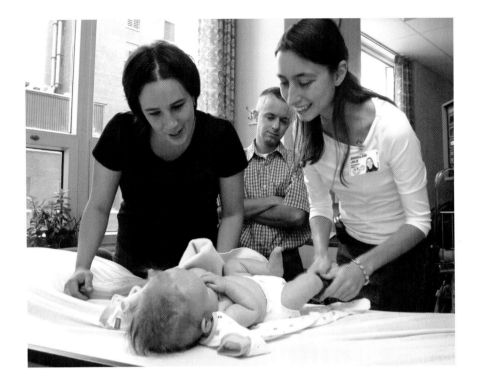

Young Thomas gets friendly attention from nurse Julie Brouillard of the Alternative Care Module, under the watchful eyes of parents Julie Bougie and Sylvain Beauchamp.

The day shift nurses arrive on the units and read their patients' charts before meeting to exchange information and discuss cases with the departing night staff. Patient care units occupy most of the 6th, 7th, and 8th floors of the C-Wing. There used to be units on the 5th floor as well, but as the proportion of outpatient services increased, and units were reorganized, they have been gradually replaced by offices.

The 9th floor houses the intensive care units—pediatric (PICU) and neonatal (NICU). As their names suggest, they are designed for children and infants requiring more intensive care, in terms of both personnel and equipment, than the other nursing units can easily provide.

The ER, the OR, the nursing units, and the clinics, while they have their peak times, are almost always busy. To reduce the pressure on these departments, and make things easier for children and families, a new unit called the Alternative Care Module was created in 1994. Located on 7C, near the surgery

units, it is open from 7:00 a.m. to 7:00 p.m. Patients who are having surgery go there a week in advance to learn what to expect, have preoperative tests, and meet the specialists who will care for them. They may also go back for surgical follow-up, such as removal of sutures or change of dressings, or for regular checkups for chronic conditions. This way, they avoid going through Emergency and spend little or no time in a hospital bed—an added advantage when demand for beds is high.

8:00 A.M.

In the clinics, children begin to arrive for appointments. By the late 1970s, clinic activity in the main buildings was being largely centralized on the B-Wing's second floor, to facilitate sharing of information and facilities. During the average year, some 165,000 young patients visit MCH clinics here.

Most come up the moving ramp from the main entrance, an innovation brought to the hospital with the B-Wing in 1977 to alleviate the long waits at elevators that had already become insufficient for the traffic level. During the 1990s, the walls around the ramp were redecorated. Frescoes beside it depict outdoor scenes and hot-air balloons. Colourful painted windows at the top, and in the ER waiting area on the first floor, record the generosity of the hospital's donors. In the main clinic waiting area, brightly coloured outdoor scenes provide cheer and diversion for concerned parents and fretful children.

The 1990s was a period during which the Children's was most active in its continuing efforts to create comforting, healing physical environments for patients and their families. This has been achieved through paint colours, artwork, games on the walls, or specialized carpentry projects such as a lighthouse housing a television and play kitchen in Day Surgery, dropped ceilings in the form of fish on the nursing units, distorting mirrors in the ER waiting area, and many more.

The impetus for these improvements was the Task Force on Pediatric Design, set up in 1989 by then

Executive Director Nicolas Steinmetz, with Board member Mary Anne Ferguson in charge.

"Design is like a drug . . . it is part of the therapy," maintains Ms. Ferguson. "A well designed environment gives patients a sense of control and alleviates stress. A lot of institutions have to be convinced that a healing environment pays off in terms of reduced medication and healing time. But we're grateful that at the Children's, Dr. Steinmetz had that vision and the architectural services and maintenance staff spent a lot of time turning our dreams into reality."

Always at a premium, clinic space is used judiciously. Many of the areas are multi-purpose, housing different clinics on different days of the week or month. Among the few exclusive clinic spaces are those located away from the main clinic area: Orthopedics (E-Wing), and Ophthalmology, on the first floor of the D-Wing. The Hematology/ Oncology Day Treatment Centre has its own, more private, space on the B-Wing's 3rd floor.

A number of outpatient clinics are held outside the main buildings. The Adolescent and Dental clinics, for instance, are held in the Gilman Pavilion, while psychiatrists and psychologists see patients in their offices at 2018 St. Catherine Street West.

By 8:15 a.m., the nursing units are lively as patient activities begin. Despite the calm, reassuring air of the people working there, the units are busy places. Family members are everywhere—in the rooms with their children, walking, or waiting in the hallways. Starting in the morning, a variety of professionals look after the children in different ways. Staff doctors do their rounds with residents. Nurses carry out their many tasks, whether administering medications, inserting intravenous lines, or advising parents. They may be accompanied by student nurses learning from the professionals.

Dietitians see to patients who need feeding tubes and pain specialists care for those who need pain relief. Lab technologists come to take blood samples. Child Life workers use play therapy to prepare children for procedures or to give them information and

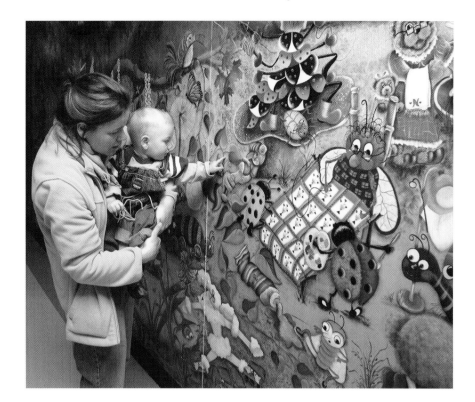

reassurance. Volunteers entertain the children, and clowns make weekly visits. Professionals from Social Services and Pastoral Services come to support children and families.

Although most nursing units have been moved into the C-Wing, there are still some important ones located in the D-Wing. The Hematology and Oncology Unit on the 8th floor is devoted to children and adolescents with leukemia and other cancers. Because of the long stays and frequent returns on this unit, a family feeling often develops among the staff, patients, and families. In fact, the unit owes many of its updated, family-friendly facilities to the support of fundraising parents.

The unit known as 7D also has its own family feeling. There, children and adolescents with psychiatric conditions engage in a wide range of activities designed to help them build and maintain healthy relationships—group games, outings, even a bazaar and bake sale held by the kids to raise funds

Brightly coloured scenes on the walls of the 2B waiting area amuse children of all ages by challenging them to find figures painted on the wall. Here, young Aimeri shows his mother, Fannie, where to find a mouse under a toadstool.

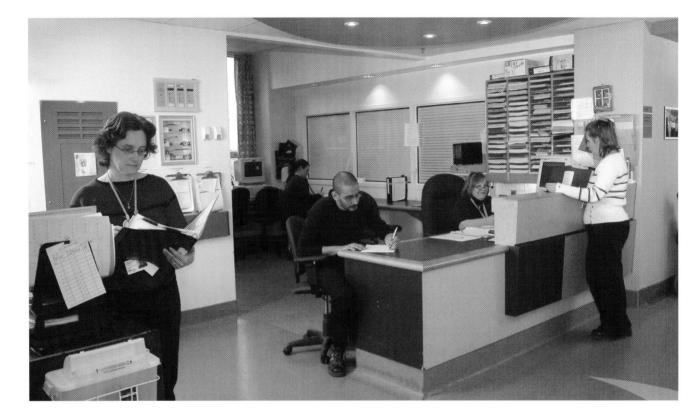

for their activities. Government policy on psychiatric care led to the closing of the unit on weekends between 1987 and fall 2004. Now, although only teenagers stay overnight, the school-aged children still share activities and communal meals during the day.

9:00 A.M.

Medications ordered throughout the day are delivered to the nursing units from the main Pharmacy on the basement level. Porters bring them up on their regular rounds, although emergency, or "stat," orders are delivered at once. By the time they reach the units, prescriptions have been through several rigorous checks to make sure that the type and dosage are appropriate for each child, and that they will not interact with any other medications he or she may be taking. This process of checking starts with the doctor who orders the prescription, then involves the pharmacy technician who makes it up, then the pharmacist who verifies it, and finally, the nurse who gives the medication to the child.

Throughout the various MCH buildings, in the main complex and the satellite buildings, most administrative and office staff arrive for work between 8:00 and 9:00 a.m. They include secretaries, clerks, managers, and people occupying dozens of other positions, who ensure that appointments are made, patients' charts prepared, supplies are ordered, personnel are paid, budgets are met, and a wide range of regulations and standards are respected.

10:00 A.M.

By now, the hospital's outpatient clinics are in full swing, the early arrivals returning from diagnostic tests and others still arriving or making follow-up appointments.

The early surgeries are wrapping up, and the CSR picks up used surgical instruments for washing and re-assembly, as it will do approximately every two hours for the rest of the day.

By the time the clinics are humming, lab technologists have completed their morning procurement rounds taking blood samples on the nursing units, and have returned to their laboratories and work-stations to carry out diagnostic testing. Many technologists work on the 4th floor of the C- and D-Wings, in the laboratories that together constitute the "Central Labs": Biochemistry, Hematology, Immunology, Endocrinology, and the Renal Function lab. They also work in the clinics doing on-the-spot blood tests for quick results. In the Central Labs and clinics, as well as in the Pediatric Test Centre on the second floor, hundreds of samples of blood, urine, and other substances are analyzed each day. The results help to determine a child's condition, its seriousness, and its susceptibility to various treatments. Results are reported back to the appropriate nursing unit, clinic, or emergency staff. The 9th-floor intensive care units, which need especially quick turnaround time on results, use the critical care satellite lab located on their own floor.

In Microbiology, the Bacteriology and Virology labs test specifically for infections. If a urine sample in the Renal Function lab reveals an infection, the sample will go upstairs for a more detailed analysis, to determine the type of micro-organism and the type and strength of drug that can combat it. These labs are located separately, on the 13th floor of the C-Wing, to minimize any risk of contamination.

Some specialized diagnostic labs are housed elsewhere. Molecular Genetics (Place Toulon) and Biochemical Genetics (A-Wing) reflect the increasingly critical importance of genetic knowledge in fighting disease and abnormalities. In the Cytogenetics lab (A-Wing), cells from the mother's uterus can help diagnose a baby's problem even before birth.

11:00 A.M.

In the E-Wing's 4th-floor kitchen, preparations are being completed for lunch. Meals for children on the nursing units have been cooked two days in advance, then chilled in a special refrigerator called a "chill blaster." On the day they are to be served, meal trays are loaded into large enclosed carts known as "retherm trucks," where they are reheated for 45–50 minutes. When the food is hot, dietary helpers deliver the trucks to the nursing units. This centralized "cook–chill" method was introduced in the mid-1990s to improve temperature control and cost-efficiency. Prior to that, meals had to be prepared the same day they were to be served, portioned hot by kitchen staff, and sent right away to the wards.

At the same time the food trucks are leaving to feed patients, heated food prepared in bulk is being sent down to the 3rd-floor cafeteria for staff and visitors.

12:00 NOON

Tables in the cafeteria start to fill up. When the cafeteria on this site first opened in 1956, it was a big step up from what staff had been used to at the Cedar Avenue buildings—one fixed meal, no choices, passed through a window over a counter. Former hospital manager Winnifred Jones remem-

TESTING AND ANALYSIS

The Pediatric Test Centre on 2D obtains blood or urine specimens from all ambulatory MCH clinic patients for analysis or culture. It also serves as a valuable resource for community physicians who can send children any Monday to Friday between 10:00 a.m. and 4:00 p.m. to have these tests done. The PTC distributes samples to the labs for analysis and communicates the results back to the referring doctors. The Pediatric Consultation Clinic (PCC) serves patients from community physicians who need to see a doctor for a specialized consultation or second opinion.

bers, "When we saw that long counter just like in a store and all the foods laid out for us to see, well, we thought we'd arrived!"

The new cafeteria became the place where medical and nursing staff met for coffee after rounds, and had lunch together. It facilitated interaction among staff and provided social opportunities. A passageway was built from the F-Wing to facilitate access from the residents' quarters.

Over the past few decades, the pace of work has become faster, and heavy schedules now mean that many people have time only to grab a sandwich and take it back to their place of work. As a result, corridors and stairwells have become places of choice for those seeking out colleagues for a quick chat.

Staff can also grab a quick sandwich at the café centrally located off the clinic waiting area on 2B operated by the hospital's Auxiliary and still familiarly known by many as the Tiny Tim snack bar. The café is also the location of choice for children and families visiting the clinics.

On many days, the attractively decorated waiting area is also the scene of cultural and fundraising activities—bake sales, bazaars, ethnic meals, and information displays.

Families and personnel from both the main complex and rented buildings take advantage of the numerous small restaurants and snack bars to be found on St. Catherine Street or in the nearby shopping plazas. At times, some of these have become unofficial secondary cafeterias, with the result that staff wanting to have private conversations have had to lunch farther afield.

DID YOU KNOW?
Including the formula room, where babies' bottles are prepared, the hospital's kitchens prepare 140 to 180 meals a day for patients. The cafeteria serves 150 to 180 meals per day—up to 220 during busy times of the year—the bulk of them during the busy lunch period.

1:00 P.M.

This is frequently a time when medical students attend teaching sessions in the amphitheatre. More formal sessions are also given at various times of the day in two rooms on 4C near the Medical Library. At other times, students may be found attending the more traditional form of "rounds" on the patient care units. For medical students alone, there is some kind of teaching going on at almost every moment of the day. When nursing students, lab technology trainees, and a wide variety of other professionals-in-training are taken into account, on any given day there are few places in the institution that are not actively preparing the next generation of caregivers. The designation of "teaching hospital" is not taken lightly.

By 1:00 p.m., crowds in the cafeteria and café have thinned out somewhat, and some staff and visitors are still out of the MCH buildings for lunch.

However, movement at the Children's never really slows during the daytime. One area that sees considerable patient traffic throughout the day is Medical Imaging, on the 3rd floor of the C-Wing near the cafeteria entrance. Concentrated here are most of the diagnostic imaging technologies: CT scanning, ultrasound, the entrance to the MRI suite, a cardiac catheterization lab and angiographic suite, as well as the X-rays that gave the department its older, and still frequently used name, Radiology. That name is soon to be made even more obsolete: X-rays, whose use dates back to the earliest days of the hospital, are about to join the digital age as this book is being written. The familiar large, grey sheets of film are being replaced by more practical digital images that are much easier to store, share, retrieve, and interpret.

2:00 P.M.

Clinic activity picks up again, and will continue until about 4:00 p.m.

While in the main complex this affects mostly the 2B area, some of the second-floor outpatient clinics overflow from the B- into the A- and C-Wings; still others are located in D and E. But they are often so close together that the transitions from one wing to another are not evident to a visitor. This can lead to unwelcome confusion for parents arriving with cranky children in tow and having as their only direction a piece of paper with a room number on it. Wayfinding is one of the biggest challenges of a complex made up of several different, interconnecting buildings.

Two o'clock is another peak time in Emergency, too, often for illnesses that have become evident as the morning progresses. This means a higher workload for housekeeping staff, who must keep the waiting, examining, and treatment areas clean between patients. When the ER is busy, Housekeeping is busy.

3:00 P.M.

While 3:00 p.m. is the time many shift workers leave, others must step up their activity levels. Mid-afternoon is when the more complicated surgeries finish in the ORs, causing small peaks in activity for Housekeeping and Laundry, as used supplies are taken away for cleaning and fresh ones ordered. Pharmacy receives a new set of prescription requests for patients leaving the ORs.

For these patients, the most essential activity occurs in the recovery room, more formally known as the PACU (Post-Anesthesia Care Unit), on the 10th floor not far from the ORs. There, they are closely monitored as they awaken after surgery.

In its early days, before the move to Tupper Street, the recovery room had only blood pressure cuffs and stethoscopes to monitor patients, usually eight patients per day. Fifty years later, the patient volume has increased to 40 per day and the technology consists of dozens of highly sophisticated devices measuring intracranial pressure, oxygen saturation, and other vital signs.

Physically, the PACU has undergone some basic changes since the MCH first moved to Tupper Street.

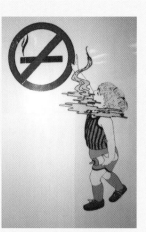

BUTTING OUT

In the early days of the hospital, no one thought twice about lighting up. As the dangers of second-hand smoke became better known, cigarettes and cigars were banished to non-patient areas, then private offices, and finally the smoking room—an area enclosed by Plexiglas—located in the cafeteria. The smoking room only lasted for a brief few years in the 1990s. Despite the special ventilation system, it became so thick with smoke that some employees quit smoking rather than use it. Determined puffers then moved to building entrances, but most have since been persuaded to use the outdoor smoking shelters provided by the hospital, or nearby park benches.

"The waiting rooms were full of smoke," said Dr. Jean-Luc Leblanc, community pediatrician and allergist, recalling the 1950s at the MCH 90th anniversary celebration. "Now, nobody would ever think of smoking in the waiting room or in the offices. Habits change because new information has come along to tell us what's right and what's wrong."

For many years, the windows were bricked up to prevent infection. Now, infection control is more sophisticated and a central air system regulates airflow and temperature. In 2001, windows were again created, allowing children to wake up to the warmth of the sunshine and the magnificent view of the city.

"We have brought in the light and replaced the white and sterile finishes with warm colors, wood finishes, and new, more comfortable furniture," says Teresa Di Bartolo, Manager of Architectural Services. "This has enabled us to create an environment that is less scary for the kids and more conducive to their healing."

FINDING YOUR WAY AROUND

Wayfinding—getting to the right place—has always been an interesting and sometimes frustrating challenge for visitors to the MCH's Tupper Street buildings. The wings, built in different decades, have different ceiling heights. As a result, the floors do not match up. For instance, it is impossible to walk from the 3rd floor of the A-Wing directly to the 3rd floor of the C-Wing. Visitors can reach the A-Wing only from the main and second floors of the B-Wing. The F-Wing can only be reached through the basement, by walking around the buildings outside, or via the walkway stretching from the 3rd-floor cafeteria in the E-Wing. So taking the wrong bank of elevators can get visitors far from where they wanted to go.

As the level of traffic increases every year, so does the need for directions. Colour-coding the wings was tried, but required a lot of specially coloured paint and could be confusing. Additional confusion was created by frequent moves of offices and clinics—a result both of chronic space shortage and development of new programs. Keeping up with the room number changes was almost impossible, so wrong information appeared as often as right. In the early 1990s, the hospital gave up listing doctors' names on main directories. That's when a discovery was made: most people don't read signs—they ask someone for directions. While this is especially true for the many visitors who read neither French nor English, it is also true for anyone looking at too much information. Generally, the more information provided, the more gets missed. So, more signs came down.

Now, a variety of solutions is used. Day surgery patients get to the operating room quite easily by following a line of blue dots on the floor. Children with clinic appointments use the newly installed wall paintings as reference points. Other visitors are guided by a reduced selection of signs and arrows. Many find the best way is still to ask a friendly staff member.

4:00 P.M.

Clinic activity draws to a close, except in Dermatology, and at the Adolescent Clinic in the Gilman Pavilion, which remain open longer to accommodate teenagers' schedules.

Administrative staff in clinical areas begin to wind up their day. Charts must be completed and in the right place; appointments must be confirmed for the next day.

5:00 P.M.

Most of the day staff have now left. However, activity in the ER remains at a high level. The late afternoon contingent of patients arrives—children who have had after-school accidents. Injuries often occur late in the day, when children are tired and less vigilant, and parents are either not home yet or tired from their own long days.

6:00 P.M.

The café and gift shop on 2B have closed and the clinic area is very quiet compared to earlier in the day. Children in all the nursing units are finishing dinner and are being settled in for the evening. Some parents and other family members linger; others have returned home to see to dinner and bedtime for their other children.

7:00 P.M.

The nursing night shift arrives and is briefed on the patients and their conditions. By now, as many post-operative patients as possible have been moved from the PACU back to the surgical units, so that they could be settled in during the day shift. The others will wait till 8:00 p.m., when the night shift is briefed and ready to take on new charges. Those whose surgeries finish late may spend the night in the PACU. However, recent developments in anesthesia have meant quicker recoveries. Also, from a purely practical viewpoint, it makes sense to move children to the nursing units quickly—if the recovery room is full, the ORs must slow down; if the ORs slow down, other children must wait longer for their surgery.

8:00 P.M.

Security locks the main entrance of the Tupper Street complex. From now until 6:00 a.m., all arrivals will be via the ER door. Activity in the other buildings has slowed, although lights shine in research labs and offices where people are working late.

By now, the ORs are shut down unless there is an emergency. The clinics are quiet. Lab capacity has been reduced to about 5% of its daytime strength. Other patient service personnel have started the lonely night shift, keeping just enough staff to handle emergencies.

Patients and families in the ER waiting room are becoming less numerous, the time for after-school injuries and illnesses having peaked. Emergency will, however, stay open around the clock. And housekeeping, security, and maintenance staff will be ready to help if needed. Its patients may sleep, but the Children's does not.

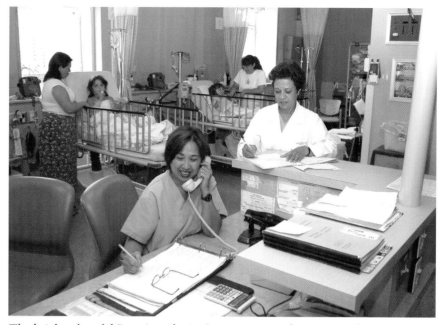

The bright, cheerful Post-Anesthesia Care Unit in early 2005 is a far cry from the dark atmosphere of the recovery room a generation earlier. Here, Assistant Head Nurse Della Rous is seated, on the phone; standing at the desk is nurse Gloria Lutchman.

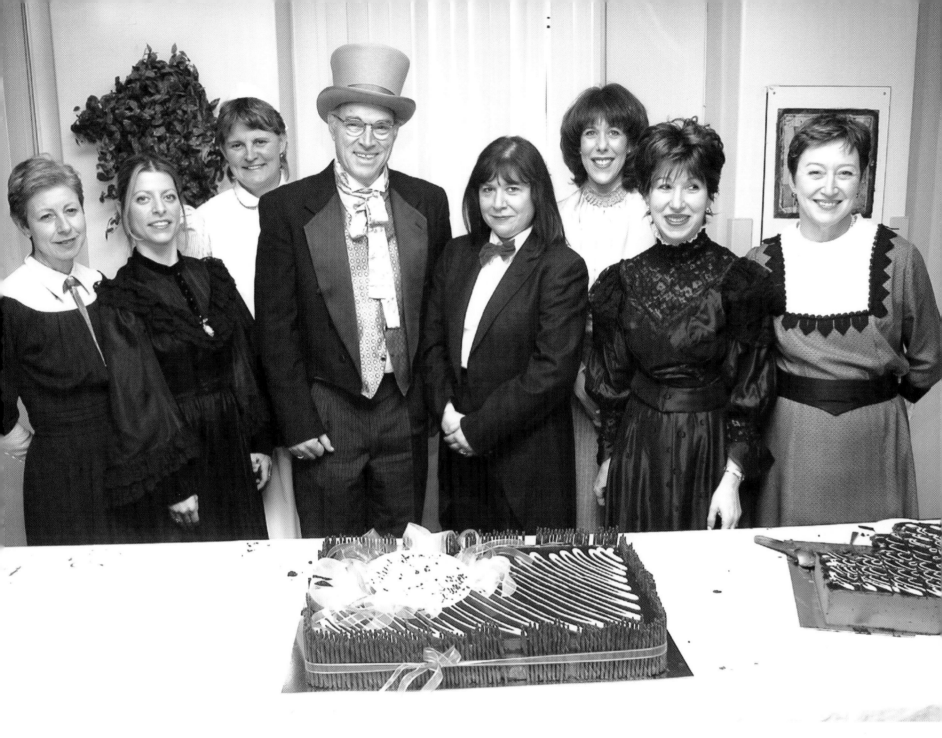

Dressed for the occasion (left to right): Ginette Manseau, Demetra Kafantaris, Diane Borisov, Dr. Nicolas Steinmetz, Teresa Di Bartolo, Patricia Kalnitsky, Marcie Scheim, and Eileen Mahoney demonstrate centennial spirit during the cake cutting at the Internal Launch of the MCH centennial celebrations.

"During the centennial year, the hospital and the Foundation
worked side by side to create a series of unforgettable events
in celebration of the Children's rich history and accomplishments
as a world leader in pediatric care."

MARC A. COURTOIS, CHAIRMAN OF THE BOARD,
THE MONTREAL CHILDREN'S HOSPITAL FOUNDATION,
AND MEMBER OF THE CENTENNIAL COMMITTEE

14

Celebrating a Century of Caring

To celebrate the MCH's centennial was to pay tribute to 100 years of excellence in pediatrics, to acknowledge the skill and expertise that have made it a world-renowned institution, and to thank all who have contributed to its success. Just as it has been since its inception in 1904, the Children's continues to be a special place that attracts exceptional people. These health-care professionals, researchers, support staff, volunteers, community groups, and, of course, patients and their families, have all contributed to the extraordinary and enduring spirit of the Children's. Centennial events celebrated not only the hospital's past, but also its present and future as a leader in pediatric health care.

HUNDREDS GET INVOLVED IN PLANNING

A wide array of academic, social, and fundraising events spanned the year, with several events each month providing opportunities for learning, laughter, and friendship for people of all ages. Reflecting the dedication and enthusiasm characteristic of the Children's, hundreds of people got involved, individually or in groups, in planning the centennial events over a period of about three years under the leadership of Centennial Committee co-chairmen Hugh G. Hallward and Martha Hallward. The Hallwards were the natural choice to take on the daunting task of planning and overseeing the year's activities. Direct descendants of two of the Montreal Children's Hospital's founders, their volunteer involve-

ment with both the hospital and the Foundation was unmatched. When approached to share the chairmanship of the Centennial Committee, they readily agreed and went on to assemble a committee of representatives from the MCH, the Foundation, and the community.

The committee's mandate was clear: to celebrate 100 years of excellence in pediatric care at the Children's and to bring the festivities to as many Montrealers as possible. Dr. Hy Goldman, who had been instrumental in planning the hospital's 90th anniversary celebrations, was named chairman of the In-House Centennial Committee. This dedicated group planned a full schedule that included academic lectures, staff activities, and an ambitious Homecoming Weekend. To keep staff informed of upcoming events, a centennial bulletin board became a permanent fixture in the second-floor outpatient waiting area, while the employee newsletter featured centennial news every two weeks.

In addition to raising funds for the hospital's ongoing needs, the Foundation assumed the responsibility of promoting the Children's centennial in the media and in the community. Chairman Marc Courtois pledged the Board's full support for a comprehensive media campaign unlike any previously undertaken. Agreements were soon struck with a number of radio broadcasters, television stations, and newspapers to provide coverage of centennial events and to create new ones. The Foundation's

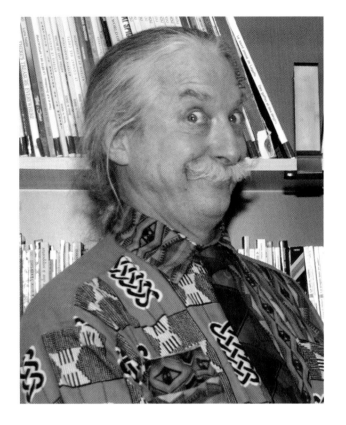

annual campaigns and major events adopted the centennial theme and volunteer groups were armed with 100th anniversary stickers, posters, and banners to display at their fundraisers. New events, such as the Official Launch, the Sports Celebrity Dinner, and the Fête Folie, were added to an already full slate of activities to create an unforgettable centennial year.

One full year in advance of the centennial, the Countdown to Launch Breakfast was held to announce the plans for the centennial year to the hospital staff and encourage their participation.

THE CENTENNIAL YEAR IS LAUNCHED

The centennial's Official Launch on January 28, 2004, began the year of celebrations. From the Internal Launch to the Gong Show; the Academic Lecture Series to the Deli/Jazz Soirée; the Centennial Awards Ball to the Sports Celebrity Dinner; the

Multicultural Gala Dinner to Family Fun Day and Homecoming Weekend; and finally closing with the Fête Folie in December, the centennial year offered something for everyone, because everyone has a reason to celebrate the Children's.

The Official Launch of the 100th anniversary celebrations was a gala evening produced by the Montreal Children's Hospital Foundation. An informative and moving multimedia presentation depicted the Children's past, present, and future in fairy-tale fashion, with the help of some well-known friends of the hospital. More than 800 guests, including donors, volunteers, and staff, gathered at the Centre Pierre-Péladeau for the sold-out show. Co-hosted by star Rémy Girard and actress and former patient Carrie Libling, the evening was studded with stellar performances by musicians Sass Jordan, Daniel Bélanger, and Grégory Charles; dancers Mariusz Ostrowski and Geneviève Guérard of *Les Grands Ballets Canadiens*; Dr. Patch Adams, the renowned physician-clown; and, most especially, patients of the Children's.

As guests departed, they received advance copies of an insert to be included in the next day's editions of local newspapers *The Gazette* and *Le Journal de Montréal*. This special section featured the hospital's historical firsts, success stories, and a calendar of events for the year. The stage was now set for a year of celebration.

Following the gala opening, members of the hospital staff welcomed their colleagues to the Internal Launch on January 30, dressed in the fashion of a century past and setting the mood for the hospital's 100th birthday celebration. A birthday breakfast presented jointly by the Foundation and the Auxiliary concluded with the cutting of a giant cake. Cards filled with heartfelt messages and birthday wishes addressed to Caramel, the hospital mascot, written by Montreal elementary school children and generous donors, were displayed at the main entrance and in the 3rd-floor cafeteria for all to read and appreciate.

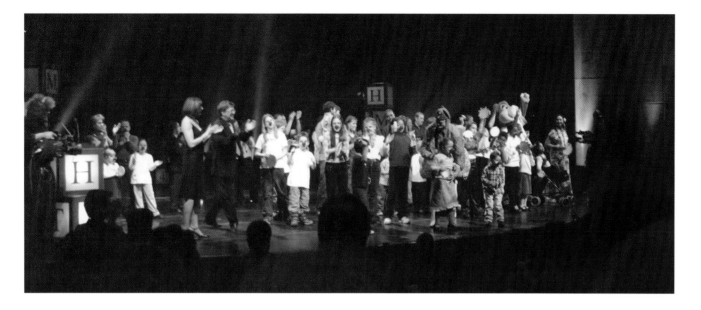

Hosts, performers, and MCH patients at the Official Launch return to the stage for the final bow and a standing ovation.

ACADEMIC LECTURES HONOUR THE CHILDREN'S

Throughout the year, Physician-in-Chief Harvey Guyda oversaw the many prestigious academic lectures hosted by the Children's in honour of 100 years of excellence in pediatrics. Health-care professionals from around the world gathered in Montreal to share knowledge and expertise. Several lectures were specially planned for this year, including the keynote Centennial Lecture on February 13, presented by Dr. Nuala Kenny, Professor of Pediatrics, Dalhousie University, on "The Future of Canadian Health Care." Other annual lectures, supported through named endowment funds honouring individuals who have made outstanding contributions to the development of the Children's, were given a centennial twist and included in the program. Many of the speakers in this special centennial edition of the Academic Lecture Series had current and prior links to the Children's.

CELEBRATING WITH BOOKS, TV, AND RADIO

Staff, parents, and patients shared memories, stories, and recipes in two books (of a series of three, including this history) published by the MCH and the Foundation for the centennial year. The first, a cookbook called *Lovin' from the Oven*, is an initiative of MCH medical laboratory technologists. It was coordinated and edited by Dr. Claire Dupont, who headed the Biochemistry Laboratory for many years before becoming Director of Professional Services in 1987. The book's sales will benefit the hospital by supporting continuing education for the technologists. This compilation of hundreds of favourite family recipes and nutrition tips was launched in March, with the help of actor and MCH spokesperson Rémy Girard and Chef Christian Brion of Provigo-Loblaws.

The second publication, *One Hundred Years of Stories*, edited by Anita Szabadi-Gottesman and Lesley Reford, is a collection of heartwarming personal accounts of life at the hospital depicted through stories, letters, and children's illustrations. The book is dedicated to the staff, volunteers, and children of the MCH, with all proceeds benefiting the hospital's pediatric intensive care unit. Renaud-Bray bookstores agreed to carry the book, featuring it prominently in displays and promotional brochures.

Global TV and TVA partnered with the hospital

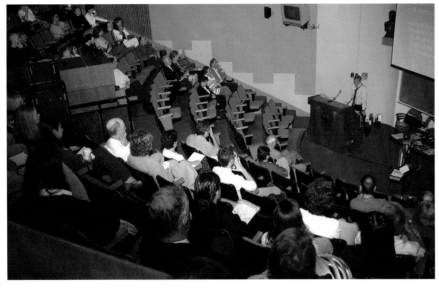

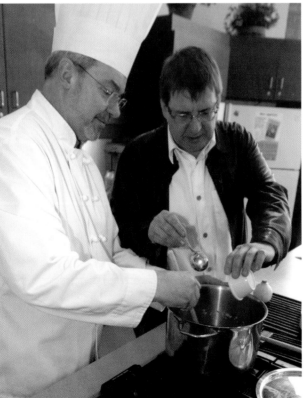

During the Centennial Academic Lecture series, numerous lectures were hosted in the Forbes-Cushing Amphitheatre. The Annual Alan Ross Lectureship on September 15, also an event of the Pediatric Medical Grand Rounds, featured Dr. Charles Larson of McGill University. In his lecture entitled "Moving from Effectiveness to Health Impact in Lesser Developed Countries: Taking a Promise and Making It a Solution," Dr. Larson acknowledged past and present contributions by the MCH to international health.

Chef Christian Brion and actor Rémy Girard prepare two dishes with recipes from the cookbook Lovin' from the Oven, *in the community kitchen of the Angus Loblaws.*

and the Foundation to produce a series of historical vignettes that aired for several months during the year. Each clip profiled an area of expertise of the Children's, such as cardiology and cardiac surgery, neurology and neurosurgery, genetics, and trauma. Specialists and medical professionals were also interviewed on popular morning shows.

Long-time Children's supporter Standard Broadcasting participated in the centennial festivities through the Foundation's first annual Caring for Kids Radiothon in early March. Broadcasting live from the hospital's cafeteria over a three-day period, radio personalities interviewed dozens of patients, families, and caregivers, encouraging listeners to join the newly created Circle of Hugs. Centennial spirits were high as $1.2 million was collected, setting a North American record for the most successful first radiothon ever held to benefit a pediatric hospital.

SHOWCASING OUR TALENTS

The first annual Gong Show, appropriately slated for April Fools' Day, was an evening of odd talents and hilarity. This variety show featured performers from throughout the hospital, in costumes ranging from shocking to delightfully ridiculous. Co-hosted by a Chicken Lady and an Elvis impersonator (a.k.a. Chantal-Mignonne Mailloux and Jack Strulovitch), the evening was an opportunity for fun and camaraderie. As staff revealed their hidden talents, whether chair-balancing, singing and dancing, or stand-up comedy, the audience more than once found itself laughing to the point of tears.

Judges selected three winning performances which best showcased the hospital staff's sense of humour and remarkable talent. Dr. Fifi (Melissa Holland) and Dr. Frogge (Alexis Roy), of the Children's own Dr. Clowns, took the title for "Most Outrageous Act;" "Funniest Act" was awarded to Terry Séguin of Public Affairs; and Drs. Chris Karatzios, staff pediatrician, and Preetha Krishnamoorthy, staff endocrinologist, won the honourable

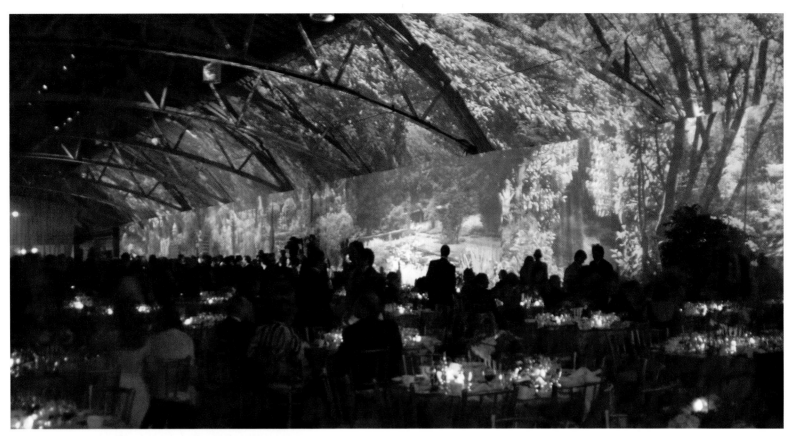

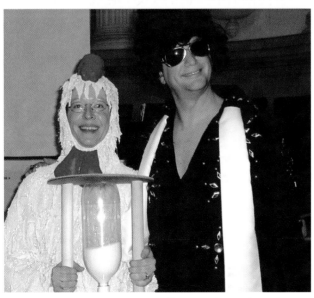

Nurse Chantal-Mignonne Mailloux and social worker Jack Strulovitch co-hosted the first MCH Gong Show.

title of "MCH Idols" for their impressive dance performance.

CENTENNIAL AWARDS BALL

The month of May brought with it the Centennial Awards Ball. The organizing committee, led by co-chairs Lyn Lalonde Lazure and Sara Provencher, adopted the theme of the Secret Garden, inspired by Frances Hodgson Bennett's classic children's tale. Lavender wisteria adorned the beautifully decorated Windsor Station, and luxuriant garden images were projected on the surrounding walls. With the added prestige of a milestone celebration, the annual fund-raiser attracted a record 800 guests, and with the help of generous contributions from four honorary chairmen, raised $700,000 to benefit the Children's.

The Ball set the stage for a special edition of the annual Awards of Excellence, first established in

Guests of the Centennial Awards Ball are seated beneath lush images of trees and greenery, enjoying the Secret Garden.

2000. Thanks to the generous support of corporate sponsors, each year up to 10 people are recognized for their remarkable work and dedication to the Children's. In recognition of his leadership and vision, Dr. Hy Goldman received the Centennial Spirit Award of Excellence, created specially for the Centennial Ball. Jack Cole was also honoured posthumously with the Community Leadership Award for his instrumental role in creating the Foundation and his unflagging support of the Children's for more than 30 years.

PEDAL FOR KIDS

The Foundation's longest running event, Pedal for Kids, presented a perfect opportunity to encourage donors to make special gifts to the hospital in honour of its 100th birthday. Event chairman Paul Normandin, in the spirit of the centennial, incorporated a vintage bicycle into the event's logo. The team captains and pedallers accepted the challenge with fierce determination, raising a remarkable $715,000 over a five-day period in early June. In particular, the HSBC team fulfilled their promise of raising more than $100,000 to mark the special milestone.

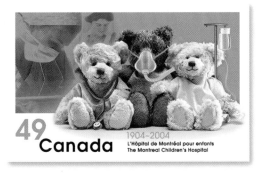

COMMEMORATING CARE

In May 2004, Canada Post launched a 49¢ stamp commemorating 100 years of compassionate care and multiculturalism at the Children's. Three teddy bears appear on the stamp in different colours and sizes, to represent diversity among the hospital's young patients. The background, illustrating health-care professionals of two very different eras, offers a sense of how significantly health care has changed in the last century. The stamp was carefully designed to convey the hospital's empathetic approach to relieving the fears of children and their families, and to helping sick children better understand and cope with their illnesses.

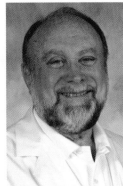

"The centennial celebration year provided a unique opportunity to highlight the Children's accomplishments as a world-renowned pediatric centre, as well as its commitment to assuring the future health of the most treasured segment of our society, our children."

DR. HY GOLDMAN,
CHAIRMAN OF THE
IN-HOUSE CENTENNIAL COMMITTEE AND
RECIPIENT OF THE CENTENNIAL SPIRIT AWARD

COMING HOME TO THE CHILDREN'S

Midway through the centennial year—concurrent with the Canadian Pediatric Society's National Conference in Montreal—the much-anticipated Centennial Homecoming Weekend, June 17 to 20, welcomed alumni from far and wide. As a show of appreciation for those who have contributed to the Children's throughout the years, the program was lively and full of opportunities to share knowledge, reminisce, appreciate the special culture of the Children's, celebrate multiculturalism, and enjoy the distinctive flavour of Montreal.

Homecoming began in true Montreal style with the Deli/Jazz soirée at the MCH. Transformed into a bistro with live jazz by the Donny Kennedy Quartet, the outpatient clinic waiting area on 2B became a hospital hot spot for meeting with colleagues and friends, both old and new. A sampler of Montreal's most characteristic flavours included smoked meat, bagels, and orange julep. Good music and great company brought back many memories and happy times in a relaxed, jazz-infused atmosphere.

During Homecoming Weekend, staff and alumni also were welcomed to the launch of the First Annual Evelyn Rocque-Malowany Nursing Symposium, in recognition of the former Nursing Director's substantial contribution to the Children's. Described as a visionary nurse leader, Evelyn Malowany broke through traditional boundaries and helped redefine the role of nursing in patient care and research. As a platform for nurses to share knowledge and experience, the Symposium will stand as a tribute to the high level of nursing expertise and care at the Children's well into the next century.

Another highlight of Homecoming Weekend was the hospital's Open House. Visitors were invited to take one or more of five hour-long guided tours through different wings of the hospital. Tailored to appeal to alumni and visitors of all ages, these tours provided an opportunity for small groups to explore the inner workings of the hospital, to visit the institution in a festive atmosphere, to ask questions, and to develop an appreciation of the hospital as a whole. The tours were also a chance for alumni to visit old haunts and even encounter former colleagues. Each tour ultimately led visitors to the outpatient clinic waiting area, where colourful and informative display booths set up by medical and nursing staff, the Auxiliary, the Foundation, and the Research Institute offered lots to explore and discuss. More than 46 departments participated in the Open House.

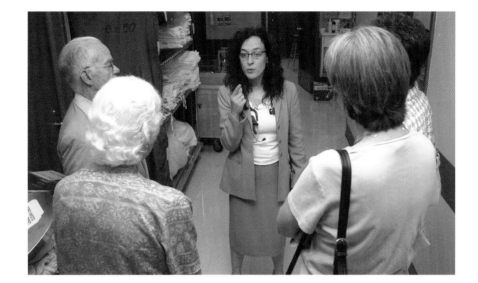

Dr. Helen Karounis played the role of tour guide for MCH alumni during Homecoming Weekend.

The Centennial Multicultural Gala Dinner, co-hosted by the Canadian Pediatric Society, was another highlight of Homecoming Weekend. At this event, the MCH honoured its own multicultural heritage as well as the multicultural spirit of Montreal. Proudly the first Canadian hospital to establish a multiculturalism program, the Children's celebrated with an evening of international cuisine,

"When I arrived at the Children's, I was aware that there was a culture here that was different from other organizations in which I had worked. Although it was child- and family-centred, I know that the leadership of people like Dr. Jack Charters, to whom I reported, was very significant in information sharing, and in creating the culture which allowed me to do the work for which I have been very generously credited.

"The real credit goes to the nursing staff who work at the bedside and in administration, teaching, and research. I was privileged to join such an organization and I have been told that I have made a contribution. I have been a very fortunate person to be able do so."

EVELYN MALOWANY,
DIRECTOR OF NURSING, 1976–1997

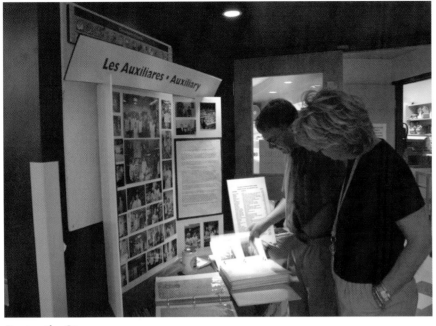

During the Open House, guided tours delivered visitors to the outpatient clinic waiting area, where this presentation by the Auxiliary was one of many elaborate and informative displays.

music, and stunning traditional dance performances. In exquisite costumes, Spanish, Indian, Irish, and Greek dance troupes graced the stage at the Centre Mont-Royal, demonstrating the beauty of diversity.

Centennial celebrations would not have been complete without honouring the children themselves—and Homecoming Weekend's largest public event, Family Fun Day, did exactly that. For this special occasion, Cabot Park, facing the Children's on Tupper Street, was transformed into a fun zone for kids and their families. Giant inflatable slides, carnival games, fun food, face painting, plenty of entertainment, and tons of laughter were all on the menu. Eighty singers from the Evangel Pentecostal Church Choir, neighbours to the MCH on Cabot Square, added joy to the atmosphere as the enormous centennial cake was served to everyone who had "played" up an appetite.

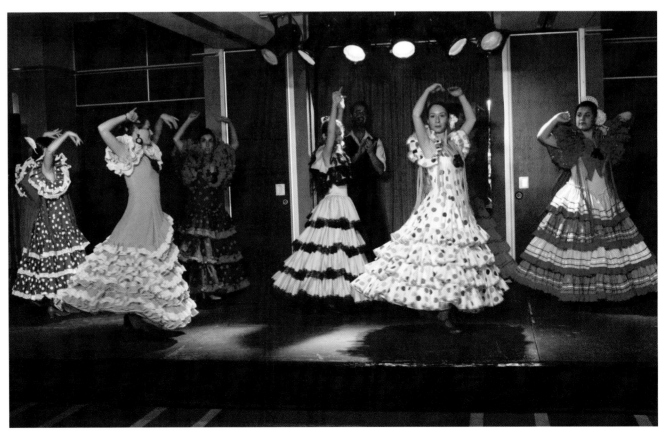

The Alegría de España dance troupe entertains guests at the Multicultural Gala.

THE CELEBRATIONS CONTINUE

Even after Homecoming Weekend, the celebrations continued. Two new additions to the MCH's collection of child-centred art were unveiled on National Aboriginal Day, June 21. A pair of unique Inuksuit—Inuit statues made of stone—representing a parent and a child honour both the MCH's long-standing ties with Quebec's aboriginal communities and the hospital's 100th anniversary. Northern food, demonstrations, workshops, and traditional music and dancing welcomed the Inuksuit to the Children's family. This special event was one of several Multicultural Days held during the centennial year.

Every September, the MCH Foundation holds its annual golf tournament at the prestigious Royal Montreal Golf Club. The organizing committee, chaired by Hugh Hallward, was intent on making the centennial edition their biggest success to date. True to their word, they raised $650,000 and even managed to avoid a rain-out by Hurricane Frances, thanks to the generosity of the golf club and the flexibility of the 56 participating teams in rescheduling the event. After chairing eight consecutive annual tournaments that raised more than $3 million, Hugh Hallward passed on the torch in 2005 to Peter Morton.

That same month saw the premiere of a documentary entitled *Courageous Kids: a Day in the Life of the Children's OR*, aired on Global TV in English and on CHTV in French. The hour-long special brought into viewers' living rooms the harrowing and uplifting stories of five brave young patients facing highly specialized and complex surgery with uncertain outcomes. Narrated by actress and hospital spokesperson Macha Grenon, Olympic ski champion Jean-Luc Brassard, and television personality Al Dubois, the production provided a rare inside look at the heroic efforts of medical professionals at the Children's and their compassionate and caring treatment of the patients and their families.

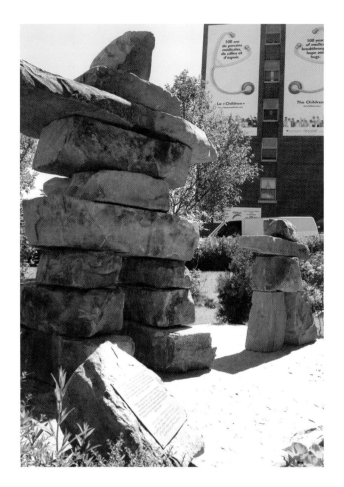

In commemoration of the MCH's 40-year relationship with Quebec's Aboriginal communities and the hospital's centennial, these Inuksuit, in the form of a parent and child, welcome visitors to the main entrance.

MCCORD MUSEUM: GROWING UP IN MONTREAL

During its first century, the Children's not only bore witness to the growth and development of the City of Montreal and its people, it was an active participant. In recognition of this role, a McCord Museum special exhibition, entitled *Growing Up in Montreal*, paid homage to the hospital's long history of important contributions. Coordinated by a committee chaired by Dr. Bruce Williams and including Dr. Victoria Dickenson, Executive Director of the McCord Museum, Hugh Hallward, Martha Hallward, Derek Price, Brian Baxter, and Deirdre Stevenson, the exhibition opened in October 2004 and was slated to run until the spring of 2006.

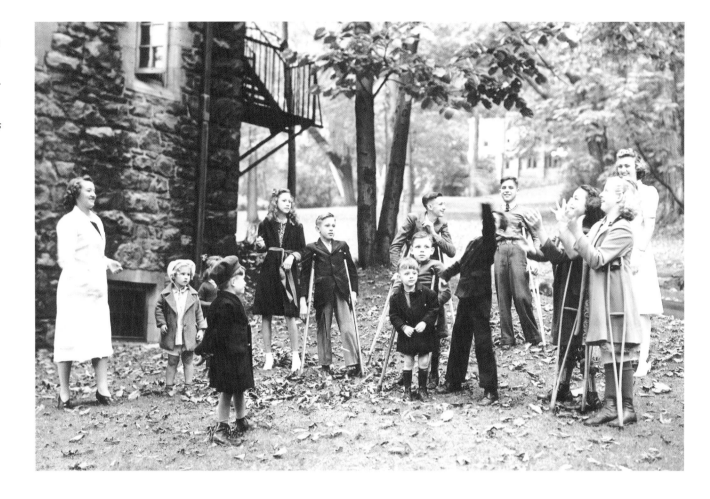

Featured in the McCord Museum exhibit Growing Up in Montreal, *this photograph—from the MCH's own extensive collection—shows children playing outside while waiting for physiotherapy treatment at the Children's Memorial Hospital in 1942.*

The photographs and artifacts selected for inclusion offered visitors a sense of what life was like for children in the 19th and 20th centuries. The exhibition recalled an era before major medical breakthroughs such as vaccines and traced the evolution of our understanding that children are not simply small versions of adults, and that in their treatment, one size does not fit all. Photographs depicted the story of the Children's as the hospital itself grew, as pediatric care developed, and as medical and nursing professionals responded to the changing needs of the city's children.

SPORTS CELEBRITY DINNER

On November 10 at the Bell Centre, sports aficionados were rewarded with the long-anticipated return of the Sports Celebrity Dinner, which had been a flagship event for the Hospital for more than 25 years. The revival of this event—a Montreal tradition from 1967 to 1993—was a major focus of the Centennial Committee, with plans set in motion almost three years earlier. Working closely with the Foundation team, event chairman Charles Matheson and his committee delivered a unique and memorable evening that improved on the original and raised $350,000 in the process. Ten world-class sports celebrities, including Olympic gold medallists, professional stars, and local legends, were honoured for their athletic and philanthropic accomplishments, to the delight of 900 fans of all ages. Highlight reels on each honouree, produced by CFCF-CTV, elicited emotion and applause from the enthusiastic crowd that included several hospital patients and their families. Autograph seekers were not disappointed as the celebrities stayed long into the night signing program books, hockey sticks, and any other items put before them.

A CENTURY OF VITAL PEDIATRIC RESEARCH

On December 3, the MCH Research Institute hosted an open house for the public in honour of the MCH centennial, to celebrate the vital role of research in the evolution of children's health care. More than 24 labs participated, preparing posters and presenting research topics related to pediatric and adolescent health and prenatal development. The event provided an opportunity for the curious to learn about the latest developments and projects of the MCH Research Institute, sharing information about research in genetics, nephrology, endocrinology, ophthalmology, surgery, mental health, and other fields.

CLOSING PARTY

The closing celebration of the centennial year was the Fête Folie – A Family Party, which welcomed hundreds of guests to the top of Mount Royal to share the magic of the Children's on December 12. A light dusting of snow settled on the mountain as the Chalet Mont-Royal filled with families of staff, patients, donors, and volunteers to celebrate the final moments of the milestone year. As the sun set and the lights of the city twinkled below, the visiting children crafted sparkling stars, conferred with Stretch the Clown, and breathed the warm scent of popcorn and cotton candy. The multigenerational crowd was mesmerized by magic and illusions, balancing acts, and gravity-defying feats.

As the family party drew to its close, Louise Dery-Goldberg, President of the Foundation, Marc Courtois, and Hugh Hallward thanked all who had contributed to the success of the centennial celebrations, as well as everyone who contributes to the Children's each year. Martha Hallward then ceremoniously cut the cake—with a toy sword! Event co-chairmen Joan McKinnon and Pat Miller, together with their dynamic committee, looked on proudly as their labour of love for the past two years marked the end of a full year of centennial festivities in grand fashion and ushered in another century of caring.

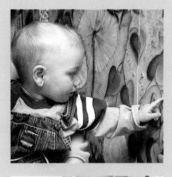
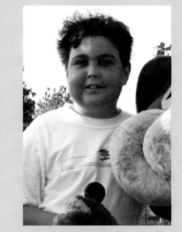
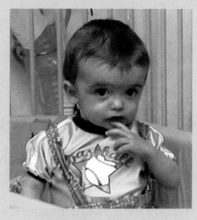
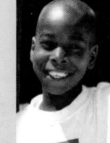

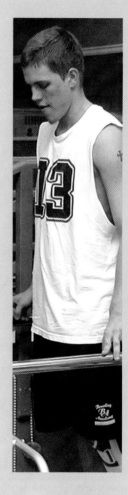
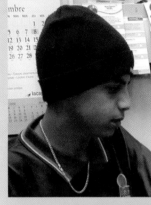
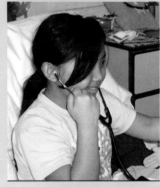
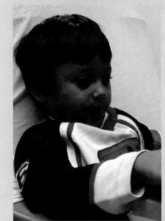
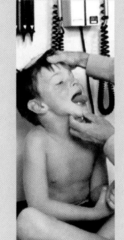
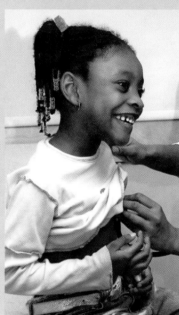
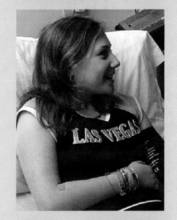
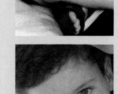
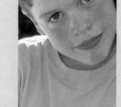
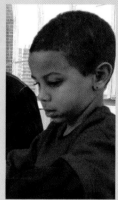
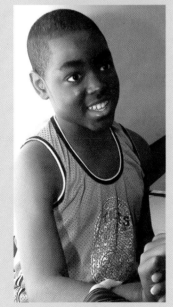
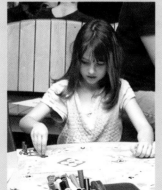
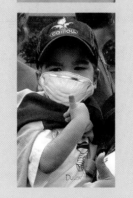
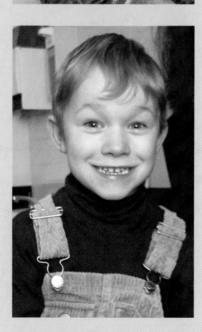
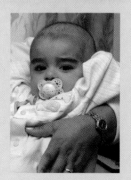

"Standing, as we do, on the shoulders of those who came before us, we have learned that nothing is impossible. We know this, because we have seen our predecessors repeatedly attempt the impossible, until it became possible."

DR. NICOLAS STEINMETZ,
EXECUTIVE DIRECTOR, 1987–1995, 2003–2004

15

"A Place Where Science and Laughter Dwell"

Looking ahead to the future is invariably a fascinating and instructive—also frustrating and daunting—exercise. The next century, and beyond, will inevitably bring continued change and many more surprises for the Montreal Children's Hospital. The only certainty is that the pace of change will continue to accelerate as new developments affect every area of the hospital's life: patient care, research, education, physical facilities, and working conditions, as well as community relations and our role within the health-care system.

As the MCH enters its second century, planning is well advanced for the move to the brand-new campus of the McGill University Health Centre (MUHC) on the Glen site near the Vendôme metro station. There, the Children's will rub elbows and share space with its adult hospital partners for the first time. During the hospital's centennial year, implementation teams for the MUHC move were announced and work began on preparing the former railway yard for its new life as a hospital campus.

The prospect of moving into a purpose-built facility has preoccupied planners for more than a decade. In 1992, the MCH and four other McGill University teaching hospitals began to explore the concept of banding together to create a medical centre that would be a new model for health care in the 21st century.

THE VIVIAN REPORT

In fact, the concept that eventually resulted in the MUHC was initially broached more than half a century ago. In the busy post-war period, a survey of the English hospitals of Montreal conducted by Dr. R.P. Vivian, Professor of Public Health at McGill University, assessed the medical needs of the community and recommended some "rethinking."

The Joint Hospital Committee, a group of professionals and laymen put together to plan the future of McGill's teaching hospitals, studied Dr. Vivian's recommendations and came up with a plan to create a McGill Medical Centre that would combine the services and activities of all of the university's teaching hospitals. After much "discussion and jealousy," the plan was rejected, as members of the hospitals feared the uniqueness of their individual institutions would be lost.

Fast forward 50 years. The merger concept has been painstakingly adapted to the very different reality of the 21st century, with much serious deliberation and extensive consultations with patients and professionals alike. The McGill University Health Centre was officially formed in 1997, merging the Montreal Children's, Montreal General and Montreal Neurological hospitals, with the Royal Victoria Hospital joining the next year. (The Montreal Chest had previously been merged into the RVH.) The move to the new campus will complete the circle. The Children's will be the first of the MUHC hospitals to rise on the Glen site, possibly as early as 2008.

COMPLEXITY AND COLLABORATION

The dozens of health-care professionals who were interviewed for this book have clearly done some hard thinking about the future of pediatrics, and of their hospital. Dr. Charles Scriver believes more fervently than ever that, as Wordsworth wrote in 1807, "the child is father of the man."

"Yes, and mother of the woman," says Dr. Scriver. "To understand the diseases that appear in middle age and old age, you really have to understand childhood and the biological basis that is laid down for those diseases when the child is developing."

Areas of pediatric medicine in which the Children's has been a leader for decades, such as neurosurgery and cardiac surgery, will continue to see exciting developments. Dr. Christo Tchervenkov, Director of Cardiovascular Surgery, says, "We're into the fine-tuning phase, making sure that what today's surgeons do is the right operation when we look at it 10, 20, 30 years down the line ... We want to improve the quality of life."

Trends that will clearly continue include the increasing complexity of patient care; developments in home care and ambulatory services; new knowledge and abilities that will lead to both more lifesaving treatments and more difficult decisions; a higher level of collaboration among staff and institutions, facilitated by the proximity of people and buildings on the new site, and by more enriched forms of communication and information flow (such as digital or video); and more revelations from the rapidly evolving field of genetics, affecting every area of health care from prevention to cure.

Gene therapy is likely to become more widely available, and treatments for many serious conditions will become more specific. Dr. Arthur Porter, Executive Director of the MUHC, believes that "genetics will bring the biggest benefits to cancer patients and children, allowing us to analyze and eventually repair conditions." By placing the accent on prevention whenever possible, and earlier treatment if prevention is not possible, we will achieve better outcomes, in many cases saving babies who in earlier times would have died in the womb or at birth.

Multidisciplinary teamwork is another trend that will be amplified in the future. "The causes of genetic diseases will be shared," says Dr. Scriver. For instance, if eye and kidney problems are part of a common syndrome, why is that? The answer may turn out to be a shared protein. "So that language gets to be shared by people who are going to each others' seminars—and it's all within walking distance [on the new site]."

With information readily available on all sides, from television, the Internet, magazines, and other media, patients and their families today are more knowledgeable. This trend will only increase in intensity, driving them to have higher expectations of the health-care system. They want answers and solutions—right away. Dr. Anne-Marie MacLellan uses a striking analogy to explain why even with sophisticated testing, sometimes a precise, instant diagnosis just isn't possible. "Do you remember black-and-white TV? You couldn't tell whether the sweater [the actress was wearing] was blue, or pink, or orange. With a lot of things in medicine, we're still in the black-and-white era."

"Through the years, hundreds of thousands of children have found happiness and health within the walls of The Montreal Children's Hospital. The hospital's story has no ending. It continues into the future, the story of a great humanitarian service to the children of Montreal."

The Children's Story
50th anniversary history, 1955

STATE-OF-THE-ART—FOR THE FIFTIES

The hospital on Tupper Street was built in and for a very different world. Many baby boomers will recall, for instance, spending a whole week in the hospital after having their tonsils removed—a once-routine surgery that is now performed only when deemed absolutely necessary and on a day-surgery basis. The 1992 Strategic Plan summary noted that 66% of the operations performed the previous year at the Children's were in day surgery, a figure that continues to rise.

The everyday realities of working in overcrowded buildings with a rabbit warren of small rooms, rigidly designed for a different era, have caused considerable frustration. Hospitals of the past were not set up for teaching, either, even though teaching and exchanging information have always been fundamental aspects of any university hospital's mission. At the Children's, medical students and other professionals frequently have no alternative but to discuss cases discreetly in hallways, elevators, or at clinic doors—obviously not optimum in terms of comfort, and especially not for confidentiality. Private meeting spaces within the new hospital will make these impromptu in-public discussions a thing of the past.

The new facility will undoubtedly play a major role in attracting health-care professionals to the Children's and the MUHC. The synergy that comes from sharing a campus with the adult hospitals and the research institute is bound to prove a potent magnet for bright students, postdoctoral fellows, and seasoned professionals alike.

The face of the medical professions is changing, too. Dr. Scriver points to a "gender shift in caregivers." While his mother, Dr. Jessie Boyd Scriver, was one of only five women in her class at medical school, today more than half of medical students are women. Many female professionals with small children are unwilling to work the long shifts of the past, leading to changes in work patterns, such as more part-time schedules.

> "The future looks rosy. We have such a great staff here, and we treat so many different conditions in so many different specialties in this hospital. The future of the Children's is in the MUHC, and the MUHC will strengthen the Children's. It's very important to keep the Children's separate. It will just be in a different location—bigger and better, clean, with bigger beds and lots of computers."
>
> DR. BRUCE WILLIAMS, SURGEON-IN-CHIEF

FLEXIBLE, FORWARD-LOOKING DESIGN

The design of the new Montreal Children's Hospital within the MUHC will correct many problems that have caused immense frustration over the years for staff, patients and families, and visitors. The goal is to create a flexible facility with a logistics flow that supports optimum care. In newer hospitals, for example, emergency services, operating rooms, and imaging technologies are now being located in close proximity to each other to speed up diagnosis and treatment, especially in cases of trauma. By bringing together services that work together, hospitals can reduce or even eliminate the running around that is now a fact of life for staff and families alike.

A planning document produced in 1997, *21st Century: A New Vision for Health Care*, described some design elements of the new hospital. "The design of inpatient accommodations will be flexible in order to meet both social and medical needs of the patient and family. For example, some families might need or request privacy, while other children whose families may not be available all the time will benefit from companionship. Moveable walls will help ... address these diverse patient needs."

Parents who have tossed and turned on a pull-out chair while keeping vigil by their child's bedside will rejoice at the facilities available in the new hospital: "Comfortable sleeping arrangements, lounges, kitchen facilities, telephones in patients' rooms, lockers, showers and laundry facilities are basic necessities for parents who stay overnight with their children for long periods of time."

Also, given that only the sickest children will be admitted to hospital, the trend is toward single-bed rooms, with a variety of built-in equipment and enough space to accommodate mobile technologies. With the miniaturization of medical technologies and the ability to capture and transmit data from most locations, it will become increasingly routine to bring diagnostic (and eventually interventional) technologies to patients, rather than the other way around. This means less disruption and displacement for sick children, better infection control, and more privacy for families and the staff supporting them.

Accommodating the equipment and technology that are so integral to a modern children's hospital—and building in the flexibility to meet currently unforeseeable needs—is another major issue. For example, operating rooms must be set up with an inventory of equipment for pediatric patients ranging in size from 500-gram neonates to 120-kilogram adolescents. Other, less visible, technologies that will find their place in the hospital's ceilings and walls will make it possible to adapt spaces more easily and rapidly from one use to another, vastly improving ventilation, infection control, and information flow.

AQUARIUMS AND ARTWORK

The development of hospital design as a respected area of architecture has resulted in an understanding of the many ways in which the physical environment can help patients feel better. Natural light, soothing colours, the presence of green spaces, reduced exposure to unpleasant odours and sounds, and private spaces where families can spend time together and discuss their child's condition with medical professionals have all been proven to reduce stress and speed healing.

The "healing environment" favoured a century ago by the hospital's founders remains a prime consideration. As described in the 1997 plan, "Patients' spaces will be personalized with flexible décor and artwork that can easily be changed or replaced to suit patient and family preferences. Positive distractions, such as ceiling artwork, aquariums, and whimsical objects, will be used to create an environment that is less intimidating. Colour, texture, and beautiful things will create an atmosphere that encourages visual interaction and interest … " Indoor and outdoor play areas and access to outdoor gardens and courtyards will provide a welcome respite for children and their parents.

These features, and many more, will be hallmarks of the new Montreal Children's Hospital.

"DISTANCE" MEDICINE

Of course, with telehealth and community outreach services, many patients will never need to pass through the doors of the new Children's at all. A collaborative and technologically integrated health-care network will link the Children's with community hospitals and clinics, CLSCs, doctors' offices, and rehabilitation centres, enabling many patients whose conditions are not life-threatening to receive non-invasive treatment in their own community.

The telehealth connection has been on the drawing board for years, ever since computers began to play a major role in communications. A 1986 case study on the Montreal Children's Hospital by Karlsberger Planning Associates recommended that "One area for implementing cost savings is the application of the new telehealth services in which health education (consumer and provider), health care delivery, and administrative functions are provided by a network of communications technology such as teletype, computer terminals, one and two way radio and video connections, telephone lines, satellites and cable television. The hospital needs to be redesigned and re-equipped, rewired to facilitate this happening."

SERVICES ACROSS THE LIFESPAN

Having all the MUHC hospitals on a single site will facilitate the sharing of medical information and ease adolescents' transition from the pediatric to the adult system. The advantages of promoting continuity of care are clear, starting with integrated maternity and infant care. Cardiologist Dr. Marie Béland, for one, eagerly anticipates the advantages for fetal cardiologists of "being close to babies being born." A fetal well-being clinic will be centralized at the new site to monitor prenatal health.

GAZING INTO THE CRYSTAL BALL

From today's vantage point, we can barely imagine the scope of the changes that will mark the Montreal Children's Hospital's second century. Children and their families, medical professionals, and society at large have embarked on a sweeping adventure. When the time comes to write that history, the Children's will be long established on its Glen campus, in buildings that will have seen many mutations and adaptations. Medical breakthroughs, surgical techniques, and new technologies and drugs will again have transformed the medical landscape, vanquishing many of today's diseases, and others we cannot yet imagine.

"High-tech" must be balanced with "high-touch," however, and this is one area where the Children's will continue to shine. Nurses will never be too busy to hold a sick child's hand or comfort a distraught parent. Caring volunteers will always be there to play a game of cards or soothe frayed nerves.

> "The MCH will definitely maintain its culture and identity. It will be a beacon of innovation, caring, and compassion that will light up the whole Glen site."
>
> DR. ARTHUR PORTER,
> EXECUTIVE DIRECTOR, MUHC

While change may be a constant, so is continuity. The unique spirit of the Children's and the qualities the hospital has always been known for—compassion, family feeling, innovation, flexibility, mutual support, collaboration, and teamwork—will not change, except to grow deeper and stronger. "I hope we can retain 'the Alan Ross MCH,'" says Dr. Béland—a friendly place where everyone is treated with equal respect.

Seeing change and complexity as stimulating challenges, the professionals at the Children's will continue not only to keep pace with but to anticipate new developments, new demands on their time, new ways to serve their community. As described by an observer in 1935, this hospital will always be "a place where science and laughter dwell."

Appendix I

The Mission of
The Montreal Children's Hospital

The Montreal Children's Hospital is the pediatric hospital of the McGill University Health Centre. This bilingual institution aims to be a leader in the care and treatment of sick infants, children, and adolescents, to be a source of support for their families, and to be an advocate for the rights of all children to reach their full potential.

In pursuing this mission,

* we combine patient care, education and research in an atmosphere of inquiry, innovation and self-evaluation that enables us to develop the qualities that lead to excellence in all we do;

* we share our expertise in the treatment of disease, in the prevention of illness or injury, and in the promotion of health with other institutions and professionals in a collective effort to solve our society's health care problems;

* we continually strengthen our relationships with all the communities we serve, based on open communication, understanding, mutual support and respect for cultural and linguistic diversity.

Every member of The Montreal Children's Hospital family shares the responsibility for treating with dignity those who turn to us and for helping them feel comforted and secure.

Appendix II

Significant Dates

1869
- Reference to a proposed Children's Hospital first appears in the minutes of a meeting of "the Committee appointed to secure the establishment of a children's hospital," cited in *The Montreal Gazette*

1902
- Committee of Organization of the Proposed Children's Memorial Hospital announces its intention to build a small hospital

1903
- Alexandra Hospital for Contagious Diseases opens in Pointe St. Charles

1904
- First patient is admitted to the Children's Memorial Hospital on Guy Street

1905
- Legislative Assembly of Quebec passes the act of incorporation of the Children's Memorial Hospital
- The Children's Memorial Hospital Training School for Nurses is founded

1907
- First school "commencement" (graduation ceremony) is held for patients who completed their schooling while in hospital
- Training School for Nurses graduates its first class
- Infant mortality rate is 262/1000 live births
- Work begins on Administration Building and Maxwell Memorial Cottage

1909
- Children's Memorial Hospital moves to Cedar Avenue
- Typhoid fever epidemic causes acute shortage of hospital beds, leads to first expansion, and creation of isolation ward

1911–13
- First floor of the Arnott Memorial Cottage opens as an isolation ward in 1911; upper floor becomes the hospital's first infant ward in 1913

1915
- School for Crippled Children (today the Mackay Rehabilitation Centre) opens on land belonging to the Children's Memorial Hospital
- Total number of inpatients for the year is 394; total outpatients (or outpatient visits—records unclear): 998

1916
- School for Crippled Children admits its first seven students
- Volunteer-run Social Services Department is established

1918
- Temporary nurses' residence is established in the Travancore building
- The great influenza epidemic generates need for an additional isolation ward
- School for Crippled Children becomes a separate organization

1920
- Children's Memorial Hospital is designated a teaching hospital of the McGill University Faculty of Medicine
- James Carruthers Memorial Building opens for outpatient clinics, including new dental clinic

1921
- Quebec Public Charities Act provides partial funding for hospitalization of the poorest patients

1922
- Dr. Alton Goldbloom co-founds the Canadian Pediatric Society
- Insulin is discovered by Banting and Best

- Dr. Jessie Boyd Scriver is one of five women to graduate from McGill medical school; she later becomes Montreal's first female pediatrician

1923
- CMH enters into affiliation with other nursing schools, providing pediatric training to their students

1924
- Kiwanis Club of Montreal finances the construction of a pavilion (Ward K) for tuberculosis patients
- Western Hospital becomes the Western Division of the Montreal General Hospital; some of its facilities are later sold by the MGH to the Children's and become part of the Tupper Street complex

1925
- Kinmond and Judah Pavilions open

1926
- Department of Social Services is officially integrated into the hospital (a first for a children's hospital)
- A second typhoid epidemic hits Quebec

1927–34
- New laboratory facilities in biochemistry, bacteriology, and pathology enable widespread expansion of research into children's diseases

1930
- American Academy of Pediatrics is founded, marking the establishment of pediatrics as a medical specialty in the U.S.
- New wing is added to the main building of the Children's Memorial Hospital

1931
- Biochemistry Department is founded
- Serious polio epidemic occurs, one of the worst in Canadian history

1932
- Montreal Foundling and Baby Hospital and Children's Memorial Hospital amalgamate
- Another serious polio outbreak inspires the development of a respirator at the CMH
- Western Division of the Montreal General Hospital constructs the buildings that will later become the D- and E-Wings of the Montreal Children's at its Tupper Street facilities

1933
- First Speech Therapy Clinic in a Canadian pediatric hospital is established at the CMH
- Allergy/Immunology Department is created

1934
- Final class graduates from the CMH Training School for Nurses

1935
- Hazel Fountaine Brown Cottage is constructed
- Total number of inpatients at the Children's Memorial, 3,198; total outpatient visits, 35,412

1936
- Occupational Therapy Department is established
- First course in use of play activities for children hospitalized at the CMH is given to nurses and volunteers

1937
- McGill University establishes a separate Department of Pediatrics

1938
- First operation in Canada to repair a congenital heart defect is performed at the CMH

1939
- First public appeal for funds results in a total of more than $1,175,000 in donations
- The Women's Auxiliary of the hospital is founded

1940
- Montreal Children's Hospital (Vipond) and Children's Memorial Hospital amalgamate
- Department of Anesthesiology is founded

1941
- Sulfa drugs become available for general use

1942
- Montreal Foundling and Baby Hospital closes; patients are transferred to the CMH

1944
- Nurses' residence opens on Redpath Crescent
- Penicillin becomes available for general use

1945
- Medical library is inaugurated at the CMH

1946
- First pediatric cardiac catheterization in Canada is performed at the CMH
- Division of Neurology is founded
- Convalescent and long-term care, most outpatient departments, and all outpatient clinics move from Cedar Avenue to St. Antoine Street (former Vipond Hospital)
- First Peter Holt House, on Redpath Crescent, becomes home to interns and residents
- First research fellowships are established in McGill's Department of Pediatrics

1947
- Cardiology Division is founded
- Hematology and Oncology Division is founded

1949
- Large number of polio cases treated, but outbreak not as bad as 1945
- CMH is first pediatric hospital in Canada to establish a Division of Medical Genetics

1950
- CMH is first pediatric hospital in Canada to establish a Psychiatry Department
- General Pediatric Surgery Division is founded
- Psychology Department is created
- Public financial campaign is undertaken jointly with the Royal Edward and Montreal General hospitals to raise money for expansion of hospital facilities

1951
- Western Division buildings are purchased from the Montreal General Hospital
- First hospital-based clinic in Canada for patients with genetic disorders is inaugurated at the Children's

1952
- Hospital appoints first full-time physician, Dr. Ronald L. Denton

1954
- Plastic Surgery Division is founded
- Polio outbreak affects the province of Quebec, similar in severity to 1949

1954/55
- Total number of inpatients at the Children's is 5,300; total number of outpatient visits, 65,000

1955
- Hospital name is officially changed to The Montreal Children's Hospital

- Ophthalmology and Dentistry divisions are founded
- Endocrine Division, Clinical Endocrine Laboratory, and Endocrine Research Laboratory are established

1956
- Hospital moves from Cedar Avenue to Tupper Street in December
- Ross Residence opens as nurses' residence (A-Wing)
- Construction completed on what is now the C-Wing
- New Peter Holt House is inaugurated on Dorchester Boulevard (F-Wing)

1957
- Specialized clinics open: Rheumatoid Arthritis, Children's Care, Convulsive Disorders, Cystic Fibrosis, Nephrology, and Pediatric Gynecology
- Rheumatology and Respiratory Medicine divisions are founded
- Neonatal Intensive Care Unit (NICU) is established
- Kiwanis Club sponsors construction of chapel in basement of D-Wing
- Camp Carowanis for diabetic children is established in Ste-Agathe-des-Monts

1958
- First open-heart surgery on a child in Quebec is performed at the MCH
- Orthopedic Surgery Division is founded
- MCH officially recognized as a Poison Control Centre for the City of Montreal
- Dedication of the Ross Residence (A-Wing) as the Atholstan Wing

1959
- Her Majesty Queen Elizabeth II and Prince Philip, Duke of Edinburgh, visit the MCH
- Dr. Alton Goldbloom publishes his autobiography, *Small Patients*
- McGill–Montreal Children's Hospital Learning Centre opens, the first Canadian pediatric hospital-based centre for children with learning disorders
- Dermatology Division is founded
- Major polio outbreak occurs in the Montreal area, the most serious since the Second World War

1961
- Quebec Hospital Insurance Plan provides free public access to acute hospital care and laboratory and radiological diagnostic services

- The divisions of Neonatology, Adolescent Medicine, Endocrinology and Metabolism, Cystic Fibrosis, and Neurosurgery are established
- MCH establishes the first outpatient clinic in Canada specifically for adolescents
- The DeBelle Laboratory in Biochemical Genetics is established

1962
- A public campaign is launched, with a goal of $500,000, to cover Outpatient Department costs
- Hospital appoints first full-time staff surgeon, Dr. J.M. McIntyre

1964
- Otolaryngology and Nephrology divisions are founded
- Home Care program is inaugurated
- Last major outbreak of rubella (German measles) occurs

1965
- Pediatric outreach program is begun in the Baffin area of what is now Nunavut
- Three-year project to establish a pediatric service in Ludhiana (India) is begun by Dr. Isobel Wright
- Urology Division is founded

1966
- First therapeutic heart catheterization in Canada on a patient of any age is performed at the MCH
- The McGill University–Montreal Children's Hospital Research Institute is founded

1967
- Alexandra Hospital for Contagious Diseases becomes a long-term care institution, under MCH management; its infectious diseases patients are transferred to the Children's
- Medical residents strike across Quebec

1968
- MCH begins to establish a pediatrics program at University of Nairobi, Kenya, a project that will continue until 1978
- Pediatric Adolescent Gynecology Division is founded

1969
- Pediatric Intensive Care Unit is created

1970
- Emergency Medicine and Infectious Diseases divisions are founded

- Medicare is implemented in Quebec under the Health Insurance Act, providing free access to physician services
- Nursing training is transferred from hospitals to CEGEPs

1971
- Pediatric Burn Unit is created at the MCH, the first in Quebec
- Quebec Network of Genetic Medicine established to screen for genetic diseases in the community

1972
- MCH establishes Montreal's first family medicine unit for the training of McGill residents
- Medical Genetics Group is created, today (2005), the longest-running CIHR-funded research program in Canada
- Quebec Public Health Protection Act establishes the right of teenagers aged 14 and over to make their own medical decisions

1973
- Montreal Children's Hospital Foundation is established
- Audiology Department is established

1974
- Gilman Pavilion is purchased to house Dentistry and Dental Hygiene

1975
- Total number of inpatients at the MCH is 12,213; total outpatient visits, 198,535
- Gastroenterology and Nutrition Division is established
- MCH sets up a screening program for scoliosis for the City of Montreal

1976
- MCH is first hospital in Canada to establish a community pediatric research program
- Owen Day Surgery Centre opens

1977
- First CT scan in a pediatric setting in Canada is performed at the MCH
- B-Wing construction is completed
- Last case of smallpox is recorded

1978
- Registration, admitting, and clinic appointments become the first services to be computerized at the MCH
- First Nursing Coordinator for Research in a Canadian hospital is appointed: Dr. Celeste Johnston

1979
- Dr. Jessie Boyd Scriver, Montreal's first female pediatrician, publishes *The Montreal Children's Hospital: Years of Growth*
- MCH institutes first intensive insulin management program in Canada for children with diabetes
- The McGill University–Montreal Children's Hospital Research Institute moves into new quarters in Place Toulon
- First child protection legislation in Quebec is introduced

1980
- Pediatric Critical Care Division is established
- MCH becomes a founding member of the Pediatric Oncology Group (POG)
- One of the first evoked potentials labs in Canada devoted to pediatrics is created in the MCH's Neurophysiology Service, allowing mapping of the brain during surgery
- First bone marrow transplant in a pediatric setting in Quebec is performed at the MCH
- Ultrasound, a painless imaging technique based on sound waves, is first used at the MCH

1981
- Adolescent Medicine services are moved to the Gilman Pavilion
- MCH's Family Medicine Unit is closed

1982
- AIDS epidemic recognized; children become infected through blood transfusions or, later, before and during birth

1984
- Clinical Ethicist position and Institutional Review Board are created

1985
- First successful liver transplant to the youngest recipient ever in Canada is performed at the MCH, in collaboration with three other Montreal hospitals, under the Pediatric Conjoint Liver Transplant Program
- Molecular Genetics Diagnostic Service is established
- Canadian Red Cross establishes testing system for blood donations

1986
- First cochlear implant in a deaf child in Quebec is performed at the MCH
- First successful treatment of a Canadian child with Ondine's disease through implantation of a phrenic nerve pacemaker is carried out at the MCH

- MCH is first hospital in Canada to set up a hospital-wide multiculturalism program
- MCH is first pediatric hospital in Canada to open a comprehensive provincial centre for sudden infant death syndrome (SIDS), the Jeremy Rill Centre

1987
- Pastoral Services Department is established
- MCH begins participating in the creation of a master's program in community health in Ethiopia

1988
- Heart transplant on the youngest recipient ever in Canada is performed at the MCH
- Alexandra Hospital closes under the direction of the MCH
- Child Development Program is established
- Psychiatry and Psychology departments move to rented quarters on St. Catherine Street West

1989
- Last major outbreak of measles occurs
- Kidney Transplant and Dialysis Program is established
- First Neurotrauma Program in Quebec is created at the MCH
- Together We Care financial campaign for the MCH is launched, which surpasses its goal and raises $44 million
- Task Force on Pediatric Design is set up to create a more attractive, healing environment in the MCH

1990
- First bone-anchored hearing device in a child in Canada is inserted at the MCH
- MCH becomes first hospital in Quebec to establish a pediatric injury prevention program, co-founding the Children's Hospital Injury Reporting and Prevention Program (CHIRPP)
- Neonatal Transport Team is created
- Asthma Centre is established

1991
- First living-donor pediatric kidney transplant program in Quebec is established at the MCH
- MCH becomes first hospital in Quebec to offer extracorporeal membrane oxygenation (ECMO)
- Palliative Care Program is established for hospitalized patients, the first such program in a Canadian pediatric hospital
- Polio is eradicated—last case is diagnosed

1992
- MCH enters into feasibility studies with four other McGill University teaching hospitals about joining forces for the future

1993
- MCH is first hospital in Quebec to develop a Pediatric Intermediate Care Unit
- Adolescent Medicine and Gynecology merge into one division
- MCH is designated a tertiary care Pediatric and Adolescent Trauma Centre for Quebec

1994
- MCH becomes first pediatric hospital in Quebec to offer magnetic resonance imaging (MRI) service, installed in new construction on third floor of the B-Wing
- MCH is first pediatric hospital in Quebec to offer transesophageal echocardiography for young children
- Alternative Care Module opens
- Palliative Care and Intensive Ambulatory Care services inaugurate an award-winning program to support parents caring for a dying child at home

1995
- Gustav Levinschi Laboratory opens, the first pediatric voice and speech laboratory in Canada
- Formal planning begins for a new hospital centre (eventually, the MUHC)

1996
- Transcultural Psychiatry Clinic opens—first in Quebec
- MCH is first pediatric hospital in Quebec to create a Short-Stay Unit
- Research institutes of the Montreal Children's, Montreal General, and Royal Victoria hospitals join the Meakins-Christie Laboratories to form the McGill University Health Centre (MUHC) Research Institute

1997
- MCH establishes Vision Centre
- MCH merges with the Royal Victoria (including Montreal Chest), Montreal Neurological and Montreal General hospitals to form the McGill University Health Centre (MUHC)

1998
- Hematology–Oncology Day Treatment Centre moves into newly constructed quarters on third floor of B-Wing

2000
- First Fetal Diagnosis and Treatment Group is developed as part of an MUHC team
- MUHC team performs first delivery in Quebec of a baby using EXIT procedure (ex-utero intrapartum treatment) at the MCH

2002
- Mechanical heart device (Berlin heart) is used successfully for the first time in Canada at the MCH as a bridge to transplant on the youngest patient ever in North America
- Neonatal Outreach Teaching Program is established

2002/03
- Total number of inpatients is 6,779; total outpatient visits, 265,337

2003
- Speech and Language Pathology Department, in conjunction with Department of Otolaryngology, pioneers the use of telehealth to provide long-distance speech therapy sessions
- Autism Spectrum Disorders Program and associated clinic are established

2004
- Children's marks its centennial year with a variety of celebrations and events
- McCord Museum exhibition, *Growing Up in Montreal*, pays homage to the MCH's first 100 years
- Canada Post issues stamp commemorating MCH centennial
- Child, Youth and Family Health Network is inaugurated

2005
- Insulin Pump Therapy Centre is established

Appendix III

Leaders over the Years

Founders
Sir Melbourne M. Tait
Dr. Alexander Mackenzie Forbes
Hugh Graham, Lord Atholstan
Mr. George H. Smithers
Mr. Robert Reford
Mr. George G. Foster, K.C.
Dr. Harold B. Cushing
Dr. Arthur A. Brown

Chairmen of the Board of Directors
1902–1917	Sir Melbourne M. Tait
1917–1933	Mr. George H. Smithers
1933–1935	Mr. W.J. Horrice
1936–1949	Mr. George G. Foster, K.C.
1949–1958	Mr. John H. Molson
1958–1963	Mr. Stuart M. Finlayson
1963	Mr. W.F. Macklair, Q.C.
1963–1964	Mr. E.A. Mackenzie
1964–1968	Mr. Elliot S. Frosst
1969–1970	Mr. Anson C. McKim
1970–1971	Mr J.C. Lessard
1971–1973	Mr. J.L. Wallace
1973–1976	Mr. G.H. MacDougall
1976–1978	Mr. W.D. Lennox
1978–1980	Mr. André E. Gadbois, Q.C.
1980–1982	Mr. Charles B. Matheson
1982–1984	Mrs. Pierrette Rayle-Gomery
1984–1987	Mr. Thompson E. Skinner
1987–1997	Mr. Eric Maldoff

Chairmen of the Council for Services to Children and Adolescents, MUHC
1997–2003	Mr. Eric Maldoff
2003–	Mr. Graham Bagnall

Executive Directors
1930–1935	Dr. Howard S. Mitchell (General Superintendent)
1936–1958	Dr. John E. deBelle (General Superintendent)
(1941–1945)	Dr. Lionel M. Lindsay (Acting Medical Superintendent)
1958–1969	Dr. Robert Ingram
1969–1970	Dr. Donald Hillman (Interim)
1970–1987	Dr. John S. (Jack) Charters
1987–1995	Dr. Nicolas Steinmetz
1995–1997	Ms. Elizabeth J. Riley

Associate Executive Directors for the Pediatric Mission, MUHC
1997	Ms. Elizabeth J. Riley
1997	Mr. Charles McDougall (Interim)
1997	Ms. Valérie Gagnon (Interim)
1997–2000	Ms. Patricia Sheppard
2000	Dr. Claire Dupont (Interim)
2000–2002	Ms. Suzanne Tremblay
2003–2004	Dr. Nicolas Steinmetz
2004–2005	Ms. Diane Borisov (Interim)
2005–	Dr. Linda M. Christmann

Surgeons-in-Chief
1904–1929	Dr. Alexander Mackenzie Forbes
1929–1933	Dr. E.W. Archibald
1933–1937	Dr. Frank Scrimger
1937–1954	Dr. Dudley E. Ross
1954–1974	Dr. David R. Murphy
1974–1992	Dr. Anthony R.C. Dobell
1992–	Dr. H. Bruce Williams

Physicians-in-Chief
1904–1905	Dr. A.D. Blackader
1905–1938	Dr. Harold B. Cushing
1938–1946	Dr. Rolf R. Struthers
1946–1953	Dr. Alton Goldbloom
1953–1968	Dr. Alan Ross
1969–1974	Dr. Mary Ellen Avery
1974–1986	Dr. Keith Drummond
1986–1996	Dr. J. Richard Hamilton
1996–	Dr. Harvey Guyda

Directors of Nursing
1903–1906	Miss Haye-Browne
1906–1910	Miss Edith McCallum
1910–1915	Miss Jessie Barnard
1915–1919	Miss Jean Giffen
1920–1925	Miss B. Willoughby
1925–1935	Miss Anne S. Kinder
1935–1938	Miss Marjorie Jenkins
1939–1958	Miss Dora Parry
1958–1976	Miss Roselyn Smith
1976–1997	Mrs. Evelyn Rocque-Malowany
1997–1998	Miss Gwendolyn Olivier
1998–	Ms. Diane Borisov

The Montreal Children's Hospital Auxiliary Presidents

1939–1941	Mrs. E.D. Christmas
1941–1943	Mrs. C.A. Gallagher
1943–1945	Mrs. C. Budge
1945–1947	Mrs. F.G. Rutley
1947–1949	Mrs. C. Nelson
1949–1951	Mrs. D. Harrison
1951–1953	Mrs. G.A. Grant
1953–1955	Mrs. R. Rollock
1955–1957	Mrs. D.S. Abbott
1957–1959	Mrs. E.T.H. Seely
1959–1961	Mrs. J.A. Woollven
1961–1963	Mrs. H. Davidson
1963–1965	Mrs. J.H. Ross
1965–1967	Mrs. H.J. Lang
1967–1969	Mrs. F.T. Denis
1969–1971	Mrs. R.L. Hoffman
1971–1973	Mrs. K.F. Waldorf
1973–1975	Mrs. F.G.S. Kelley
1975–1977	Mrs. K.F. Hofman
1977–1979	Mrs. B. Culver
1979–1981	Mrs. J.E. Roche
1981–1983	Mrs. Ann Trott
1983–1985	Mrs. Sue Gledhill
1985–1987	Mrs. Ellen Wallace
1987–1989	Mrs. Irene Martin
1989–1992	Mrs. Jean Heuser
1992–1993	Mrs. M. Roche
	Mrs. K. Saunderson
	Mrs. Jean Heuser
	Mrs. Esther Scriver
1993–1995	Mrs. Esther Scriver
1995–1998	Mrs. Pen Bridgman
1998–2000	Mrs. Patricia Hamilton
2000–2002	Mrs. Marcie Scheim
2002–2005	Mrs. Irene Pothitos
	Mrs. Sandy Maheu
2005–	Mrs. Sylvia Piggott

McGill University–Montreal Children's Hospital Research Institute

Chairmen of the Board of Governors

1966–1969	Mr. John H. Molson
1969–1972	Mr. Peter Bronfman
1972–1990	Mr. H. Arnold Steinberg
1990–	Mrs. Gretta Chambers

Chairmen of the Research Committee

1966–1968	Dr. Richard Goldbloom
1968–1976	Dr. Charles Scriver
1976–1980	Dr. Harvey Guyda
1980–1987	Dr. Michael Whitehead
1987–1988	Dr. Barry Pless
1988–1989	Dr. Michael Kramer

Scientific Directors

1981–1987	Dr. Michael Whitehead
1987–1988	Dr. Barry Pless
1988–1989	Dr. Cynthia Goodyer
1989–1999	Dr. Roy Gravel

Montreal Children's Hospital Research Institute of the MUHC Research Institute

Scientific Directors

2000–	Dr. Rima Rozen

The Montreal Children's Hospital Foundation

Chairmen of the Board

1973	Mr. R.C. Legge (provisional)
1973–1975	Mr. J.L. Wallace
1975–1986	Mr. John (Jack) Cole
1986–1992	Mr. Carl Otto
1992–1994	Mrs. Martha Hallward
1994–1996	Mr. Graham Bagnall
1996–1999	Mr. Ronald T. Riley
1999–2000	Mr. J. Robert Doyle
2000–2002	Mr. Claudio F. Bussandri
2002–	Mr. Marc A. Courtois

Honorary Chairman

1986–2004	Mr. John (Jack) Cole

Presidents

1988–1994	Ms. Thérèse Gaudry
1995–1998	Ms. Marie-Claire Morin
1998–	Ms. Louise Dery-Goldberg

Appendix IV

Centennial Committees

Centennial Committee

Co-Chairmen
Hugh G. Hallward
Martha Hallward

Members
Marc Courtois
Louise Dery-Goldberg
Jonathan Goldbloom
Dr. Hy Goldman
Dr. Harvey Guyda
Charles Matheson
Derek A. Price
Dr. Nicolas Steinmetz
Dr. Bruce Williams

Support staff
Valerie Frost
Coleen MacKinnon

In-House Centennial Committee

Chairman
Dr. Hy Goldman

Members
Tatiana Aparicio
Diane Borisov
Connie Cloutier
Louise Dery-Goldberg
Dr. Claire Dupont
Lisa Dutton
Valerie Frost
Harriet Greenstone
Dr. Harvey Guyda
Dr. Richard Haber
Irwin Haberman
Coleen MacKinnon
Emmanuelle Rondeau
Dr. Aimee Ryan
Marcie Scheim
Dr. Bruce Williams

Photo Credits

All photographs taken by Medical Multimedia Services of the Montreal Children's Hospital or supplied by the Montreal Children's Hospital archives, with the following exceptions:

Page 8 Robert Derval, Medical Multimedia Services, Montreal General Hospital

Page 11 The Montreal Children's Hospital Foundation

Page 13 (top) The Montreal Children's Hospital Foundation

Page 22 Bertrand Dupuis

Page 23 (left) Dr. Stephane Schwartz

Page 23 (right) Courtesy of Ricardo Cesar and family

Page 25 The Montreal Children's Hospital Foundation

Page 30 The (Montreal) Gazette, Gordon Beck

Page 31 Courtesy of Hanna Strawczynski

Page 33 The Montreal Children's Hospital Foundation

Page 49 Sherilyn Ami

Page 76 The (Montreal) Gazette, Taillefer

Page 82 The (Montreal) Gazette, Pierre Obendrauf

Page 86 The (Montreal) Gazette, Vincenzo D'Alto

Page 98 (left) Courtesy of Dr. Bernard Rosenblatt

Page 99 The Montreal Children's Hospital Foundation

Page 110 McGill University Archives PL006304

Page 124 The Montreal Children's Hospital Foundation

Page 135 The (Montreal) Gazette

Page 137 The Montreal Children's Hospital Archives. Original source: McDougall Smith & Fleming, Architects

Page 152 Christos Calaritis

Page 153 (left) The Montreal Children's Hospital Foundation

Page 156 The Montreal Children's Hospital Foundation

Page 179 MP-1979.131, Notman Photographic Archives, McCord Museum of Canadian History, Montreal

Page 184 Camp Carowanis

Page 186 MP-1984.105.19, Notman Photographic Archives, McCord Museum of Canadian History, Montreal

Page 191 (bottom) Courtesy of the Northern and Native Child Health Program of the Montreal Children's Hospital

Page 196 Courtesy of the Montreal Children's Hospital Pediatric and Adolescent Trauma Program

Page 197 (both) The (Montreal) Gazette

Page 199 Harold Rosenberg

Page 201 The Montreal Children's Hospital Foundation

Page 203 ODCPhoto.com

Page 208 The Montreal Children's Hospital Foundation

Page 209 The Montreal Children's Hospital Foundation

Page 210 ODCPhoto.com

Page 230 ODCPhoto.com

Page 231 ODCPhoto.com

Page 232 (bottom) Canadian Press

Page 233 (top) ODCPhoto.com

Page 233 (bottom) Courtesy of Chantal-Mignonne Mailloux

Page 234 (bottom) The Montreal Children's Hospital Foundation

Page 234 (top) © Canada Post Corporation, (2004). Reproduced with Permission.

Page 236 (bottom) Ulric Garriguet

Page 241 Collage of details from photos credited above

Index

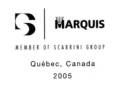

MEMBER OF SCABRINI GROUP

Québec, Canada
2005